HEALTH
in elementary schools

A CONCEPT OF HEALTH

Health is personal; it is individual and variable in its nature.

Health is complex; it relates to the total person and involves physical, psychological, social, and spiritual components.

Health is dependent on self-actualization; it necessitates internalization by the individual.

Health is the result of personal decisions; it involves selection from positive and negative alternatives, the assessment of consequences, and risk taking.

Health is a frequently changing phenomenon; it is the result of the interaction of the individual with a multiplicity of experiences in the environment.

Health is necessary for effective learning and living; it is a means to an end.

HEALTH
in elementary schools

HAROLD J. CORNACCHIA, Ed.D.

Professor of Health Education, San Francisco State University,
San Francisco, California

WESLEY M. STATON, Ed.D.

Palm Springs Unified School District, Palm Springs, California;
formerly Coordinator of Health Science, New Mexico State University,
Las Cruces, New Mexico

FIFTH EDITION

with **62** illustrations

The C. V. Mosby Company

ST. LOUIS • TORONTO • LONDON   1979

FIFTH EDITION

Copyright © 1979 by The C. V. Mosby Company

Previous editions copyrighted 1962, 1966, 1970, 1974

Printed in the United States of America

The C. V. Mosby Company
11830 Westline Industrial Drive, St. Louis, Missouri 63141

Library of Congress Cataloging in Publication Data

Cornacchia, Harold J
   Health in elementary schools.

   Bibliography: p.
   Includes index.
   1. School hygiene. 2. Health education
(Elementary). I. Staton, Wesley Morgan, 1920-
joint author. II. Title.
LB3405.C58 1979   372.3'7   78-21076
ISBN 0-8016-1062-1

GW/CB/B 9 8 7 6 5 4 3 2 1   02/B/245

Preface

Since the first edition of this book there have been a number of important changes in the health sciences, elementary education, and health education. We have seen a long overdue heightened interest in health education in the nation's schools. With the mounting evidence clearly demonstrating the human and financial values of prevention—above and beyond the restorative contributions of hospital and medical care—educators, health professionals, health insurers, and the general public increasingly support health education as an essential part of general education. Nowhere is this more significantly applicable than in the education of children in the elementary school.

One reflection of this favorable attitude and increased awareness is seen in the growing national trend toward state legislation calling for comprehensive health education for all students, K through 12.

Such authoritative and influential professional organizations as the National Education Association, the American Medical Association, the American Academy of Pediatrics, the American Public Health Association, the National Association of Elementary School Principals, the American Association of School Administrators, and most voluntary health agencies continue to urge that quality programs of health education be available to all elementary school children.

Since good health is more and more recognized as an essential thread in the fabric of quality living, it follows that teachers—especially at the elementary level—need an understanding and appreciation of the values inherent in sound, forward-looking school health programs.

Hence, as in previous editions, this revision is designed to help meet present and future demands for elementary classroom teachers and supervisors who are prepared to take advantage of the many opportunities to protect, maintain, and improve the health of young children. To this end the book continues to deal with the basic aspects of school *health education*—curriculum, values, methods and strategies, human and material resources—*health services*, and *healthful school environment*.

While the book is designed primarily for prospective and in-service teachers, it should also be of interest and value to school health coordinators, curriculum coordinators, principals, superintendents, school board members, and health specialists now serving or working with elementary schools. Public health workers should find the book helpful in clarifying certain problems of educational organization, objectives, curriculum development, supervision, and teaching methods and materials as they relate to the elementary school health program.

The book has three broad purposes: (1) it seeks to help elementary school teachers recognize more clearly their responsibilities and their many opportunities for protecting and improving the health of their pupils; (2) it provides the information that teachers want and need to improve their contribution to the health service program in raising the

v

level of healthful school living in those elementary schools in which they serve; and (3) it is concerned with developing understanding and skill in curriculum development, teaching methods, and source materials that will help classroom teachers make a major contribution to the improvement of health in youngsters by doing a better job of health education.

Every effort has been made to present the latest and best in research, practice, and pioneer thinking in school health in light of what is feasible and practical in most elementary schools throughout the nation. While keeping documentation at a minimum for better readability and conceptual clarity, we have attempted to provide a synthesis of those fundamental principles of health education, health services and guidance, and healthful environment that research and experience indicate are best for elementary schools. The book is divided into six parts.

Part One is concerned with fundamental concepts of the elementary school health program, including orientation, and the classroom teacher's role in health instruction, health services, and healthful environment.

Part Two deals with the physical and emotional aspects of a healthful elementary school environment. Attention is focused on the influence of the school environment on the child's total health and safety.

Part Three emphasizes the importance of school health services, including health appraisals, counseling and guidance, safety, and mental health in protecting and improving the health of pupils.

Part Four highlights the increasing need for health education, its place in the modern curriculum, administrative problems, and organizing for health teaching.

Part Five elaborates on the methods and materials useful in health teaching—behavior modification, the principles of learning, the application of methods, over 1,200 teacher-tested techniques categorized into 17 health areas, and up-to-date materials and resources for better health education. Specific sources of health teaching materials are provided.

Part Six concentrates on the place of evaluation and measurement in the school health program.

The Appendices provide a handy communicable disease summary for teachers, the compulsory immunization law requirements by states, and a device for evolving the total school health program.

Throughout the book we have pointed up the importance of cooperative effort on the part of teachers, parents, community health agencies, physicians, nurses, dentists, eye specialists, and others concerned with child health and safety. These mutually favorable reciprocal relationships are essential in translating good elementary school health program theory into actual practice. Our underlying belief is that anything as fundamental as the health of children calls for the highest possible level of partnership among school, home, and community.

The book provides the specific competencies needed by teachers to carry out their responsibilities in health education, health services, and the healthful school environment. It gives appropriate attention to problems and possible solutions of the deprived, the poor, and the ghetto children of different racial and ethnic backgrounds, such continuing needs of young people as venereal disease, drugs, sickle cell anemia, epilepsy, nutrition, safety on buses, learning disabilities or perceptual problems, drug counselors, and nurse practitioners.

The text continues to include the new concept of health (wholistic or holistic health) and adds a spiritual dimension (values, moral issues, and humanism) to the usual physical, social, and psychologic aspects. This concept has received specific application to eleven illustrative partial units (Chapter 9). These units, together with Chapters 10 and 11 on behavior modification and methods and techniques in health teaching, provide curriculum guidelines that will enable teachers to plan and organize for health instruction in their individual classrooms.

New and updated material has been introduced in each of the areas of school health. Recent developments and trends in child health and education have focused attention on humanistic education—especially values clarification and decision making, parent education and involvement, school-community relations, preventive medicine and health self-care, new state immunization requirements for pupils, health problems of minority and poor children, battered children, child alcoholism and other drug abuse, mental health—suicide and death education, and related issues and problems in educating for better health.

Several additional features found in the fifth edition of the text include an emphasis on informal health education (Chapter 5 especially), curriculum material for use in special education, Head Start, and fire safety programs (a nationwide development of the National Fire Protection Association), change of Chapter 10 from "The Learning Process in Health Education" to "Behavior Modification in Health Education," combining of former Chapters 11 and 12 into one chapter entitled, "Methods and Techniques in Health Teaching," and updating of Chapter 12, "Material Aids in Health Teaching."

It has been our task to design a text that not only identifies the known principles and practices for health in elementary schools but also makes them operational and functional for school personnel use. It remains for teachers, administrators, and other concerned persons to implement these measures in schools throughout the country.

If we help bring about just one favorable change in the health program of one elementary school, if we lead one classroom teacher to recognize the powerful potential influence she has for child health, if we provoke one principal to take a critical look at his school's health program, if we but touch the conscience of one superintendent or school board member, if we pique the curiosity of a health department or a voluntary agency, or—above all—if we in some way indirectly enrich the life of an elementary school boy or girl, this will be reward enough.

Finally, we are grateful to all those people and organizations who have helped us to make this edition of *Health in Elementary Schools* a better book. We are especially indebted to those classroom teachers and our students who offered stimulating and useful suggestions.

Harold J. Cornacchia
Wesley M. Staton

Contents

PART FIVE

Methods and materials in health education

10 Behavior modification in health education, 229

11 Methods and techniques in health teaching, 245

12 Material aids in health teaching, 350

PART SIX

Evaluation

13 Evaluating the school health program, 377

Appendices

PART ONE

The elementary school
health program

Improved school health programs will be a key element in the comprehensive national child health policy which I will ask the Public Health Service to develop for the Department. . . . Effective health education early in life can help to prevent the major diseases of adulthood. . . . As children grow older we must teach them how to become responsible informed consumers of health care.
I recognize that interest in improving school health programs has been spotty over the years. . . .
I believe that the time has come again to forge ahead in expanding and improving these programs.

JOSEPH A. CALIFANO, Jr.,
SECRETARY OF THE U.S. DEPARTMENT OF HEALTH, EDUCATION, AND WELFARE,
NATIONAL SCHOOL HEALTH CONFERENCE,
MINNEAPOLIS, MINN., MAY 12-13, 1977

1 School health

ITS NATURE AND PURPOSE

After many years of struggle and growing support it now appears that both the educational community and the general public are aware of the vital significance of *prevention* in the protection, maintenance, and improvement of the nation's health. Although debate and controversy continue over whether health care programs should be financed by government or by individuals and families through private insurance, one basic fact has become increasingly clear: most of the costs of medical and hospital care can be avoided, minimized, or postponed by better *health education*. More important, we now realize that health and the quality of life depend mainly on one's life-style, behavior, and environment rather than on medical science and hospital care.* Nowhere is this more apparent than in the realm of child and adolescent health and safety.

If we can bring to our schools and our students the best of what we now know about personal, family, and community health and safety, we will lengthen the strides already taken to make major positive changes in the lives of children, youth, and adults.

Authorities agree that the best time for building the foundations for better health is early in life. It follows then that one of society's largest—and potentially most influential—organizations offers vast opportunities for raising the health of the individual, the family, and the community. Obviously, we speak here of the 80,000 elementary schools dotting the cities, suburbs, towns, and countryside of America. We think too of the almost limitless ways in which elemen-

tary teachers and school administrators—with the help of health specialists *and* the support of the community—can favorably affect the health of 30 million boys and girls in schools across the land. This is through enlightened *health teaching, health services,* and a *healthful school environment.* Fig. 1-1 outlines the main activities of the entire school health program.

But our schools are in trouble. Teachers, prospective teachers, educational administrators, legislators, parents, education faculty in colleges and universities, taxpayers, and the news media have all become increasingly concerned about our schools. As problems continue to pile up, cluttering the road to quality education for all children, it is plain that bold measures must be taken if we are to give more than lip service to repeated statements of lofty objectives and high ideals for America's schools.

Our schools and our society are beset with the harsh reality of economic, political, and other social problems that affect the quality of life. The question of tax sources for the equitable and adequate support of our schools has become a critical one. Piled atop the money problems are the tangled issues of busing, collective negotiations between teachers and school boards, health and safety conditions for pupils and teachers, selection and purchase of up-to-date quality textbooks, lock-step versus performance pay raises, certification standards for teachers, school lunches for all pupils, state legislatures and their influence on school policies and practices, employment opportunities and educational goals, conflicts in administrative and learning theories, and "accountability" procedures for both pupils and teachers.

However, since this is a book about ele-

---

*America's doctors: a profession in trouble, U.S. News and World Report **83:** Oct. 17, 1977.

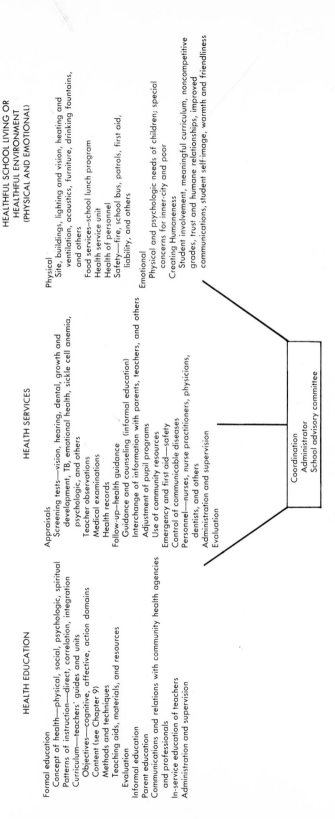

Fig. 1-1. Elementary school health program.

HEALTH EDUCATION

Formal education
  Concept of health—physical, social, psychologic, spiritual
  Patterns of instruction—direct, correlation, integration
  Curriculum—teachers' guides and units
    Objectives—cognitive, affective, action domains
    Content (see Chapter 9)
    Methods and techniques
    Teaching aids, materials, and resources
  Evaluation
Informal education
Parent education
Communications and relations with community health agencies
  and professionals
In-service education of teachers
Administration and supervision

HEALTH SERVICES

Appraisals
  Screening tests—vision, hearing, dental, growth and
    development, TB, emotional health, sickle cell anemia,
    psychologic, and others
  Teacher observations
  Medical examinations
  Health records
Follow-up—health guidance
  Guidance and counseling (informal education)
  Interchange of information with parents, teachers, and others
Adjustment of pupil programs
Use of community resources
Emergency and first aid—safety
Control of communicable diseases
Personnel—nurses, nurse practitioners, physicians,
  dentists, and others
Administration and supervision
Evaluation

HEALTHFUL SCHOOL LIVING OR
HEALTHFUL ENVIRONMENT
(PHYSICAL AND EMOTIONAL)

Physical
  Site, buildings, lighting and vision, heating and
    ventilation, acoustics, furniture, drinking fountains,
    and others
  Food services—school lunch program
  Health service unit
  Health of personnel
  Safety—fire, school bus, patrols, first aid,
    liability, and others
Emotional
  Physical and psychologic needs of children; special
    concerns for inner-city and poor
  Creating Humaneness
    Student involvement, meaningful curriculum, noncompetitive
    grades, trust and humane relationships, improved
    communications, student self-image, warmth and friendliness

Coordination
  Administrator
  School advisory committee

mentary schools and their health programs, we cannot properly analyze all those forces that tend to shape our culture and our schools. Nevertheless, the need for *preventive* health care has never been more critical, and its advocacy is increasing substantially each year. Authorities are beginning to realize that it is not only necessary but also economically more feasible and desirable to reduce the incidence of health problems. The schools have a vital role to play in such action.

Yet, school health does not exist in a vacuum. The school health program is part of the lifeblood of America's better schools, and like all aspects of good schools, it is sensitive to significant thinking and events in the community in which it thrives. In a very real sense the school reflects the character of its community—local, state, and national. Health instruction must be closely related to day-to-day problems of health and safety; school health services depend in large measure on the community's health resources; and the healthful school environment is in itself part of the community.

It is the basic thesis of education that the thinking and the behavior of people can be changed for the better. We assume with the confidence that grows out of research and experience that good teaching in a favorable setting will raise the quality of living for pupils. By enriching the lives of millions of children, elementary education cannot help but contribute to forming a better society.

This "better society" and "the good life" have challenged man for thousands of years. Along with the family, the church and temple, and the community in general, schools have continuously sought to help people live better individually and in groups. Although there have been shifts in philosophy from time to time, the ultimate purpose of our schools has remained constant. From the log cabin of colonial times to the ultramodern structures of contemporary suburbia, the nation's schools have always been concerned with helping boys and girls to live better lives.

In the old days the Three R's made up the curriculum. Teaching methods were characterized by the "boss teacher" and his history stick. In sharp contrast today's pupils enjoy the advantages and opportunities of a broad curriculum that includes the Three R's *plus*. Modern elementary school teaching stresses working *with* children to help them learn and want to learn those things that are necessary for a happy useful life in our modern democratic society.

Of course there are poor, unimaginative teachers today just as there were at the turn of the century. Not all school buildings are of modern design with safe and functional facilities, nor are they all set in spacious, pleasant surroundings; children still strive to learn in small frame structures in the country and in dark ancient buildings in the inner city.

Yet, like business and industry, science, the military, and government, education has sharpened its tools and streamlined its techniques to keep in step with a dynamic society. As with these other fields of human interests and effort, education has not always found the road to improvement a smooth one. There are still areas of honest controversy in curriculum; much remains to be found out about how pupils learn; democratic administration and supervision are not always practiced; many schools are overcrowded and understaffed; too many children spend their school days in buildings that must frankly be considered firetraps, and perhaps above all, really good teachers are hard to find and harder to keep in communities where money for schools is limited.

In the main, however, progress in education has outrun its problems. Elementary school pupils today have a better chance than ever before to prepare to "live most and serve best."

The curriculum now includes substantially more than the Three R's. This does not mean that such basic subjects as reading, writing, spelling, arithmetic, social studies, and science are being neglected. It simply reflects the concern of elementary school administrators and teachers as well as most parents for such important areas of learning as health and safety, music, art, physical education, and foreign language.

Elementary school teachers today are better prepared than ever before to help pupils learn. Prospective and in-service teachers each year are better informed on the latest research in the psychology of learning. National and local studies on pupil achievement generally indicate significant improvement in the teaching-learning situation in elementary schools.

With better understanding of the complex nature of educational leadership, there has been a comparable increase in the application of democratic principles in the administration of our schools. The autocratic, dogmatic principal appears to be fading from the modern educational scene.

Because the schools are doing a better job of public relations and because parents seem to have more accurate information on the aims of elementary education, it is likely that more state and federal funding will be available for our schools. Passage of Proposition 13 in 1978 sharply reduced local property taxes in California and drew attention to the shift in school financing from local to state and federal sources. Actually, this trend had been developing gradually in other states during the 1970s.

WHY SCHOOL HEALTH?

Schools exist to improve society. Educational activities, therefore, are worthwile only to the degree that they contribute to social betterment. Since one of the basic characteristics of a free democratic society is the high value placed on human life and health, it follows as a natural corollary that our schools have both a *responsibility* and an *opportunity* to help protect, maintain, and improve the health of pupils. While these objectives are shared with the home, the health department, voluntary health agencies, and family health advisors, the obligation of the school is luminously clear.

The schools have both a legal and a moral responsibility for providing a safe and healthful environment for pupils and school personnel. Most schools today require that elementary pupils spend approximately 6 hours a day for some 180 school days per year in the school and its environs. To do less than provide an optimally safe and healthful home away from home is to shirk our responsibility as educators and as citizens.

Since there is a consensus of authoritative opinion supporting the view that general education includes those understandings, attitudes, and skills that contribute to better individual, family, and community health, the obligation of our elementary schools for health instruction is apparent. As we shall see, it is through the health instructional phase of the school health program that the most substantial and far-reaching effects on human health may be realized. Obviously, it matters little how much a child has learned in arithmetic, language, science, or history if that child dies or becomes ill because of a lack of the knowledge necessary for making wise choices and intelligent decisions for safe and healthful living.

If children are to get optimum benefit from their elementary school learning experiences, they must be healthy. The child who is frequently absent because of illness, the pupil who needs glasses, the emotionally disturbed troublemaker, the malnourished or frankly undernourished child, the child who is always a bit tired, the "battered child"—these and others like them—are simply not able to learn most efficiently and effectively even with the best kind of teaching. The American Academy of Pediatrics* identifies these endogenous factors that contribute to underachievement in pupils: chronic and frequently recurring physical problems; specific sensory defects (vision, auditory, speech); neurologic and neuromuscular problems (brain defects, epilepsy); psychosocial problems (passive-aggressive behavior, fears, anxieties); and mental retardation. Therefore, by making available medical examinations, screening tests, teacher health observations, dental inspections, and other health services, the school is helping to assure maximum efficiency in the education of its pupils.

---

*American Academy of Pediatrics: School health; a guide for health professionals, Evanston, Ill., 1977, Committee on School Health.

As we will learn, the school's health service and guidance efforts are in no way intended to alter the *fundamental assumption that parents have the primary responsibility for the health of their children*. Rather, the health service activities of the school along with those of the pediatrician, the dentist, the eye specialist, the local health officer, the public health nurse, and others concerned with child health, are essentially concerned with helping parents recognize and carry out their basic responsibility. Perhaps the best example of this principle is the recent crisis of inadequate immunizations of elementary school children in Detroit and other cities—large and small—around the country.

WHAT ARE THE HEALTH PROBLEMS OF CHILDREN?

One of the central purposes of education is to minimize or eliminate defects in our society. Although varying levels of positive health cannot always be identified or measured, we do have much specific data on illness, injury, and death. These figures (vital statistics, illness surveys, accident facts, and results of school health examinations) all contribute to the bookkeeping of humanity.

Indisputably the most blunt evidence of society's health needs is presented each year in the grim list of the nation's top killers. Table 1-1 shows the leading causes of death in the United States during 1900 and 1975. Although this list of the country's major causes of death does not pinpoint problems identified chiefly with boys and girls of elementary school age, it does serve to point out the most serious threats to life among the general population. These problems may directly affect the child, or they may influence his life by involving a member of his family; they may touch his life today, tomorrow, or in the distant future. Hence, it is logical and proper for schools to be concerned with these facts of life and death in America.

Since it is the 5- to 14-year age group

Table 1-1. Leading causes of death in the United States: then (1900) and now (1976) (death rates per 100,000 population)*

1900		1976	
Cause	**Rate**	**Cause**	**Rate**
Tuberculosis	194.4	Heart diseases	388.6
Pneumonia	175.4	Cancers	174.6
Diarrhea and enteritis	142.7	Stroke	88.1
Heart diseases	137.4	Accidents	46.8
Stroke	106.9	Motor vehicle (21.3)	
Kidney diseases	88.6	All other (25.5)	
Accidents	72.0	Pneumonia and influenza	29.3
Cancers	64.0	Diabetes	16.3
Diseases of early infancy	62.6	Cirrhosis of liver	14.5
Diphtheria	40.3	Arteriosclerosis	13.4
		Other blood vessel disorders	12.5
		Suicide	11.7
		Causes of death in early infancy	11.6
		Emphysema, bronchitis, asthma	11.1
		Homicide	8.8
		Birth defects	6.4
		Kidney diseases	5.8
		Peptic ulcer	2.9
		Hernia and intestinal obstruction	2.8
		High blood pressure	2.8
		Tuberculosis	1.5
		Gall bladder disease	1.3

*Adapted from data from the National Center for Health Statistics, U.S., Washington, D.C., 1978, Public Health Service.

with which we are specifically concerned in the elementary school, causes of death for children of this segment of the population have more immediate implications. Table 1-2 delineates the leading causes of death for children of elementary school age. As with the list for the total population, it is apparent that accidents and chronic diseases make up the bulk of the serious health problems. It should be painfully obvious that the major threat to life and health of our elementary school pupils is accidents. Yet the "time bomb" health crises for most of them will occur in later life.

Still, many of these children die needlessly each year because schools and society fail to bridge the gap between what we know about accident and disease prevention and what we actually do to prevent or postpone these deaths.

What are the safety hazards for pupils?

Data from the National Safety Council's *Accident Facts* show that each year some 8,400 children from 5 to 14 years of age lose their lives in accidents. Although the rate for this school-age group has been substantially reduced over the past 35 years, a yearly loss of more than 8,000 boys and girls is both tragic and unnecessary. Most of these accidents are not only predictable but also preventable.

Table 1-2. Major cause of death probabilities for elementary-age children in the United States*

Rank	White male	White female	Black male	Black female
Ages 5 to 9				
1	Motor vehicle accidents	Motor vehicle accidents	Motor vehicle accidents	Motor vehicle accidents
2	Accidental drowning	Leukemia	Accidental drowning	Fire-related accidents
3	Leukemia	Pneumonia	Homicide	Pneumonia
4	Firearm-related accidents	Cancerous brain tumors	Fire-related accidents	Accidental drowning
5	Machine-related accidents	Circulatory birth defects	Pneumonia	Cancerous brain tumor
6	Circulatory birth defects	Accidental drowning	Firearm-related accidents	Circulatory birth defects
7	Pneumonia	Fire-related accidents	Leukemia	Leukemia
8	Cancerous brain tumors	Cystic fibrosis	Circulatory birth defects	Homicide
9	Fire-related accidents	Strokes, blood vessel disorders	Anemia	Anemia
10	Strokes, blood vessel disorders	Congenital hydrocephalus	Machine-related accidents	Rheumatic heart disease
Ages 10 to 14				
1	Motor vehicle accidents	Motor vehicle accidents	Motor vehicle accidents	Motor vehicle accidents
2	Accidental drowning	Pneumonia	Homicide	Homicide
3	Suicide	Leukemia	Accidental drowning	Pneumonia
4	Firearm-related accidents	Suicide	Firearm-related accidents	Accidental drowning
5	Machine-related accidents	Strokes, blood vessel disorders	Pneumonia	Fire-related accidents
6	Homicide	Homicide	Fire-related accidents	Strokes, blood vessel disorders
7	Leukemia	Circulatory birth defects	Machine-related accidents	Leukemia
8	Pneumonia	Accidental drowning	Leukemia	Anemia
9	Accidental falls	Cancerous brain tumors	Suicide	Cancerous brain tumors
10	Circulatory birth defects	Fire-related accidents	Kidney disease	Kidney disease

*Adapted from the Geller-Gesner Tables, Indianapolis, 1974, Methodist Hospital of Indiana.

In a recent year 4,110 children of elementary school age were killed in motor vehicle accidents (the tragic truth here is that so many were killed as innocent passengers in cars driven by uninformed or careless parents); 900 of these resulted from collisions between motor vehicles, 520 from collisions between motor vehicles and bicycles, 550 as a result of the motor vehicle overturning or running off the roadway, 100 from collisions between railroad trains and motor vehicles, 120 from collisions with fixed objects, and 20 from other types of collisions. Some 1,900 children were killed by motor vehicles in pedestrian accidents.

Public nonmotor vehicle accidents accounted for approximately 2,500 deaths in the 5- to 14-year age group; 1,200 of these were by drowning, 150 were associated with small boats and other water transportation, 100 resulted from falls, 100 were attributed to firearms, 40 occurred in air transportation, 70 in railroad accidents (except for those involving motor vehicles), and 800 in a variety of miscellaneous public accidents such as fires, burns, and bicycle accidents other than collision with motor vehicles.

Sixteen-hundred children of elementary school age were killed in home accidents; 600 of these by fires and burns, 300 by firearms, 250 by mechanical suffocation, 120 by falls, 110 by suffocation by ingesting objects, 60 by poison gases, 50 by ingesting solid or liquid poisons (usually aspirin or petroleum products), and 110 by other types of home accidents.

Work accidents claimed the lives of 200 children, an understandably low figure since so few boys and girls of this age group are classified as workers by accident statisticians. Of course, a significant number of these deaths were among children engaged in farm work. Leading types of fatal farm accidents are tractor and other machinery accidents, injury by animals, falls, vehicular accidents, burns, and lightning.

Although most of the accidental deaths of elementary school pupils have relatively little implication for the health service program, there are painfully clear meanings for

safety education in the health instructional program and for the maintenance of a safe school environment. The relationship to curriculum content in health teaching is obvious and will be dealt with in detail in Chapters 6 and 9.

The death and injury of pupils and teachers in school fires should leave no doubt about the moral responsibility of every community to provide fire-safe buildings, including automatic warning systems, and to establish firm policies for periodic fire drills, inspections, and other fire safety procedures.

School bus tragedies have motivated school boards throughout the nation to take stock of their policies and procedures for school bus operation. Warning devices at grade crossings, careful selection of drivers, better bus maintenance, safe routings, and an additional adult to accompany drivers are some of the primary considerations for safer transportation of pupils by bus. Since two out of three pupils killed in school bus accidents were either approaching or leaving a loading zone, more emphasis should be given to education of motor vehicle operators regarding school bus laws.

Although accidents are by far the leading killer of elementary school children, like illnesses, most childhood accidents are not fatal. Yet, since there are about 100 disabling injuries for each death by accident, we cannot afford to overlook those environmental hazards that impair the health of pupils. Most school accidents occur in what the National Safety Council classes as "unorganized activities." Such accidents usually take place on the school playground or other areas outside the school building. Other locales of school accidents are the gymnasium, classrooms, auditoriums, playground apparatus, and traveling to and from school.

Fortunately, except for accidents going to and from school, most of the school accidents are not of a serious nature. Most involve abrasions, cuts, contusions, and minor bone and joint injuries.

Many of the accidents occurring in "unorganized activities" could be prevented if more schools would conduct organized, supervised programs of physical education rather than simply permitting pupils to run about on the school playground with little or no supervision.

What conditions commonly affect pupils?

Although the mortality rates for the nation and for the 5- to 14-year age group help us to focus on the major threats to life and health, these are not the problems that most frequently confront the classroom teacher in day-to-day relationships with children. By way of illustration, cancer kills more school-age children (10.57 per 100,000 population) than any other disease. Fortunately, the elementary school child's group shows a crude death rate less than one-half that of the 1- to 4-year and the 15- to 24-year groups. But the teacher and the school nurse deal with a variety of illnesses and accidents that are quite common in the daily routine of the elementary school.

These common health problems—with the exception of specific emotional disturbances—are outlined and ranked in Table 1-3. Of

Table 1-3. Common health problems contributing to short-term disability and school absenteeism in elementary-age children*

Rank	Condition
1	*Respiratory conditions:* including the common cold, sore throat, earache, bronchitis, influenza, asthma, and related conditions
2	*Infectious diseases:* including—despite readily available vaccines—measles, chickenpox, German measles, and mumps; skin infections; venereal diseases among upper grade students
3	*Injuries:* including motor vehicle, bicycle, moped, pedestrian, home, farm, and school accidents; assault by other children or adults in the school-neighborhood environs; physical-emotional injury resulting from child abuse by parents or guardians
4	*Digestive disorders:* including viral and bacterial intestinal infections, food allergy, constipation, and appendicitis

*Adapted from data from Current estimates from the health interview survey; United States, 1976, Vital Health Statistics (10) **119:** Nov., 1977.

course, it would be both difficult and naive for teachers to attempt to assess the emotional and educational implications of health statistics relating to elementary-age boys and girls. Yet there can be little question that many of these day-to-day illnesses and injury incidents can have at least temporary effects on a child's ability to learn and to relate to teacher and classmates.

From this and other health surveys it is obvious that the elementary school classroom teacher and the school nurse can expect to deal with colds and coldlike conditions, communicable diseases of childhood, ear and throat infections, accidental injuries, headaches, stomach upsets, and allergies on a rather regular basis. It is estimated that 1,600,000 under 16 years of age have asthma.* To provide a handy reference to common childhood illnesses, we have included the Appendix the *Communicable Disease Summary for Teachers* prepared by the Colorado State Department of Public Health. Many state health departments provide similar material for use in the school health program. Additional detailed information is usually available from local or state health departments.

Recent surveys have shown that less than half of elementary pupils studied have had all of their basic immunizations required for school attendance. This, of course, is an average, with some communities showing much better records and others—chiefly among inner city children—much worse. The problem continues and has prompted the Immunization Division of the Public Health Service's Center for Disease Control to launch an intensive public education campaign urging parents to have their children properly protected. Appendix B provides updated information on immunization required or recommended for school enrollment in the various states.

It is estimated that 2½ million children who live in areas where there is great risk of lead poisoning, approximately 400,000 to

*McGovern, J. P.: Allergy problems in children, Journal of School Health **44:** May, 1974.

600,000, will have elevated lead levels in the blood that may be toxic. The condition causes brain damage that results in learning disabilities and hyperactivity.*

What about mental health? There is a lack of detailed evidence on the nature and extent of personality disorder and emotional disturbance among elementary school children, but authorities in the field of mental health as well as most educators and health specialists agree that such disorders represent a leading problem for this age group. Several studies indicate that one child in ten is sufficiently disturbed to require professional help. The American Academy of Pediatrics† estimates that 5 million school children have moderate to severe emotional problems. They state that suicide is the third most frequent cause of death in adolescents. The rate is small below the age of 10 years but increases considerably in late adolescence.

A panel of experts concentrated on the mental-emotional fitness of children and youth of school age at the Eighth National Conference on Physicians and Schools. Serious concern was expressed on three problems: (1) the lack of mental health education in the professional preparation of teachers, (2) the failure to utilize fully the limited measures currently available for mental health screening of future teachers, and (3) the inadequacy of facilities for student counseling in mental health. Subsequent reports and surveys have reaffirmed the observations and recommendations of that American Medical Association conference. Home, community, and school must cooperate to the optimum if the mental health of children is to be protected and improved. The message here for our elementary school health programs should be vividly apparent.

Drugs at this age? The drug problem appears to have leveled off but remains high. We live in a drug-oriented society. We take drugs to wake up, to go to sleep, to keep alert, to escape from reality, to relax, to calm our nerves, to ease pain, and for numerous other reasons. Many people are using, misusing, and abusing legal as well as illegal drugs. Alcohol, tobacco, aspirin, laxatives, coffee, glue, solvents, and other chemicals are readily available to anyone who wishes to purchase them, while such illegal drugs as marijuana, PCP ("angel dust"), and LSD are obtainable if desired.

The chief concern of most parents, educators, psychologists, and law enforcement people centers on the high school and college populations, but there is sufficient evidence that drugs are available and being used by elementary school children. Most, if not all, adolescents use drugs in some form at some time in their lives. (However, not many who use drugs develop problems.) Certain legal drugs, such as aspirin and laxatives, are frequently given to young children by parents and adults; tobacco and alcohol are reaching youths in the fourth and fifth grades, and illegal drugs are being used by seventh and eighth grade students. Recent reports suggest that 10% to 15% of 12- to 13-year-olds have used marijuana. In addition, surveys show that alcohol, amphetamines, barbiturates, LSD, and more recently, PCP are drugs being used with varying degrees of frequency among upper elementary grade pupils. The illegal drug problem used to be one of the inner-city ghetto areas, but this is no longer true. Middle and upper class children and youths have been and are becoming increasingly involved in the use of such drugs.

The use of legal as well as illegal drugs poses a major challenge to schools and elementary classroom teachers. Preventive efforts are needed. Prevention is the essence of the objectives of drug education as an integral part of health instruction.

In analyzing the dilemma of increased educational emphasis with little or no demonstrable results, Cornacchia points out*:

---

*Does your state have a free lead testing program for children? Journal of School Health **46:** June, 1976.
†American Academy of Pediatrics: School health; a guide for health professionals, Evanston, Ill., 1977, Committee on School Health.

---

*From Cornacchia, H. J., Smith, D. E., and Bentel, D. J.: Drugs in the classroom; a conceptual model for school programs, St. Louis, 1978, The C. V. Mosby Co.

Parents, legislators, and the community have expected schools to help in the resolution of the drug problem among young persons . . . schools and school districts have made sincere efforts to comply by developing programs with unclear guidelines and models needed for direction, and without qualified leadership. . . . The result has been that numerous fragmented, piecemeal, "crash," poorly planned, misguided, and frequently uncoordinated programs have been developed. Is it any wonder that schools have been . ineffective?

What is their level of dental health? One of the most common child health problems today is dental neglect. Available data indicate rather conservatively that the average kindergarten pupil has one *permanent* tooth already decaying. The rate of decayed-filled-missing teeth increases sharply during the elementary grades with figures of five, nine, and twelve reported for typical fourth, sixth, and eighth graders. Most frequently decayed and lost are the 6-year molars, which many parents and even some teachers mistakenly regard as baby teeth. The urgent need for better dental health education and services in our elementary schools cannot be overstated.

What do they eat? As with dental problems, nutritional inadequacies are common among elementary pupils, especially among students from low-income families. Studies of dietary habits of boys and girls consistently show that a substantial percentage of children are not getting the foods necessary for optimum growth and health. Many have a meager breakfast or no breakfast at all. Frequent shortages in pupils' diets involve vitamins A, C, D, and certain B-complex vitamins; calcium, iron, and complete proteins are also found to be lacking. Perhaps most significant is the general finding that pupils' diets become poorer as they get older, with the major inadequacies occurring among girls. Obesity is common among adolescent girls (15%). From the overwhelming statistical evidence, it is clear that there is good reason for elementary schools to renew their efforts to improve child nutrition through education, periodic evaluation of pupil growth, and support of sound school lunch programs, particularly for needy children.

How well do pupils see and hear? Studies show that approximately 20% of the elementary school population have visual problems requiring professional care. Most of these pupils have errors of refraction (nearsightedness, farsightedness, astigmatism) or eye muscle imbalance (strabismus, or crosseye, and other eye deviations).

Some 15 million Americans suffer impaired hearing. About 1 in every 20 children has some loss of hearing. Many cases of hearing loss in elementary school pupils contribute to psychologic problems as well as to retarded development of normal speech and language. Most of these are caused by some obstruction of sound passing from the outer ear to the inner ear.

Much can be done through education to prevent certain of these eye and ear defects. Proper lighting in classrooms may help in some instances. Screening tests for vision and hearing will help assure prompt medical attention and greater likelihood of improvement in children who have eye or ear problems.

How fit are they? Since Dr. Hans Kraus, a New York specialist in physical medicine, and his colleagues stunned the American public two decades ago with data indicating that our children were far inferior to European boys and girls in certain tests of muscle fitness, there has been a mounting concern for physical fitness programs in our schools. Although follow-up studies with the Kraus-Weber tests showed that American youngsters were not as unfit as had first been indicated, it was obvious that there was much to be done in this area of health.

National fitness norms for school children have now been established as a result of the 1958, 1965, and 1975 classic studies conducted for the U.S. Office of Education by Dr. Guy G. Reiff and the late Dr. Paul A. Hunsicker, both of the University of Michigan. These studies revealed that significant gains were made by most age levels tested between 1958 and 1965. Yet the 1975 results showed little significant improvement over

1965 measures. Girls scored slightly higher, but boys' performance remained the same or, for some tests, dropped slightly. This may be a result of the decline of national interest in physical fitness following the Kennedy administration emphasis, economic stringencies limiting school physical education programs in some school districts, or the continued trend toward "soft living" by America's children and youth. Probably all three factors have been of some influence.

The study continues with the next two phases, examining the physical education programs in public schools and testing boys and girls from grades 6, 8, and 10 from the twelve largest central cities in the nation. This latter sample will include children from poverty schools and will be compared with the 1975 national norms.

Although no one would propose that physical fitness represents the most important aspect of total health, it is recognized by medical and other scientific authorities that physical fitness is indeed essential if children and adults are to lead full, vigorous, happy lives.

Venereal disease among elementary pupils?

Each year two million cases of gonorrhea and one-half million cases of syphilis are reported in the United States. Surprising to most people is the fact that a growing proportion of these occur among upper grade elementary school children. This is especially true in the inner-city schools and other schools where the majority of pupils come from poverty level families. The need for basic information on venereal disease for elementary pupils in the intermediate and upper grades is obvious. Both prevention and, where necessary, prompt treatment depend largely on the inclusion of such content in the unit on communicable disease.

What about teenage pregnancies?

One million teenagers become pregnant each year and 30,000 girls are under 15 years according to the Planned Parenthood Feder-

ation of America.* These young people are biologically immature for effective childbearing. Adolescent pregnancy is a serious threat to the life and health of young women. Babies of young teens are more likely to die in the first year of life at a rate that is two or three times higher than for older women. Toxemia and anemia are the worst health hazards to these young mothers.

Special health problems for minority groups?

In recent years increasing attention has been accorded the unusually high rate of illness among such minority groups as black Americans, Mexican Americans, and American Indians. Poverty and ignorance are the common contributory causes of these higher disease rates. Poor diet, inadequate medical and dental care, unhealthful housing, health misconceptions and superstitions, and lack of adequate childhood immunizations are major reasons for the generally subpar health of minority families.

Some of the health problems of minority groups are based on genetic variances (such as sickle cell anemia in blacks and Tay-Sachs disease in Jewish and other groups of Middle East origin), whereas others appear to be related to life-style and environment (such as alcoholism among Irish Americans and high blood pressure among black Americans). Migrant and seasonal farmworkers and their children, most of whom are black or Chicano, suffer severely under the burden of poverty, poor housing, inadequate diets, discrimination, occupational accidents, emotional problems, and exposure to agricultural pesticides. Among American Indians these conditions are prevalent: tuberculosis, high death rates, dental decay, alcoholism, drug abuse, accidents, and a variety of emotional problems.

Again, the school health program can be a

*The Alan Guttmacher Institute: Eleven million teenagers; what can be done about the epidemic of adolescent pregnancies in the United States? New York, 1976, The Research and Development Division of Planned Parenthood Federation of America.

potentially favorable influence if funding and leadership are made available and if school health education is correlated with that of other community agencies. Yet our schools still have the opportunity to improve the health of minority children and, indirectly, that of their families.

TERMINOLOGY IN SCHOOL HEALTH

There is frequent misunderstanding concerning the exact meaning of words and terms used to describe various phases of the school health programs. Numerous individuals, groups, and organizations have attempted at times to define the health terms commonly used. Although these attempts to universally clarify health terminology have been helpful, rapid progress and changing conditions and situations operate to change and alter the meaning of rigidly defined terms.

The most recent report of the Joint Committee on Health Education Terminology was a product of health education authorities representing the American Academy of Pediatrics; American Alliance of Health, Physical Education, and Recreation; American College Health Association; American School Health Association; American Public Health Association; and the Society for Public Health Education. From this authoritative document the following definitions—germane to our concerns here—have been selected*:

health education A process with intellectual, psychological, and social dimensions relating to activities which increase the abilities of people to make informed decisions affecting their personal, family, and community well-being. This process, based on scientific principles, facilitates learning and behavioral change in both health personnel and consumers, including children and youth.

school health education That health education process associated with health activities planned and conducted under the supervision of school personnel with involvement of appropriate

community health personnel and utilization of appropriate community resources.

school health education curriculum All the health opportunities affecting learning and behavior of children and youth in the total school curriculum. These health experiences are gained in both school and community settings as the individual interacts with his environment, including other students, school personnel, parents, and community members.

school health educator An individual with professional preparation in health education or health science who is qualified for certification as a health teacher and for participation in the development, improvement, and coordination of school and community health education programs.

health instruction The process of providing a sequence of planned and spontaneously originated learning opportunities comprising the organized aspects of health education in the school or community.

school health program The composite of procedures and activities designed to protect and promote the well-being of students and school personnel. These procedures and activities include those organized in: school health services, providing a healthful school environment, and health education.

school health services That part of the school health program provided by physicians, nurses, dentists, health educators, other allied health personnel, social workers, teachers and others to appraise, protect and promote the health of students and school personnel. Such procedures are designed to (a) appraise the health status of students and school personnel; (b) counsel pupils, teachers, parents and others for the purpose of helping pupils obtain health care and for arranging school programs in keeping with their needs; (c) help prevent and control communicable disease; (d) provide emergency care for injury or sudden illness; (e) promote and provide optimum sanitary conditions and safe facilities; (f) protect and promote the health of school personnel; and (g) provide concurrent learning opportunities which are conducive to the maintenance and promotion of individual and community health.

healthful environment The promotion, maintenance, and utilization of safe and wholesome surroundings, organization of day-by-day experiences and planned learning procedures to influence favorably emotional, physical and social health.

*From Report of the 1972-1973 Joint Committee on Health Terminology, Journal of School Health **44:** Jan., 1974. Copyright, 1974, American School Health Association, Kent, Ohio 44240.

Definitions are often stated in somewhat stilted and cumbersome phrases that may tend to overwhelm the student by the apparent complexity of the various professional terms. However, as we shall see, each of these dictionarylike definitions has significant functional application to health programs in our elementary schools.

WHAT IS GOOD HEALTH FOR PUPILS?

Everything we do in the elementary school health program is aimed at the protection and improvement of child health. It is important, therefore, that we understand the basic concept of health.

Most children and adults give little thought to their health until they lose it through illness or injury. Consequently, barring disease or accident, we tend to think we are healthy. This, of course, represents the negative viewpoint of health. We know that the human organism is protected and, in a sense, maintained by its avoiding or minimizing the stress of disease or injury. Yet, above and beyond this defensive concept of health lies a vast potential for building an optimal personal fitness. In this light the true meaning of health takes on many shadings and degrees of quality. Two elementary school pupils may both be well in that they are not ill or disabled, yet one may be merely existing at a marginal level of health while the other child is enjoying brimful living characterized by maximum physical, mental, and emotional fitness and efficiency.

Perhaps the most widely quoted and affirmed definition of health is that set forth by the then young World Health Organization in 1947. This scientific group defined health as "a state of complete physical, mental and social well-being, and not merely the absence of disease or infirmity." Some years ago at a national meeting of the American Public Health Association in Detroit, Dr. Howard S. Hoyman of the University of Illinois emphasized the dynamic, shifting nature of health and presented a five-point scale: *health, wellness, minor illness, major illness,* and *critical illness.* His definition of health is the following: "optimal personal fitness for full, fruitful, creative living." Surely classroom teachers can regard their pupils as being healthy only when they are living at the highest possible levels of physical, mental, and emotional fitness commensurate with their inborn capacities.

A new concept of health

After years of research and observation it seems obvious that our old definitions and ideas of "good health" must be somewhat altered. A modified concept of health is shown in Fig. 1-2.

Here we see that health is a composite of *physical, psychologic, sociologic,* and *spiritual-philosophic* dimensions. All these facets of the complex of human health are inseparably bound up in each of us. It is not easy to diagram such forces and their outcomes. Yet, working each day with elementary school boys and girls, we may see possibilities for applying these shifting concepts to our plans for objectives, content, methods and materials, and appraisal of results in health education in our elementary schools. To show how this concept can be realistically applied and involved as an integral theme of quality health instruction, we have included specific examples in the units in Chapter 9.

Although most of us are familiar with the physical, psychologic, and social aspects of health and healthful living, perhaps the spiritual-philosophic phase is not so clearly understood. Yet it is this component of the health determinants that is so often the decisive one. The use of the word "spiritual" here is not used in the religious sense so much as it is used to focus attention on the importance of values, moral issues, humanism, and the self-image in making health choices and decisions. As we shall see in forthcoming chapters, it is this force that so often makes the difference between health and illness, quality living and mere existing, and—all too often—between life and death.

How can you tell if pupils are healthy?

Of course, the classroom teacher is not able to diagnose illness or to make a clinical

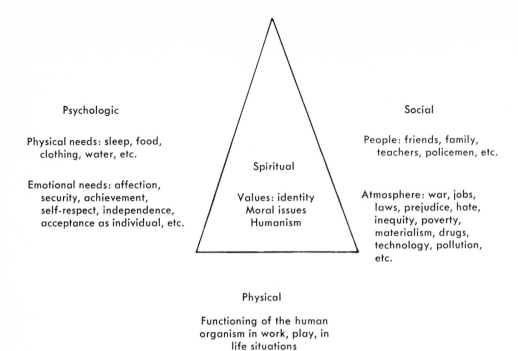

Psychologic

Physical needs: sleep, food,
    clothing, water, etc.

Emotional needs: affection,
    security, achievement,
    self-respect, independence,
    acceptance as individual, etc.

Spiritual

Values: identity
Moral issues
Humanism

Social

People: friends, family,
    teachers, policemen, etc.

Atmosphere: war, jobs,
    laws, prejudice, hate,
    inequity, poverty,
    materialism, drugs,
    technology, pollution,
    etc.

Physical

Functioning of the human
organism in work, play, in
life situations

Fig. 1-2. A modified concept of health. (Adapted from Cornacchia, H. J., Smith, D. E., and Bentel, D. J.: Drugs in the classroom; a conceptual model for school programs, ed. 2, St. Louis, 1978, The C. V. Mosby Co.)

assessment of pupil health. However, some specific characteristics distinguish healthy children from those who are not healthy. Actually, these attributes help spell out a definition of good health. To be able to enumerate, albeit roughly and incompletely, the more basic telltale clues of good health is to be better prepared to recognize and promote buoyant health among your pupils. Here are some of the things you should look for in the healthy child:

1. He is able to carry out routine learning activities in school and in homework assignments without undue fatigue or emotional upset.
2. He is able to participate regularly in physical education and other physical activities in the school curriculum.
3. He demonstrates skill in games and basic body movements appropriate to his age, sex, body type, and motor learning experiences.
4. He shows progressive gains in weight and height without unusually wide deviations.
5. He has enough energy to do the things that most children of his age and sex want to do.
6. His skin is smooth and clear, without discoloration, eruptions, or excessive dryness or oiliness.
7. His appetite is good, and he has regular habits of elimination and excretion.
8. He has no more frequent illnesses or accidents than are typical of his age and sex groups.
9. He is interested in and enthusiastic about most activities that are popular with his classmates.
10. He has confidence in his own abilities yet enjoys working and playing with others.
11. He is able to control his emotions about as well as most of his classmates can.

12. He is honest, truthful, and sincere in his relations with adults and age-mates.

Refer also to Chapter 4.

What factors influence pupil health?

A child's health is determined by three basic factors: *heredity, environment*, and *behavior*. Each boy and girl, as an individual personality, is a product of these fundamental forces.

Your pupils differ in many ways. Some are tall and slender, others are short and stocky, some are just plain big, others are tiny, and the rest are distributed in between. Some are fair skinned with blue eyes; others are olive skinned with brown eyes. Some have blond hair, some brown, some black, and a few red. Differences in their facial features are readily apparent, even to the casual observer. As a teacher you find that some learn quickly, others slowly; some show rapid rates of physical growth while others lag behind, at least temporarily. Some learn motor skills easily and quickly; others seem never able to quite "get the hang of it" when a new physical skill is taught. All these and more are evidences of biologic traits transmitted from parents to children. All these are proof of the miracle of heredity.

It is *heredity* that sets up a child's health endowment fund. What is passed on to the child by the genes and their constituent deoxyribonucleic acid (DNA) and ribonucleic acid (RNA) molecules from the parents, grandparents, and more distant ancestors has much to do with the child's capacity for good health. All experienced teachers have seen the pupil with a strong constitution. This is the boy or girl who is alert, vigorous, seemingly indefatigable, and relatively free from illness. Similarly, teachers are familiar with his opposite—the weak, sickly child who seems always to be perched precariously on the figurative fence dividing health and illness. Often both children are exposed to essentially the same environment and follow much the same daily routine. In the absence of other explanations, such as previous illness or impairment, these health variances must be considered as being significantly influenced by heredity.

Environment has a direct bearing on the health of pupils. Boys and girls must interact with and adjust to an environment that is physical, biologic, and social. *Physical* factors, such as weather and climate, housing, soil, water and food supply, medicines, radiation, clean or polluted air, recreational facilities, automobiles, hospitals, school buildings and sites, and many more physical things around us can affect health for better or worse. *Biologic* influences include germs, plants, animals, and other people. These, too, may be helpful or harmful to health. For example, a pupil may catch a cold from his father. At the same time the father provides shelter, food, clothing, medical care, and other necessities that serve to maintain and improve the boy's health. Some "friendly" germs in the intestinal tract manufacture certain vitamins that help prevent deficiencies; other germs are capable of causing disease and death. *Social* or *cultural environment* comprises all the interactions between and among people. These complex human relationships influence and are themselves influenced by patterns of culture at a given time and place. Hence, boys and girls are constantly exposed to the beliefs, attitudes, ideals, values, and customs of family, neighborhood, school, church, and the general community (local, state, national, and world) in which they live. In terms of nationwide values there remains little doubt of the influence of vigorous and persuasive advertising through television and other mass media on the thinking of children and adults. These cultural forces can directly or indirectly, for better or worse, affect the physical, mental, or emotional health of elementary school pupils.

To a far greater extent than either heredity or environment, *behavior* is generally the most influential factor in pupil health. Properly guided and motivated, each of us can make the most of his or her hereditary endowment and overcome or adjust to limitations or defects. We can usually change or adapt ourselves to the environment in ways that will enhance opportunities for safe and healthful living. For instance, a child may be nearsighted as a result of hereditary influences; without proper eye care and glasses, the child, living in the blurred world of the myopic would be more likely to have an accident while crossing a street or in other potentially dangerous situations. Moreover, this nearsighted child could well become increasingly withdrawn from his social group and eventually present a psychologic problem. On the other hand, with proper treatment and glasses the child could probably avoid both the physical and emotional hazards and live a happy, normal life.

Thus, what children *do* or *do not do* will usually have substantially more effect on their health than will biologic traits of inheritance or the nature of their surroundings. This is why we increasingly talk about *knowledge, attitudes,* and *behavior* as inseparable goals for health education. The significance of this "package deal" of health instructional outcomes is analyzed and discussed in more detail in later chapters.

WHERE DO WE STAND NOW?

A recent national survey* gives us a picture of the current status of health education at the elementary school level. An increasing number of states are mandating appropriate time for health instruction at all levels of the public schools.

Those states requiring specified periods of time for health instruction within the elementary school curriculum include Delaware, Florida, Hawaii, Indiana, Kentucky, Maine, Minnesota, New Jersey, North Carolina, North Dakota, Ohio, Oklahoma, Rhode Island, South Carolina, and Texas. These and other states have mandated time for health education at the junior and senior high school levels. Six states have optional comprehensive health education, and sixteen have mandated safety education.

---

*Castile, A. S., and Jerrick, S. J.: School health in America; a survey of state school health programs, Kent, Ohio, 1976, American School Health Association.

WE BELIEVE

In summing up the role and responsibility of elementary schools for the health and safety of our children, we can say with assurance that one of the most significant and encouraging trends in modern American education has been the increasingly prominent placement of health among the broad objectives of elementary education.

If we believe in something strongly enough, there are few obstacles that can deter us from our goal. We all tend to live by what we believe and feel. If teachers throughout the land have the necessary understandings and the firm beliefs about school health and safety, there is no telling what may be the limits of their influence on the health of the nation.

Principals, teachers, and parents, in the last analysis, however can never say, "Our health and safety education program is complete." It is one program that needs constant attention, revision, and observance.

Above all, though, it needs action.

QUESTIONS FOR DISCUSSION

1. How have changes and trends in the elementary school curriculum affected school health programs?
2. Why do elementary schools have a clear responsibility to provide health instruction, health services, and a safe and healthful environment for pupils?
3. What are the five leading causes of death in the United States?
4. What are the five leading causes of death for children in the 5- to 14-year age group?
5. What are the major types of accidents that cause death among children in the 5- to 14-year age group?
6. What are the ten leading causes of illness or impairment of health among boys and girls in the 5- to 14-year age group?
7. Which conditions affect boys more often than girls? Which affect girls more often than boys?
8. What are three major problems in protecting and improving the emotional health of children in elementary schools?
9. What is the general status of dental health among elementary school children?
10. What is the nutritional status of children of elementary school age?
11. What is the extent and nature of ear and eye problems among elementary school children?
12. What is the general status of physical fitness among boys and girls in elementary school and what is being done about it?

ics of the

health and how do

status?

15. What are three basic aspects of the school health program?
16. What are five major trends in school health today?
17. What is the nature and purpose of school health instruction?
18. What is the nature and purpose of school health services?
19. What is the nature and purpose of healthful school living or environment?
20. What is the meaning of the new concept of health, and can you illustrate how it may be applied to health education?

SUGGESTED CLASS ACTIVITIES

1. Prepare a list of statements of general objectives for elementary schools and tell how these aims are related to the school health program.
2. Obtain the latest statistics on children's death rates from the National Center for Health Statistics* and compare them with similar data for 1940, 1950, and 1960.
3. Obtain from the National Safety Council† the annual one-page summary of *Accident Facts* and discuss the trend for each type of accidental death in terms of implications for elementary school health programs.
4. Obtain from your state department of health the latest figures on deaths and reportable illnesses for the 5- to 14-year age group and compare these with similar statistics for the entire nation.
5. Make a list of factors in the environment that can have significant influence on a child's health.
6. Conduct a simple survey of what children in an elementary school class eat for breakfast each day for 1 week. Report on the results, showing what food groups are most often skipped or slighted by boys and girls.
7. Administer the AAHPER Fitness Tests‡ to one or more elementary school classes and report the results to your school health class.
8. Select an elementary school that is well known to you. Obtain a copy of the school's stated objectives and policies for school health. Tell how these statements could be improved.
9. Prepare a report illustrating the application of the new concept of health to several of the health areas in the instruction program.
10. Visit the health department and obtain data regarding the nature and extent of health problems among ghetto children.

*U.S. Public Health Service, Washington, D.C. 20025.
†125 North Michigan Ave., Chicago, Ill. 60611.
‡American Association for Health, Physical Education, and Recreation: Youth fitness test manual, Washington, D.C., 1961, The Association.

REFERENCES

American Academy of Pediatrics: Report of the Committee on School Health, Evanston, Ill., 1966, The Academy.

American Alliance for Health, Physical Education, and Recreation: Professional preparation in safety education and school health education, Washington, D.C., 1974, The Alliance.

American Alliance for Health, Physical Education, and Recreation: Why health education in your school? (Report of the Joint Committee on Health Problems in Education of the National Education Association and the American Medical Association), Washington, D.C., 1974, The Alliance.

American Alliance for Health, Physical Education, and Recreation: Suggested school health policies (Report of the Joint Committee on Health Problems in Education of the National Education Association and the American Medical Association), Washington, D.C.: 1966, The Alliance.

Cornacchia, H. J., Smith, D. E., and Bental, D. J.: Drugs in the classroom; a conceptual model for school programs, St. Louis, 1978, The C. V. Mosby Co.

Haag, J. H.: School health program, Philadelphia, 1972, Lea & Febiger.

Hanlon, J. J.: Public Health Administration and Practice, St. Louis, 1974, The C. V. Mosby Co.

Lee, P. R.: A new perspective on health, health planning, and health policy, Journal of Allied Health, winter, 1977.

Mayer, J.: Health, New York, 1974, D. Van Nostrand Co.

Miller, C. A.: Health care of children and youth in America, American Journal of Public Health **65:** April, 1975.

National Health Council: Two-hundred ways to put your talent to work in the health field, New York, 1974, The Council.

National Safety Council: Accident facts, Chicago, 1977, The Council.

Nemir, A., and Schaller, W.: The school health program, Philadelphia, 1975, W. B. Saunders Co.

Pollock, M. B., and Oberteuffer, D.: Health science and the young child, New York, 1974, Harper & Row, Publishers, Inc.

Read, D. A., and Greene, W. H.: Creative teaching in health, New York, 1975, Macmillan, Inc.

Read, D. A., Simon, S. B., and Goodman, J. B.: Health education; the search for values, Englewood Cliffs, N.J., 1977, Prentice-Hall, Inc.

Staton, W. M., Irwin, L. W., and Williams, E. K.: Health for better living, Columbus, Ohio; 1972, Charles E. Merrill Publishing Co.

Warshofsky, F.: The Control of Life; The twenty-first century, New York, 1969, The Viking Press.

Wilner, D. M., Walkley, R. P., and Goerke, L. S.: Introduction to public health, New York, 1973, Macmillan, Inc.

2 The teacher's role in school health education

Few stand in a place of more potential influence on a child's health than does the elementary classroom teacher. Teachers have contact with boys and girls during some of their most sensitive years—a precious time when what they know, what they think, and what they do can be significantly affected. Often the teacher sees and communicates with a child for more hours each day than do the parents. This reality becomes increasingly important in light of recent Department of Labor reports showing that over half of the mothers of school-age children hold down regular jobs.

What teachers do with this combined opportunity and responsibility depends on whether they are ready, willing, and able to assume a prominent role in school health, especially classroom health instruction.

To better understand the ways that teachers can contribute to child health and safety, let us look again at the three basic aspects of the total elementary school health program: health education, health services, and healthful school environment (see Fig. 1-1).

Through *health teaching* we seek to encourage and develop those understandings (cognitive), attitudes (affective), and behavior (action) that contribute to the highest possible levels of individual, family, and community health.

Health services include all those school activities aimed at protecting, maintaining, and improving the health of elementary boys and girls.

Healthful school living (or *environment*) includes just that—all of your school's plans, procedures, locale, facilities, equipment, and psychologic atmosphere that can affect the physical and emotional health of your pupils.

Although we tend to categorize these three phases of a good school health program as instruction, services, and environment, the broad program should be viewed as school health. It is clear that health services—including guidance—and healthful environment offer rich opportunities for health *education* in the broadest sense as a catalyst for classroom health instruction.

Quite obviously the classroom teacher has the greatest responsibility and most opportunity to contribute to child health through health instruction; yet, these teachers are not without influence in the areas of healthful school living and health services and guidance. In fact, most teachers have many excellent opportunities—if only they will take advantage of them to contribute to these aspects of the total program. Not only can they add to the effectiveness of health services and healthful environment, but, equally important, they can provide the thread of relationship and coordination among the three parts of the program.

The elementary school classroom teacher has often been called a jack-of-all-trades by educators and laymen alike in recognition of the diversity of talents possessed by good elementary teachers. Few people in the entire field of education, or in any of the other professions, for that matter, need to have as many understandings or to develop such a variety of competencies as does the elementary classroom teacher. He or she is by turns grammarian, mathematician, psychologist, space-age scientist, nutritionist, editor, art and drama critic, geographer, health educator, sociologist, agricultural expert, historian, recreation leader, zoologist, anthropologist, safety specialist, chemist, economist, and more. The teacher serves at times as leader, discussant, counselor, resource person, learner, coordinator, researcher, expediter, evaluator, committee member or chairman, observer, organizer, public relations authority, nurse, baby-sitter, pseudo-parent, and arbiter. As we shall see, the teacher's part in the elementary school health program is both strategic and decisive.

WHAT COMPETENCIES DOES THE ELEMENTARY TEACHER NEED?

While we do not expect each classroom teacher to be a specialist in health education, a recent list of competencies developed by a committee of the California School Health Association provides an additional source for self-evaluation and improvement. A committee headed by Dr. John Fodor of California State University at Northridge recommended that education students majoring in health science should be able to*:

1. Identify and make provisions for the health needs of children and youth from various socioeconomic and cultural levels.

2. As health needs are identified, refer the child to aid through appropriate channels.

3. Describe the effect of the school environment in the mental-emotional and physical well-being of children and youth.

4. Describe the role of the teacher in providing for a safe and healthful school environment.

5. Provide for the growth and development characteristics of children and youth in the teaching-learning situation.

6. State factors that influence or determine health behavior and incorporate such factors in planning for health instruction.

7. Plan and organize activities that facilitate physical, emotional, and social development of children and youth.

8. Promote the physical and emotional health of children and youth through varied experiences in the school and community setting.

9. Identify a variety of community health

resources that serve children and yo___ well as other family members.

10. Explain the role of the family and ___ community in health education.

11. Communicate health needs of the child to parents without belittling or being critical.

12. Utilize community health agencies in planning and implementing the curriculum.

13. Identify socioeconomic and cultural conditions in the community that affect the health of the individual.

14. Identify criteria for determining the content of health instruction.

15. Demonstrate a command of the fundamental concepts related to:
Drug use and misuse
Family health
Nutrition
Diseases and disorders
Environmental health hazards
Mental-emotional health
Community health resources
Consumer health
Oral health, vision, and hearing
Exercise, rest, and posture

16. Apply the fundamental concepts relative to sociology, psychology, human anatomy, and physiology in teaching about health.

17. Select important concepts to be taught relative to health problem areas.

18. Write behavioral objectives relative to health concepts being emphasized.

19. Effectively evaluate the progress students make toward achieving behavioral objectives.

20. Develop inquiry skills relative to the modification of health behavior.

21. Interrelate health concepts among health problem areas.

22. Develop strategies for making health decisions that can favorably modify health behavior.

In addition to specific competencies (see pp. 22-23) the teacher should (1) realize that health education requires the use of a different approach, (2) understand the controversial nature of some health topics, (3) appreciate the special need for the consideration of individual pupil differences, (4) be familiar

---

*Ad Hoc Committee of the California School Health Association: Suggested competencies for health science teaching majors, May, 1974 (mimeographed).

COMPETENCIES

General

The teacher understands and appreciates:
1. The meaning of health as a multidimensional state of well-being that includes physical, psychologic, social, and spiritual aspects.
2. That health of individuals is influenced by the reciprocal interaction of the growing and developing organism and environmental factors, and is necessary for optimal functioning as productive members of society.
3. The significance of children's and youth's health problems on learning.
4. The importance and the need for the school health program in today's society.
5. The nature of the total school health program.
6. The role of the teacher in each of the school health program components—services, environment, and instruction.
7. The need for basic scientific information about a variety of health content areas including dental health; drugs (alcohol, tobacco, and other drugs); care of eyes, ears, and feet; exercise, fitness, rest, and fatigue; prevention and control of diseases and disorders (communicable and chronic); safety and first aid; family health; consumer health; community health; environmental health; nutrition; mental health; anatomy; physiology.

Health instruction

The teacher:
1. Can identify and utilize a variety of techniques and procedures to determine the health needs and interests of pupils.
2. Is able to organize the health instruction program for the grade being taught around the needs and interests of students and can develop effective teaching units.
3. Is able to stress the development of attitudes and behaviors for healthful living based on scientific health information.
4. Can distinguish between the various patterns of health instruction and attempts to utilize the direct approach in teaching whenever possible.
5. Realizes that health education must receive time in the school program along with other subject areas.
6. Possesses current scientific information about a variety of health content areas.
7. Can utilize a variety of stimulating and motivating teaching techniques that are derived from fundamental principles of learning.
8. Is able to identify and utilize "teachable moments" or incidents that occur in the classroom, in the school, or in the community.
9. Utilizes a variety of teaching aids in the instructional program and is familiar with their sources.
10. Is familiar with the sources of scientific information and the procedures necessary to keep up to date with current health information.
11. Is able to provide a variety of alternative solutions to health problems to enable students to make wiser decisions.
12. Can integrate health into other phases of the curriculum, such as social science, science, and language arts.
13. Uses a variety of evaluative procedures periodically to (a) assess the effectiveness on students and (b) determine the quality and usefulness of teaching aids and materials.

COMPETENCIES—cont'd

Health services

The teacher:

1. Is familiar with the characteristics of the healthy child and can recognize signs and symptoms of unhealthy conditions.
2. Is familiar with the variety of health appraisal procedures used in schools and utilizes them to enrich the health instruction program.
3. Acquires limited skill in counseling and guiding students and parents regarding student health problems.
4. Understands the value and purposes of teacher-nurse conferences.
5. Is familiar with the variety of health personnel found in schools, their functions, responsibilities, and usefulness to the teacher.
6. Is able to utilize information contained on health records
7. Can identify and follow the policies and procedures in schools in regard to such matters as emergency care, accidents, disease control, and referrals, exclusions, and readmittance of pupils.
8. Can administer immediate care when accidents or illnesses to pupils occur, or can act promptly to obtain sources of help within the school.
9. Is able to adjust the school program to the individual health needs of students.
10. Is able to relate the health services program to the health instruction program.

Healthful environment

The teacher:

1. Is familiar with the standards for hygiene, sanitation, and safety needed in schools to provide a safe and healthful environment.
2. Is familiar with the physical and emotional needs of students and adjusts classroom activities to help students satisfy these needs whenever possible.
3. Understands the nature and importance of the food services program and is able to relate it to the instructional program.
4. Is able to recognize hazardous conditions on the playground, in the classroom, and elsewhere in the school and takes appropriate action to eliminate or correct such conditions.
5. Is cognizant of the effect of teacher health, personality, biases, and prejudices on student health and learning and is concerned with the humane treatment of pupils.

Coordination

The teacher:

1. Understands the need for school health councils or committees and is willing to participate as a member if requested to do so.
2. Realizes the importance of a coordinator, consultant, or a person with administrative responsibility being in charge of the school health program.

with a variety of sources of current scientific health information, and (5) be able to select health problems and the time needed for instruction.

Health teaching is different

Although in many ways health teaching is much like all other teaching, it does differ in certain crucial respects. In the first place, although much of the content in health education is basic to the biosocial development of the child, motivation is often difficult. It is the nature of the normal, healthy child to be blithely unconcerned about his health and safety. In fact, if the public apathy toward the value of auto seat belts and the serious danger of cigarette smoking is any criterion, we may conclude that many youths and adults demonstrate a rather perverse antagonism toward certain established facts of safe and healthful living. Quite possibly this is because we failed to build the essential knowledges and favorable attitudes a decade or more ago when these people sat in our elementary classrooms. In any event, the classroom teacher faces special challenges in the influential motivation of pupils in health education. At the same time we must avoid fear psychology, vague exhortation, and the possibility of developing an unhealthy overconcern for health among pupils. The balance is often a most delicate one.

Second, health teaching is inextricably bound up in our cultural patterns of thinking and doing. Perhaps no other area of learning in the elementary school depends so heavily on influencing attitudes and behavior. Our actions are rooted in our feelings, and our feelings are colored by our experiences and understandings. Even though children may come to school without any preconceived notions regarding reading or arithmetic, they often already have begun to develop some false ideas, poor attitudes, and harmful practices in health and safety. Altering these unsound patterns of thinking and acting is frequently difficult because of the rigidity of family and community culture and its powerful influence on the child.

Third, health science is constantly changing. What was unknown yesterday will be commonplace tomorrow; what was true last year is false this year; what was an apparently insurmountable problem a decade ago is now relegated to the museum of scientific antiques. Moreover, health science is not a simple listing of pure "blacks and whites." Whereas some concepts are clearly and unalterably established by research, others are supported in varying degrees of authenticity by the available evidence. The classroom teacher, therefore, must prepare pupils for scientific change without developing a negative skepticism; must lead children to understand the scientific method and, from this understanding, to be able to weigh the facts at hand and to make choices and decisions accordingly. And decide they must, for unlike most other subject-matter areas, health and safety demand that children be participants, not merely spectators.

Health teaching can be controversial

Some of the topics in health education may occasionally provoke emotional reactions among pupils, parents, and other concerned persons or groups in the community. Such areas of instruction include sex education, venereal disease, fluoridation, tobacco, alcohol, and other drugs, the choice of a health advisor, and medical care plans. While those who object to the teaching of certain concepts in these areas are in the distinct minority, they are sometimes highly vocal and can be disturbing to principals, superintendents, and school board members.

Of course, sex education and tobacco and alcohol instruction have certain moral and religious implications. Yet, the evidence clearly indicates that despite the hue and cry of small vocal groups, the majority of parents and religious leaders generally favor school instruction in these areas. Fluoridation of public water supplies has been associated with emotionally tinged publicity in some communities; despite the fact that every responsible scientific organization has endorsed fluoridation as safe and effective in reducing tooth decay, there is still occasional criticism of this topic. Members of some healing professions and others may take exception to the generalization that diagnosis and treatment are best performed by licensed doctors of medicine and osteopathy. A few citizens may urge that an ultraliberal view of medical care, barely short of socialized medicine, be presented in class; their opposite numbers may question any approach that suggests medical care plans beyond the traditional fee-for-service agreement between physician and patient.

Because health education is so intimately related to the cultural patterns of any community, teachers can expect that now and then some objections may arise. Neither teachers nor administrators should be intimidated by sporadic criticism of this kind. However, to be sure of standing on firm ground in these provocative areas, the teacher should do the following:

1. Maintain a scientific, unbiased approach.

2. Avoid getting involved in partisan politics or personalities.

3. Follow course and unit outlines recommended or approved by local school officials.

4. Seek the help of resource people and groups in the community (for example, local medical and dental societies, the PTA, representative religious leaders, and public health officials) in preparing units of study.

5. Wherever possible, use materials that have been prepared by such reputable organizations as the American Alliance for Health, Physical Education, and Recreation; American Medical Association; American Dental Association; National Education Association; U.S. Public Health Service; local or state health department; American Social Health Association; National Council on Alcoholism; American Red Cross; and other recognized scientific groups.

6. Use a textbook that is up to date and scientifically sound (detailed criteria are discussed in Chapter 12).

7. Maintain adequate records of pupil activities, questions, interests, and problems.

Teacher-pupil planning of units and participation by parents and other citizens in curriculum study and development are procedures that help assure public understanding and acceptance of what is taught in the schools. Increasingly closer ties among school, home, and community tend to lessen substantially the possibility of any misunderstandings regarding teaching concepts in controversial areas.

Sources of current scientific information

Many teacher education institutions today recommend or require that prospective elementary teachers take a course in personal and community health, one in school health, and others. This is minimal preparation for health teaching but may be necessary because of the crowded curriculum for elementary education majors. In any event, most teachers need and want to keep up to date with new trends and developments in the everchanging health field, subject matter, methods and materials, and other aspects of the elementary school health program. However, the sources of reliable and new information as well as the methods to be used to assess such information are problems not readily or easily resolved. There are no simple or definitive ways to discover with certainty whether material contained in publications is truthful and accurate. There are several reasons for this difficulty: (1) data is limited or inconclusive regarding the cause, treatment, or cure of many conditions, such as arthritis, cancer, and obesity; (2) research data published are frequently in conflict; and (3) a number of so-called authorities, including scientists, nutritionists, and physicians, who may be disseminating misinformation may have motived not always in the best interests of people. Therefore, it is important that teachers attempt to determine the validity of health information they read. These guidelines should be helpful in the evaluation of publications and other printed materials*:

---

*Adapted from Cornacchia, H. J.: Consumer health, St. Louis, 1976, The C. V. Mosby Co.

1. What is the *purpose* of the printed material? Is it produced to sell products, make money, or present factual information in order to make a professional contribution?
2. Is it presented in an educational or scientific manner, or does it use exaggerated claims and make misleading and inaccurate statements?
3. Is the author qualified by way of educational background and professional experiences?
4. Are the data based on appropriate research and experiences of experts in the health field or on the opinions of a few individuals?
5. Are the research data acceptable by medical, dental, public health, and other authorities and organizations?
6. What evidence exists to support or refute conflicting claims about health information? Has the claimant generalized from a particular incident or from broad research?

Specifically, here are some of the things teachers may do to obtain current health information:

1. Keep up with new developments in school health by regularly reading one or more professional journals, such as the *Journal of School Health* (American School Health Association), *Health Education* (American Alliance for Health, Physical Education, and Recreation), the *American Journal of Public Health* (American Public Health Association), and *Health Values* (Charles B. Slack, Inc.). These journals provide abstracts of the latest and best research and information in school health and safety.

2. Keep in touch with the progress in the health sciences taking place by reviewing *Family Health* (joined with *Today's Health* and formerly published by the American Medical Association), *Nutrition Today* (Nutrition Today Society), *FDA Consumer* (Federal Food and Drug Administration), *Consumer Reports* (Consumers Union), and other such magazines.

3. Read the health sections of *Time, Newsweek*, and *U.S. News and World Report* as well as local newspapers and popular maga-

zines for new developments announced in the health sciences.

4. Use current basic college health texts on the health sciences as references.

5. Obtain up-to-date health pamphlets from government agencies (National Clearinghouses for Alcohol Information, Drug Information, and Smoking and Health), professional associations (American Medical Association and American Dental Association), voluntary health organizations (Lung, Cancer, and Heart), and business firms.

6. Elect health education courses in the college program for certification or advanced degrees and, whenever possible, attend school health workshops, institutes, conferences, and conventions.

7. Make full use of the teacher's manual that publishers provide to accompany elementary health texts and readers.

Providing for individual differences

Providing for individual differences including cultural and ethnic differences is something we talk about a great deal in education. Doing much about it becomes increasingly difficult with each passing year. Overcrowded schools and oversized classes make individual guidance of pupil learning more a theoretic goal than an accomplished fact. Yet, there are things that classroom teachers can do to get better results in providing for pupil differences.

There are numerous ways teachers can learn more about their pupils. Of course, school records furnish significant information on a child's intellectual capacity, status, and progress. Often these records also contain data on a pupil's social and emotional development. Well-kept cumulative health records should provide information on illnesses, injuries, surgical operations, allergies, health examination findings, dental health, physical growth, and teacher observations from previous years. These, combined with notes and recommendations of school nurse and physician, can be most helpful to the teacher in understanding the health status of each child and the implications such status may have for learning.

Beyond the variances in the health and

growth of pupils there are important differences that relate to each child's environment. Most important of these is the home background. Economic conditions, cultural level, parental attitude toward the school, social position, marital status, value systems, leisure time activities, occupation of the head of the household, and racial, or ethnic origins of parents—all these, and more—tend to leave their mark on the child. Children's purposes, interests, and values will tend to align themselves with those of their parents. Thus, while one child comes from a home where meals are carefully planned and medical and dental care are readily available, a classmate each morning leaves a home where a full stomach is the only measure of good nutrition and where the physician or dentist is seen only for the most extreme conditions, if at all. Surely the needs and interests of these two pupils are far removed in many respects.

In the same classroom there are usually pupils whose neighborhoods vary widely. While some live in the town or city, others are transported to school from outlying rural areas; some enjoy a pleasant suburban neighborhood, while others live in the shadow of factories, railroad yards, or commercial sections, or in the ghettos. Home, family, and neighborhood influences will shape the kinds of out-of-school experiences a pupil has. Travel, work, and recreation also play a part in contributing to differences among boys and girls.

In doing our best to adapt teaching-learning situations and experiences to fit the needs, concerns, and abilities of children, we must also bear in mind that they are maturing at different rates. What is appealing and important to one fifth grader is, at the moment, beyond the understanding and interest of a classmate. We know that children grow and mature according to a general pattern, yet each child sets his or her own unique schedule. Perhaps this is the most important concept for teachers to recognize as a result of their studies in child development.

Finally, teachers should remember that effective learning also takes place in a group situation; therefore, we must try to maintain a balance between individual guidance and group learning activities. The very nature of these human differences often provides the raw materials with which a good teacher can actually mold a superior setting for health education. Although there is much more likeness than unlikeness among children at the same age and sex, the fringe areas of variance constitute both a stimulating challenge and a rich opportunity for alert teachers to achieve effectiveness in two fundamental functions of good teaching (1) providing learning experiences suited to individual purposes, needs, concerns, and interests and (2) providing opportunities for pupil sharing of diversified experiences relating to safe and healthful living.

Teachers must choose

Perhaps the most significant function of the classroom teacher is deciding how much time and emphasis to give to various health and safety topics. Even with textbooks, courses of study, teaching units, and lesson plans as guides, the classroom teacher has considerable latitude in selecting content at a given grade level. Moreover, the teacher usually must decide just how much stress to place on subtopics within a broad unit. More detailed information is provided in Chapters 8 and 9.

THE TEACHER AS COUNSELOR AND GUIDANCE WORKER IN SCHOOL HEALTH

Although we must recognize that the primary responsibility and function of the teacher is to teach, there are many other ways to favorably influence the health and learning of children. As we show in Chapter 5, the teacher has an important part in the elementary school's health guidance program.

As we shall see, the classroom teacher assumes the role of counselor and guidance worker mainly in connection with the health service program.

The teacher's role in school health services

The reader should recall that school health services are designed to conserve, protect, and improve the health of pupils and school personnel. This broad purpose is achieved through the combined, coordinated efforts of teachers, school nurses, administrators, physicians, dentists, dental hygienists, eye specialists—and parents. Once again, teachers must remember that their part in the elementary school's health service program is to supplement, not to substitute for, the contribution of parents to the health of their children. In some communities certain civic or social organizations may take part in activities where nonprofessional assistance is feasible. Generally, however, it is best that teachers or health specialists assume responsibility for the various functions and duties that are dealt with at some length in Chapter 4. These include health examinations, daily observations of pupils, screening tests for vision and hearing, utilization of health records, disease control, emergency care, health conferences, and psychologic testing.

THE TEACHER AS A LINK WITH THE COMMUNITY IN SCHOOL HEALTH

As school and community join more closely in their efforts to improve education, many reciprocal advantages accrue. Opportunities for benefits to the school health program are abundantly evident. To capitalize on these opportunities and to serve as a link with community is to achieve new gains for the elementary health program.

In all three aspects of the program—health education, health services, and healthful school living—the teacher has many occasions to work with resource people in the community. Beyond this the teacher must establish and maintain good rapport with parents, cafeteria personnel, janitors, and social workers who can have an influence on the health program in the school.

Community organizations and people who are capable of providing cooperative assistance include the following:

Medical societies and individual physicians
Dental societies, individual dentists, and dental hygienists
Local and state health departments
Local and state voluntary health agencies

Parent-teacher associations
Police and fire departments
Community health and safety councils
Child guidance clinics, individual psychiatrists and clinical psychologists
Red Cross
Service clubs
Departments of education
Departments of welfare
Youth councils
Boy Scouts and Girl Scouts
YMCA, YWCA, YMHA, CYO, 4-H Clubs, Future Farmers of America, and other youth organizations

A new teacher in a community may be at a temporary disadvantage. In the first place, each community is characterized by cultural patterns that give it the stamp of individuality. For a time any teacher is bound to be somewhat less effective in a new setting. Teachers must rather quickly seek information on the health resources, businesses, topography, history, racial and nationality backgrounds, and general tenor of the community. Such information can be of high value in teaching and in serving other objectives in the total school health program.

SCHOOL HEALTH COUNCILS

One of the best ways to fully use the personnel resources of the community is through the school health council. Membership of the school health council can include representatives from the following groups:

Teachers
Pupils
Parents
Medical society
Dental society
Health department
Voluntary health agencies
Food service and custodial staffs
School administrators (principal and school health coordinator)
School nurses and physicians

Of course membership of the council will vary, depending on the size of the school and the nature of the community. However, even in small rural elementary schools, council membership can include the principal or a delegated representative, parents, pupils, classroom teachers, and custodians. In some communities an advisory health council is established for all schools in the area; in others each school has its own council. Regardless of the size or makeup of the school health council, it has three basic functions (1) to discover health and safety problems of pupils and school personnel, (2) to study these problems, and (3) to make recommendations to the school administration for solution of the problems. In most instances the council is not responsible for taking direct action. The classroom teacher who may be appointed to the council has an excellent opportunity to directly or indirectly further relationships between school and community through many of the council activities that involve local groups and individuals.

THE TEACHER AS A MEMBER OF THE SCHOOL STAFF IN HEALTH MATTERS

As we have already seen, teachers do many things with and for pupils beyond the routine classroom learning activities. We have considered the teacher's role as counselor in the various health services, and we have illustrated several ways in which a teacher provides a link between school and community. In many of these activities the teacher also serves as a member of the school staff.

However, in the role of staff member, the elementary classroom teacher also has the responsibility for taking part in committee work and other organized efforts aimed at improvement of the school health program. The school health council is a good example of the teacher's dual role as a link with the community and as a school staff member. Certainly, as a member of the school health council the teacher is making a major contribution, as a staff member, to one phase of the overall school program.

Beyond this, the teacher may serve on committees concerned with textbook selection, curriculum development, civil defense, special events planning, safety patrol, school clubs, building and grounds, audiovisual aids, and food service. The work of certain committees, particularly the health council and the proper concern of all teachers, frequently relates to the safety and health of the school environment.

The teacher and the school nurse

The classroom teacher should make every effort to work closely with the school nurse in matters of pupil health. Some school nurses are employed by the schools; others are employed by local or state health departments. In any case, it is a fundamental school staff function of the classroom teacher to offer full cooperation to the nurse serving the school. One of the most difficult problems in assuring close rapport between teachers and nurses is that of finding time for personal conferences. Often the lunch hour offers the most practical time for discussion of matters of mutual interest. Administrators, teachers, and nurses usually find that this opportunity for productive yet informal meetings tends to conserve the time of both teachers and nurses. Yet ideally, the principal should arrange for released time for teachers so that the lunch hour remains duty free. Further information is given concerning teacher-nurse conferences in Chapter 4.

The teacher and the health coordinator

A coordinator or supervisor of school health should be employed on a systemwide basis. This person generally is a specialist in school health and health education and plays a key role in helping teachers. It is desirable that the coordinator have a major in school health education as part of his professional preparation. The health coordinator can help teachers through group work, individual guidance, communication, and research and curriculum development.

Group work. Through staff and committee meetings as well as workshops and institutes the supervisor of health education can help teachers to (1) interpret philosophy, (2) agree on objectives, (3) decide on curriculum and unit content, (4) consider new methods and techniques in health teaching, (5) assist in rating and selecting health texts and readers and other learning materials for pupils, (6) utilize community resources and personnel, and (7) recognize strong and weak points in the school's health program.

Individual guidance. Through planned conferences and informal talks the supervisor can help teachers analyze and solve the problems that relate to their own classroom situations. Much of this is concerned with evaluation of the teaching-learning process. The conference may be based on classroom observation by the coordinator. Such observation is concerned with helping the teacher do a better job, *not* with personal criticism of the teacher.

Refer to Chapter 5 for detailed information on guidance and informal education.

Communication. To bring helpful information and ideas to teachers is one of the chief functions of the school health coordinator. Elementary classroom teachers cannot possibly keep up with all the important literature in school health. Through bulletins or newsletters the health coordinator can draw the teacher's attention to especially helpful books, articles, pamphlets, television specials, films, or other materials dealing with child health and the health program. Helpful suggestions, notices of meetings, pertinent data on the community's health resources, and encouragement of teacher creativity can all be communicated through such bulletins. Over and above the advantages of disseminating information is the significant contribution such communiqués make to the teacher's sense of professional pride and confidence as a member of the school health team.

Research and curriculum development. An important but often overlooked, function of the health coordinator is that of stimulating and guiding teachers in research projects. Of course, most teachers cannot be expected to carry out extensive investigations in addition to their normal teaching load. Yet, with help and guidance from the supervisor, significant problems can be selected and delimited for worthwhile study in an elementary school. Important data can often be collected within the framework of the routine classroom activities. Policy and procedures based on objective evidence offer far more likelihood of success than those predicated on empirical opinion.

The teacher and the administrator

Technically speaking, education is a function of the state. The Tenth Amendment to the Constitution of the United States clearly places on each state the responsibility for the education of its children and youths. The Supreme Court has interpreted this part of the Constitution as meaning that final authority resides with state government. In the main, however, local school districts hold the power to almost completely control the educational policies and programs in their schools. This situation works well when the school district is strong and well financed but poorly in those districts where population and money are insufficient to provide adequate schools and educational services.

Even good local school districts cannot provide certain services that make for better schools. These include distribution of state school funds, professional preparation of teachers, and certification of teachers. Then, too, there is a legal provision in almost all of our 50 states that requires that certain aspects of health instruction—notably alcohol, tobacco, and drugs—be included in the curriculum. However, most of these are antiquated statutes couched in heavy, stilted terms. Actually, they serve mainly as echoes from the past, reminding us of the bygone era of "blood and bone" health teaching with its emphasis on moralizing and preachment.

The majority of states now require that pupils be immunized against diphtheria, whooping cough (pertussis), tetanus (lockjaw), polio, measles, and German measles. Smallpox vaccination is no longer generally required.*

Since the state health department is the supreme power in matters of public health, the school is legally bound to conform to cer-

---

*Garcia, E. M.: Immunization requirements for school enrollment by states, 1975-1976, Las Cruces, New Mexico, 1976 (unpublished report), New Mexico State University.

tain standards of sanitation and communicable disease control. Yet, few of these legal powers are actually brought to bear on a local school system. Most states promote school health programs by providing consultative service and guidance through school health specialists in departments of education and departments of public health at the state level.

Administrators and school board members who understand the problems and appreciate the values of school health and health education are essential to an effective program. Experience with health programs in elementary schools has shown with vivid clarity that the success of any such program is basically dependent on the attitude of school administrators and school board members. When administrators favor and support a sound health program it is more likely to be initiated and carried out successfully. Fortunately, in recent years the leading professional societies of administrators have recommended that school health programs be established for all schools. However, teachers may need to encourage administrators to take active leadership in providing effective school health programs.

At the superintendency level this leadership often takes shape through stimulation of school evaluations by professional groups and citizens advisory committees. Specific suggestions for evaluation of the school health program are discussed in Appendix C in some detail.

As the official leader in an individual elementary school, the principal has strong influence on the health program. Through concern for a sound program, encouragement of teachers, efforts to secure textbooks and other learning materials, consistent interest in the many activities, the principal helps classroom teachers assume their responsible roles in school health.

THE TEACHER AS A MEMBER OF THE PROFESSION IN SCHOOL HEALTH

A good teacher tries constantly to improve the health instruction by better methods and by keeping up with the literature in a variety of fields, including school health. As has been suggested earlier, many teachers will conduct surveys and experiments in connection with their health teaching or other school health work. This, too, is the mark of a professional person.

Through membership in national and state educational associations the elementary teacher takes part in the profession to a fuller extent. National and state societies generally make provision for school health concerns through member associations, divisions, or sections. Organizations specifically concerned with school health include the American Alliance for Health, Physical Education, and Recreation (NEA), the American School Health Association, the American Public Health Association (School Health Section), as well as regional and state branches of such groups.

All in all, the life of elementary school classroom teachers is indeed a diversified one in regard to school health. As we have seen they must live up to a reputation as jack-of-all-trades if they are to make contributions in the three basic phases of the health program. Although many teachers-to-be approach their first position with some trepidation, all the evidence and experience indicate that the great majority of classroom teachers can and do make substantial contributions to school health and health education. All they need is a bit of confidence and an understanding of the fundamental concepts of health instruction, health services, and healthful school living. The raw material is America's richest resource; the product is a healthier nation.

QUESTIONS FOR DISCUSSION

1. What are the competencies or skills, that elementary school teachers must have?
2. What are three characteristics of health teaching that makes it significantly different from other phases of elementary education?
3. What are the common areas or topics in health teaching that can be controversial? What can teachers do to make their teaching in these areas more effective?
4. What can elementary teachers do to keep up with new developments in school health and health education?

5. What are some of the ways teachers can find out about the individual differences in health status among pupils?
6. What are the basic objectives of elementary school health education?
7. What are the fundamental purposes of the health service program in elementary schools?
8. What are the basic purposes and makeup or membership of the typical school health council?
9. How and why should teachers work closely with school nurses?
10. What are four ways in which the school health coordinator can help classroom teachers?
11. What is the nature of the elementary school health program?

SUGGESTED CLASS ACTIVITIES

1. Observe an elementary classroom teacher, and make a list of all the things he or she does over a period of several days that relate to child health.
2. Prepare a unit on a controversial area of health teaching and show how criticisms, objections, or problems could be avoided.
3. Read a recent article on child health or school health and prepare an abstract of from 300 to 500 words, summarizing the main points of the article and telling how you could use the information in an elementary school health program.
4. Prepare an agenda for an elementary school health council meeting, listing two or three key problems and telling how you think the council might deal with them.
5. Make a list of some of the health problems that might provide the basis for pupil-teacher conferences, teacher-nurse conferences, and teacher-parent conferences in an elementary school.
6. Select an elementary school that is well known to you. Visit the school, interview the principal, the school nurse, and at least two teachers on the matter of health service activities conducted in or by the school. Report on these to your school health class.
7. Read an article in the professional literature that deals with the functions of a school nurse. Tell how her activities relate to those of the classroom teacher in working for better pupil health.
8. Visit an elementary school, and make a survey of the specific kinds of activities and environmental factors that contribute to healthful school living. Report to your class on the status quo and tell how you might make certain improvements.
9. Interview an elementary school principal, and report on his or her philosophy and policies on school health; indicate any variances between these beliefs and policies and those recommended by authoritative individuals or groups.

REFERENCES

American Association of School Administrators: Curriculum handbook for school exectuvies, Washington, D.C., 1973, The Association.

Association for Supervision and Curriculum Development: Perceiving, behaving, becoming; a new focus in education (yearbook), Washington, D.C., 1962, National Education Association.

Berman, L.: New priorities in the classroom, Columbus, Ohio, 1968, Charles E. Merrill Publishing Co.

Bruner, J.: Towards a theory of instruction, Cambridge, Mass., 1966, Harvard University Press.

Charles, C. M.: Individualizing instruction, St. Louis, 1976, The C. V. Mosby Co.

Denver Public Schools: The health interests of children, Denver, 1954, Denver Public Schools.

Joint Committee on Health Education Terminology: New definitions, New York, 1973, Society for Public Health Education.

Joint Committee on Health Problems in Education: Why health education in your school? Washington, D.C. and Chicago, 1974, National Education Association and the American Medical Association.

Levy, M. R., Greene, W. H., and Jenne, F. H.: Competency-based professional preparation, School Health Review, July-Aug. 1972.

Ludwig, D. J.: Teacher preparation in health education, School Health Review, Sept./Oct., 1972.

McCormack, P.: Report card grades teachers, Boston Herald American, June 13, 1976.

National Commission on Community Health Services: Health is a community affair, Cambridge, Mass., 1966, Harvard University Press.

Oberteuffer, D., Harrelson, O., and Pollock, M. B.: School health education, New York, 1972, Harper & Row, Publishers, Inc.

Read, D. A., and Greene, W. H.: Creative teaching in health, New York, 1975, Macmillan, Inc.

Read, D. A., Simon, S. B., and Goodman, J. B.: Health education; the search for values, Englewood Cliffs, N.J., 1977, Prentice-Hall, Inc.

Sliepcevich, E. M.: School health education study; a summary report, Washington, D.C., 1964, School Health Education (also health education; a conceptual approach to curriculum design; St. Paul, Minn., 1967, 3M Education Press).

Staton, W. M.: Monday morning at the movies, School Health Review, Jan.-Feb. 1975.

Valett, R. E.: Humanistic education, St. Louis, 1977, The C. V. Mosby Co.

Walker, J. E., and Shea, T. M.: Behavior modification, St. Louis, 1976, The C. V. Mosby Co.

Willgoose, C. E.: Health education in the elementary school, Philadelphia, 1974, W. B. Saunders Co.

PART TWO

Healthful school living

3 Healthful school environment

PHYSICAL AND EMOTIONAL

When we by law require children to spend so many of their formative years in our schools, we assume a legal and moral responsibility to provide safe and healthful buildings, equipment, facilities, and services.

Even though this obligation is accepted and the concept understood in our educational literature and professional pronouncements, tens of thousands of American schools fail to meet minimal health and safety standards for students. Many schools are considered by experts to be firetraps; others maintain overcrowded classrooms, some are hotbeds of violence; still others carry tenured teachers who are emotionally unstable; many are not meeting the emotional needs of students; many have questionable water and sewerage systems; most are operating unsafe school buses; and few provide a sanitary, nutritious food service.

A physically and emotionally healthful school environment is essential to the highest quality of education in our schools. The quality of life cannot be enriched for students who are forced to strive to learn and grow in schools that fail to provide a pleasant, conducive atmosphere.

WHAT IS A HEALTHFUL SCHOOL ENVIRONMENT?

Healthful school living . . . embraces all efforts to provide at school physical, emotional, and social conditions which are beneficial to the health and safety of pupils. It includes the provision of a safe and healthful physical environment, the organization of a healthful school day, and the establishment of interpersonal relationships favorable to mental health.*

---

*Joint Committee on Health Problems in Education of the National Education Association and the American Medical Association: Healthful school environment, Washington, D.C., 1969, The Associations.

Specific components of healthful school living include site and building construction, safety policies and procedures, lighting and acoustics, heating and air conditioning, water supply and waste disposal, food services, school bus safety, fire prevention and protection, and emotional climate.

HOW DO SITE AND BUILDINGS AFFECT STUDENT HEALTH?

Of course, teachers have no choice in school site or construction unless they are among the few who have the opportunity to serve on a school plant planning committee for a new school. Hence, we must make the very best of what we inherit. Whatever the age or other problems of school site, buildings, and facilities improvements can be affected by concerned administrators, teachers, school nurses, and others involved with the health and safety of students. School health councils are especially effective as instruments in bringing about favorable change.

Every school building in America should be maintained in accordance with state and local standards of safety, sanitation, and educational utility. Regular inspections of school buildings and facilities should be made by school administrators, local building inspectors, fire inspectors, health department sanitarians and safety experts, and other qualified personnel. Principals, teachers, custodial staff, food service personnel, school nurses, and others in the school should be alert each day for unhealthful or dangerous conditions in the building and on the school grounds.

SCHOOL FOOD SERVICES: ARE THEY ADEQUATE?

School feeding is big business. It is also big politics. And it certainly is "no small potatoes" when it comes to the nutrition and health of millions of American children and youth.

Since its beginnings under the National School Lunch Act of 1946 the program has frequently been at the center of political and social legislation controversy. Yet for millions of America's students the school breakfast, school lunch, or both is their only chance for a nutritious meal during the day. Repeated surveys show that many school-age children and youth, from *all* socioeconomic levels, are subsisting on diets that are nutritionally marginal if not frankly deficient. Many parents —rich and poor alike—have little understanding of the critical importance of quality nutrition for health, growth, and efficient learning at school. Hence, there is a pressing need for better school lunches and expansion of the school breakfast program.

School lunch program

Some 30 million students in elementary schools across the nation represent an important segment of our total population. With a daily average absenteeism rate of 10%, there are about 27 million students in school on any given day. About 13 million school lunches are served daily to elementary pupils. Thus, less than half of the students have the opportunity for a nutritious school lunch.

The overall cost of school lunches is almost $3 billion a year—about what it cost us each month during our full participation in the Vietnam war. About half of the cost is divided between federal and state governments, and the other half comes from "lunch money" from parents. Half of the federal contribution is in the form of food commodities.

The federal government contributes to each school meal at the following relative rates*:
1. *All lunches*—8 cents (statewide average) reimbursement for all lunches
2. *Free*—40 cents additional for free lunches (for needy children)

---

*Subject to increases in food costs.

3. *Reduced price*—40 cents less amount of child's payment (for needy children)
4. *Breakfast*—5 cents for paid breakfast; 20 cents for free breakfast (for needy children); 15 cents for reduced price breakfast (for needy children).

For schools with a high proportion of "especially needy" students, federal assistance may be paid for the full cost of meals: up to 60 cents for lunch, 30 cents for free breakfast, and 20 cents for reduced-price breakfast.

School breakfast program

Because of recognition of the urgent need for many elementary and secondary children to have the opportunity to eat a well-balanced breakfast, pilot breakfast programs have been initiated with the support of the U.S. Department of Agriculture. As in the school lunch program, all public and nonprofit private schools may participate in the breakfast program.

Study and experience have shown that, as with the lunch program, when students participate in a school breakfast program, they learn better, have fewer complaints of headache and stomach ache, and have fewer behavior problems.

To meet the U.S. Department of Agriculture nutrition standards, breakfasts must serve as often as possible fruit or juice, milk, bread or cereal, and a meat or meat substitute.

The problems

A number of problems have become painfully apparent over the years since the National School Lunch Act was passed during the Truman Administration over 3 decades ago. The program has made substantial contribution to the health of millions of American students, but critics from the field of nutritional science and the congressional arena continue to point up these problems:

1. The *quantity* of food, affected by the changing availability of farm surplus commodities, does not necessarily assure a *quality* diet for growing children and youth.

2. Increasing financial burden has fallen

on parents since, by implicit Congressional sanction, states can count student's lunch payments as part of the matching formula. The result has been a tendency to favor children whose parents can provide lunch money while at the same time limiting the nutritional opportunity of pupils whose parents cannot afford even the modest matching lunch cost.

3. Economic eligibility guidelines—who pays how much for what students—have contributed to administrative, political, social, and—for the student—psychologic problems.

4. Nutritionally superior school lunches are the exception, not the rule. Studies show that many school lunches are deficient in complete proteins and in vitamins A, B_1 (thiamine), B_6 (pyridoxine), C (ascorbic acid), and D.

5. More than half of the nation's schools still do not offer school lunches or other food service programs.

6. U.S. Department of Agriculture regulations now permit vending machines in school lunchrooms to provide students with competitive foods equal in nutrition to meals served in the standard school lunch. Sharp criticism has been leveled at this modification of the national school lunch program since it opens the door for students to pass up the school lunch for more appealing, but less nutritious, "junk" foods. However, an increasing number of school systems are limiting vending machine sales to milk, fruit juices, and nutritious foods.

7. Food and labor costs are causing a financial crisis for schools and parents in providing nutritious school lunches and breakfasts. A recent U.S. Department of Agriculture study revealed that just a 5-cent increase in meal price resulted in a *10% decrease* in the number of students able to pay for school lunches.

Too much too soon?

A growing body of evidence indicates that high serum cholesterol levels are a major risk factor in the development of coronary heart disease and premature fatal heart attack. It has also been clearly established that this buildup of blood cholesterol accelerates during adolescence, especially among boys.

In a recent classic, carefully controlled, study at Saint Paul's School in New Hampshire, researchers were able to substantially lower the serum cholesterol of approximately 500 boys by substituting polyunsaturate foods for those high in saturated fats.* These Harvard School of Public Health investigators modified students' dining hall diets by substituting low-fat milk for whole milk, using polyunsaturate vegetable oil in baked products and for frying doughnuts, replacing butter and regular margarine with a soft margarine, and serving whole eggs just once a week and a low-cholesterol egg mix twice. Other dietary modifications were made with the same purpose in mind—reduction of cholesterol and other hard fats.

Compounding the problem of high cholesterol and coronary heart disease is the hard fact that obesity continues to be a serious threat to health and a high quality of life for millions of American parents and their children. Obesity and malnutrition often go hand in hand—too many calories with too few essential nutrients.

We also have learned that most cases of adult obesity have their beginnings in childhood and adolescence. Yet we continue to serve school lunches and breakfasts dangerously high in saturated fats and starches. Surveys of large samples of schools throughout the nation confirm this. Under current standards such hard-fat foods as regular peanut butter, whole-fat milk, processed cheese, fatty meats, frankfurters, and regular margarine or butter qualify for federal reimbursement under the national school lunch program.

Thus, boys and girls are fed each day on those high-cholesterol foods as a result of financial expediency and lack of understanding of the role of dietary fats in human health. For the most part, neither school administrators, teachers, food service personnel, nor

---

*Stare, F. J., editor: Atheroselerosis, New York, 1974, Medcom, Inc.

parents have any idea of the potential danger of these fatty foods. One baked product that meets U.S. Department of Agriculture specifications and is served in many school breakfast programs is very high in both fat and sugar. This piles the problem of increased dental caries atop the added risk of adult atherosclerosis and obesity.

Too little too late

As previously mentioned, repeated studies show that many school lunches are deficient in complete proteins, iron, and vitamins A and C. More than a few schools also fail to provide adequate amounts of such important nutrients as thiamine, pyridoxine, vitamin D, and magnesium. All of these are needed for optimal growth and development during childhood and adolescence.

To underscore the critical need for more nutritious school lunches and breakfasts, we need only look at the 1968 U.S. Department of Agriculture report, *Dietary Levels of Households in the United States.* This survey of some 7,500 American families revealed that half were subsisting on diets that were frankly deficient in at least one important nutrient. More disturbing was the finding that the quality of diets among American families had steadily declined over the 10-year period of the study.

Streamlining school food services

Perhaps like America's railroad dining car —a nostalgic financial failure—our school lunchrooms need to move into the jet age of airline-type central food service.

Evidence is mounting that the planning and operation of school food services is best done by organizations experienced in large-scale meal delivery systems. Studies show that for the same worker cost centrally located kitchens can provide three times the number of meals that can be served under the existing unit kitchen system where meals are prepared in each individual school.

Recent experience in over 200 school districts has verified the heightened efficiency of the application of new food industry technology to school feeding programs.

The chief drawback to a central kitchen system is the high initial cost. Though such systems usually become economically stable in a year or 2, many school districts cannot afford the original financial outlay. The possibility of federal money here is a gleam of hope for the future of better school food services.

Needed legislation

Although government involvement in school feeding programs has been characterized by legislative and bureaucratic patchwork, progress during the past decade has been significant. Despite a seeming reluctance on the part of national administrations, both the House and Senate have favored bills to improve school lunch and breakfast programs.

Typical of this support and concern was the 1974 recommendation of the United States Senate Committee on Agriculture and Forestry. That report urged four alternatives to the present school feeding program:

1. *Poverty program* would offer federal support only for those children most in need. Most schools would continue to offer food services to students whose parents are able to pay.

2. *Poverty plus expanded reduced-price program* would call for withdrawal of 15 cents of federal support from paid lunches to provide more reduced-price meals for the near poor—families earning less than $8,500 a year.

3. *Universal reduced-price lunches* would extend reduced-price lunches to all currently paying pupils. This could increase the number of students participating in the program.

4. *Universal free lunch program* would raise the federal subsidy to cover the full cost of meals for all school children and youth. A sharp increase in pupil participation should result.

In 1975 Congress considered House Bill HR 4222, which would make the school breakfast program permanent, provide for a 25-cent lunch, and generally upgrade the delivery of quality meals to students. At the same time Bill S. 850, the National School

Lunch and Child Nutrition Act Amendments of 1975, was introduced to the Senate. However, these and other bills were either stalled in committee or compromised for political reasons, economic reasons, or both.

Improving school food services

Regardless of the merits or limitations of new school feeding legislation, teachers, school board members, administrators, and others concerned with student health can get information and assistance from these organizations: the United States Jaycees Center for Improved Child Nutrition (4 West Twenty-first St., Tulsa, Okla. 74102), the Child Nutrition Division of the U.S. Department of Agriculture (Washington, D.C. 20250), and the American School Food Services Association (P.O. Box 10095, Denver, Colo. 80210). In addition, teachers and those directly concerned with providing school food services can write or call their state—or District of Columbia—office listed in Appendix E for specific information.

At local and state levels there is continuing need for studies to determine the most efficient methods—lowest cost and highest nutrient meals—for raising the important contribution of the school feeding program to the health of elementary and secondary school children and youth. An up-to-date list of state offices for school lunch and breakfast programs is provided in Appendix E.

School feeding and nutrition education

Certainly one of the chief advantages of the school lunch or breakfast is the opportunity it provides for relating classroom information on healthful diets to school feeding programs. Teachers can have students keep daily records of what they eat, including school meals, and discussions can be a significant part of a unit on nutrition. Of course, any diary records from students must be anonymous if reliable responses are to be obtained.

A recent news story told about an elementary school principal, who distressed at food wastage in the lunchroom, had pupils take inventory of what had been thrown in trash cans 1 day. A pupil-prepared report disclosed that students had discarded the following items: forty-one sandwiches, two cartons of milk, two whole pieces of chicken, three bags of potato chips, nineteen apples, thirteen oranges, one piece of cake, an untouched carton of chocolate pudding, four whole carrots, two boxes of raisins, nineteen pieces of candy, and fourteen cookies! Obviously, simply offering food to children does not ensure that they will eat it.

Without sound nutrition education students may discard nutritious foods from the school lunch or breakfast, buy calorie-rich nutritionally poor foods from vending machines, or patronize one of the quick-food commercial establishments in the neighborhood. Again, health education appears as the crucial influence in choices and decisions of students whatever the environmental situation.

WHAT ABOUT SCHOOL BUS SAFETY?

School buses are part of the school environment because once the child steps aboard the bus he or she is under the jurisdiction and responsibility of the schools. The child's health and safety on the bus is just as important as it is when that child is in any other school facility or activity.

Each year about 100 students lose their lives in school bus accidents—35 as passengers and 65 while getting on or off the bus. Every day more than 300,000 school buses carry over 20 million boys and girls to and from school. All in all, the school bus is safer for children than the family or personal car, but there is substantial room for improvement. Unfortunately, parents and the general public usually are apathetic except for brief transient periods of emotional concern following a tragic accident killing large numbers of students.

The National Transportation Safety Board recently reported that 90% of America's school buses are unsafe for one reason or another. The National Highway Traffic Safety Administration has proposed new, tough requirements for all public transport buses, including school buses. Chief among these is the provision for padded, high-backed seats and safety belts for all passengers.

Congressional legislation, in the face of powerful lobbying and bureaucratic inertia, offers the promise of safer school buses. One of the better recent proposals in the U.S. House of Representatives included these new national standards:

1. Seating systems including proper padding, firm anchoring to the floor, approved passenger belts, and higher seat backs
2. Improved emergency exits
3. Interior protection for passengers
4. Greater floor strength
5. More crash-resistant bodies and frames
6. Safer vehicle operating systems
7. Improved safety glass for windshields and passenger windows

Safety experts also believe that school bus transportation can be made safer by careful selection and training of drivers, skilled mechanical maintenance, nationwide uniformity of exterior color and bus stopping requirements, and avoidance of overcrowding and unruly pupil behavior.

ARE OUR SCHOOLS FIRETRAPS?*

Not too many years ago some fire safety experts estimated that approximately 30,000 schools in America could be classified as firetraps. Many magazine articles, continued public education by the National Safety Council and local and national fire officials, such popular films as *Towering Inferno*, and the Kentucky nightclub fire in 1977 have tended to increase public concern for fire prevention and protection.

Still, many schools lack automatic fire alarm systems, and very few have automatic sprinkler systems. Such systems should, at least, be installed in shops, chemistry laboratories, boiler rooms, supply rooms, and other fire-hazard areas. Local fire inspectors should be consulted by school administrators

for regular inspections and recommendations for eliminating any existing dangerous conditions. The cost of alarm and sprinkler systems is a small price to pay for protecting the lives of children and youth in our schools.

The American Insurance Association urged that the following school fire-hazard conditions be checked and, when necessary, immediately corrected*:

1. Buildings where the walls or ceilings of exit corridors are surfaced with highly combustible finishes
2. Buildings with wood floors and masonry walls, especially if the pupils in the upper floors have no means of exit other than through stairs open to lower stories
3. Buildings of wood construction with pupils housed above the second story
4. Buildings with unventilated space below them where gas may collect and explode
5. Buildings with exit doors to the outside that cannot be readily opened from the inside
6. Buildings in which pupils on upper floors have no means of exit except down stairs that are open to lower stories having combustible walls and finishes or contents in storage that are combustible

With the increasing use of electrical current for audiovisual and other equipment in schools, careful periodic inspection by professionals should be made for faulty or overloaded wiring systems, a major fire hazard.

Monthly fire and disaster drills should be held for students and school personnel. Fire extinguishers should be approved by local fire officials, inspected regularly, and their location and operation understood by teachers and other school personnel. All school personnel and students should be aware of the location of manually operated fire alarms in the school and of regular fire alarm boxes near the school.

As with other aspects of a safe and healthful school environment, health instruction of students is essential for optimal fire prevention and protection.

---

*See the fire safety unit in Chapter 9 for use in educational programs.

*American Insurance Association: Safe schools, New York, 1968, The Association.

first aid chart for athletic injuries

FIRST AID, the immediate and temporary care offered to the stricken athlete until the services of a physician can be obtained, minimizes the aggravation of injury and enhances the earliest possible return of the athlete to peak performance. To this end, it is strongly recommended that:

ALL ATHLETIC PROGRAMS include prearranged procedures for obtaining emergency first aid, transportation, and medical care.

ALL COACHES AND TRAINERS be competent in first aid techniques and procedures.

ALL ATHLETES be properly immunized as medically recommended, especially against tetanus and polio.

Committee on the
Medical Aspects or Sports
AMERICAN MEDICAL ASSOCIATION

to protect the athlete at time of injury, FOLLOW THESE FIRST STEPS FOR FIRST AID

STOP play immediately at first indication of possible injury or illness.

LOOK for obvious deformity or other deviation from the athlete's normal structure or motion.

LISTEN to the athlete's description of his complaint and how the injury occurred.

ACT, but move the athlete *only* after serious injury is ruled out.

BONES AND JOINTS

fracture Never move athlete if fracture of back, neck, or skull is suspected. If athlete *can* be moved, carefully splint any possible fracture. Obtain medical care at once.

dislocation Support joint. Apply ice bag or cold cloths to reduce swelling, and refer to physician at once.

bone bruise Apply ice bag or cold cloths and protect from further injury. If severe, refer to physician.

broken nose Apply cold cloths and refer to physician.

HEAT ILLNESSES

heat stroke Collapse—with dry warm skin—indicates sweating mechanism failure and rising body temperature.
THIS IS AN EMERGENCY; DELAY COULD BE FATAL. Immediately cool athlete by the most expedient means (immersion in cool water is best method). Obtain medical care at once.

heat exhaustion Weakness—with profuse sweating—indicates state of shock due to depletion of salt and water. Place in shade with head level or lower than body. Give sips of dilute salt water. Obtain medical care at once.

sunburn If severe, apply sterile gauze dressing and refer to physician.

IMPACT BLOWS

head If any period of dizziness, headache, incoordination or unconsciousness occurs, disallow any further activity and obtain medical care at once. Keep athlete lying down; if unconscious, give nothing by mouth.

teeth Save teeth, if completely removed from socket. If loosened, do not disturb; cover with sterile gauze and refer to dentist at once.

solar plexus Rest athlete on back and moisten face with cool water. Loosen clothing around waist and chest. Do nothing else except obtain medical care if needed.

testicle Rest athlete on back and apply ice bag or cold cloths. Obtain medical care if pain persists.

eye If vision is impaired, refer to physician at once. With soft tissue injury, apply ice bag or cold cloths to reduce swelling.

MUSCLES AND LIGAMENTS

bruise Apply ice bag or cold cloths and rest injured muscle. Protect from further aggravation. If severe, refer to physician.

cramp Have opposite muscles contracted forcefully, using firm hand pressure on cramped muscle. If during hot day, give sips of dilute salt water. If recurring, refer to physician.

strain and sprain Elevate injured part and apply ice bag or cold cloths. Apply pressure bandage to reduce swelling. Avoid weight bearing and obtain medical care.

OPEN WOUNDS

heavy bleeding Apply sterile pressure bandage using hand pressure if necessary. Refer to physician at once.

cut and abrasion Hold briefly under cold water. Then cleanse with mild soap and water. Apply sterile pad firmly until bleeding stops, then protect with more loosely applied sterile bandage. If extensive, refer to physician.

puncture wound Handle same as cuts; refer to physician.

nosebleed Keep athlete sitting or standing; cover nose with cold cloths. If bleeding is heavy, pinch nose and place *small* cotton pack in nostrils. If bleeding continues, refer to physician.

OTHER CONCERNS

blisters Keep clean with mild soap and water and protect from aggravation. If already broken, trim ragged edges with sterilized equipment. If extensive or infected, refer to physician.

foreign body in eye Do not rub. Gently touch particle with point of clean, moist cloth and wash with cold water. If unsuccessful or if pain persists, refer to physician.

lime burns Wash thoroughly with water. Apply sterile gauze dressing and refer to physician.

EMERGENCY PHONE NUMBERS		
Physician		Phone:
Physician		Phone:
Hospital	Ambulance	
Police	Fire	Other

Fig. 3-1. From Bucher, C. A.: Administration of health and physical education programs, including athletics, ed. 6, St. Louis, 1975, The C. V. Mosby Co.

WHAT ABOUT PHYSICAL EDUCATION AND SPORTS?

Since a 1974 nationally televised ABC special on the hazards of football in senior and junior high schools, parents and school administrators have become more concerned with sports injuries.

First and foremost as a problem underlying injuries in athletics and physical education is the disturbing fact that many states do not require certification for coaches and teachers in these areas. Only *nine* of our fifty states have certification requirements for athletic coaches. Team physicians and certified trainers are still a rarity even at the secondary school level.

Until and unless parents, the general public, school administrators, and state legislators become aware of and actively involved in the problem, little improvement can be expected.

The situation is somewhat better in physical education where most schools today employ qualified, state-certified physical educators—many with a health education minor—who have had university courses in physiology of exercise, kinesiology, first aid, athletic training, and prevention of sports injuries.

The Committee on the Medical Aspects of the American Medical Association has prepared a *First Aid Chart for Athletic Injuries*, which should be of value to both coaches and physical educators. The chart, reproduced in Fig. 3-1, is available from the American Medical Association.

Though much can be done to improve the school environment with regard to athletics and physical education through removing and controlling hazards, the key factor in the problem remains; too few schools are hiring qualified physical educators, coaches, and supervisors for children's sports participation.

HOW CAN WE IMPROVE THE EMOTIONAL CLIMATE?

There is much being said and written of late about the effect of schools and school personnel on the emotional health and mental development of children. Most of us have heard the dismal estimate by some psychologists that the average child is exposed to two emotionally unstable teachers during his school years. Some of us might consider this estimate too conservative.

In any case, the teacher is the person children see day after day during the school year. Next to the parent the teacher probably has more influence on most students than any other persons in their young lives. What a challenge this is; yet what an opportunity!

Practically all certified teachers have had at least some background of study in the field of mental health. Still, teachers find it difficult to effectively deal with the emotional problems presented from time to time in the classroom and in extracurricular settings. The reason for this in most instances is that we know so little about mental health and emotional development. One of the things we do know reasonably well is that people need to be motivated, to have perceivable goals if they are to learn, perform, and develop as individual personalities capable of coping with and contributing to their world.

One of the pioneers in the field of motivational psychology is the late Abraham Maslow. His works lie behind much of the "hidden persuader" Madison Avenue advertising techniques we see every day on television commercials. Obviously they are quite effective.

Some years ago Maslow, in his classic text *Motivation and Personality*, proposed five levels of basic human needs:

1. *Physical*—the need for air, water, food, sleep, sex, and other physiologic essentials.
2. *Safety and security*—the need to be "safe" and secure in one's environment, family, job, school, social circle, and other facets of human activity and interaction.
3. *Love and affection*—the need for being liked and loved by parents, siblings, classmates, teachers, and others whom one respects.
4. *Esteem*—the "status seeker's" need to be respected and highly regarded as an individual.
5. *Self-actualization*—the need to establish oneself as a person, the self-image or

identity, and becoming what one's potential offers.

Certainly every aspect of the daily life in elementary school offers multiple opportunities for teachers and other school personnel to contribute to situations and conditions that help students fulfill these basic human needs. To do less is to fail in our obligation and opportunity to enrich the emotional lives of our students.

A more detailed discussion of these and other concepts relating to the emotional atmosphere of the school is included in Chapter 7.

QUESTIONS FOR DISCUSSION

1. What are the aims of a healthful school environment?
2. What considerations are included in a good program for healthful school living?
3. How can teachers and other school personnel help make improvements in old school buildings and poor school sites?
4. Why are school food service programs important to student health?
5. What are some of the major problems still existing in developing better school lunch and breakfast programs?
6. Why are central food service facilities considered to be better than individual school food preparation facilities?
7. What nutrients are often found lacking in many school lunch programs? What nutrients may be served in excess and too often?
8. What organizations can help start a new school feeding program or improve an existing one?
9. Why are so many school buses considered by safety experts to be dangerous?
10. What changes need to be made in the construction of school buses to make them safer?
11. What changes need to be made in the operation of school buses to make student transportation safer?
12. What are the chief fire dangers in today's schools?
13. How can school administrators and teachers improve programs of fire prevention and protection?
14. Why do so many injuries occur in physical education classes? Why do so many occur in free play in the school yard?
15. Why do experts consider that too many serious injuries occur each year in varsity athletics?
16. How can injuries—for boys and girls—in competitive athletics be reduced?
17. How can teachers help students deal with emotional stresses and problems?
18. What are the basic emotional needs of children and youth? How might failure to meet these needs relate to student alienation, unrest, and even violence?

SUGGESTED CLASS ACTIVITIES

1. Using the California criteria in Appendix C, arrange to visit an elementary school and evaluate its environment.
2. On the basis of your evaluation, prepare a report listing needed changes, and suggest ways in which these changes may be brought about.
3. Hold a round-table discussion and debate the relative merits of a food service program run by a commercial catering organization and one operated by the schools.
4. Interview an elementary school administrator and find out what he considers to be the most difficult problems in the physical-emotional setting of his school.
5. Conduct a round-table discussion on the influence of administrative policies, teacher personality, subjects, teaching methods, and classroom appearance on the human environment.
6. Interview a local fire official and report to the class on the recommendations made for fire safety in elementary schools.
7. Prepare a report that might be used to convince a school board that safety is more important than economy in the purchase and maintenance of school buses.

REFERENCES

Bard, B.: The school lunchroom; time of trial, New York, 1968, John Wiley & Sons, Inc.

Commission on School Buildings of the American Association of School Administrators: Schools for America, Washington, D.C., 1967, The Association.

Cornacchia, H. J., Smith, D. E., and Bentel, D. J.: Drugs in the classroom, ed. 2, St. Louis, 1978, The C. V. Mosby Co.

Committee on the Medical Aspects of Sports of the American Medical Association and the National Federation of State High School Athletic Associations; Tips on athletic training, Chicago, 1969, American Medical Association.

Dunbar, L.: School lunches for hungry children; an urgent unmet need (editorial), Parents' Magazine **48:** April, 1973.

Egan, R.: Congress weighs safety standards for school buses, National Observer **48:** May 19, 1973.

Hanlon, J. J.: Public health administration and practice, St. Louis, 1974, The C. V. Mosby Co.

Joint Committee on Health Problems in Education; Healthful school environment, Washington, D.C., 1969, National Education Association and the American Medical Association.

Maslow, A. H.: Motivation and personality, New York, 1954, Harper & Row, Publishers, Inc.

National Safety Council: Accident facts, Chicago, 1977, The Council.

Randall, H. B.: The teacher's responsibility for mental health in the classroom, Journal of School Health **37:** Nov., 1967.

Select Committee on Nutrition and Human Needs of the U.S. Senate: Hunger in the classroom; then and now,

Washington, D.C., 1972. U.S. Government Printing Office.

Staton, W. M.: School lunch; pupils, politics, and peanut butter. Paper presented at the Forty-first Annual Meeting of the Southwest District, American Alliance for Health, Physical Education, and Recreation, Albuquerque, New Mexico, April, 1975 (mimeographed).

Young, W. R.: Crime in the classroom, Reader's Digest, May, 1976.

PART THREE

Health services

4 Health appraisals of school children

Questions frequently asked by the teacher with health appraisal responsibilities include the following:

"Why must I be concerned with the health of boys and girls in my class?"

"How can I find out about the health status of children in my room?"

"Is the failure of children to learn related to their health problems?"

"Can the nurse help me to know more about the health of my pupils?"

"Why must children have periodic vision and hearing tests?"

"What is the teacher's responsibility in preparing children for vision testing, hearing testing, dental inspections, health examinations, and other appraisals?"

"Should I be concerned about a child with a runny nose or a skin infection or one who is always extremely fatigued?"

"What can I do about the overly active, fidgety, aggressive child in class?"

"Why are health records used in schools?"

"What should I do about children in my class who are diabetic or epileptic or who have heart problems?"

Although educators and medical specialists generally believe the home has the primary responsibility for the health of children, schools need to maintain strong supportive programs (1) because of the relationship of good health to effective learning, (2) because there are hazards associated with communicable diseases, and (3) because numerous parents fail to, or do not know how to, accept their responsibilities for maintaining high levels of health in their children. Boys and girls with measles, mumps, tuberculosis, or poliomyelitis may transmit these conditions to others. Children who cannot see or hear well may have difficulty in acquiring an education. Students with emotional problems may have trouble learning to read. Pupils who fail to eat breakfast or who are malnourished may not have sufficient stamina to endure the daily classroom activities. Dental health problems may be of sufficient severity or degree to cause young people constant pain or emotional upsets, which adversely affect their concentration and attention to learning. Children who are diabetic, epileptic, or rheumatic need to be identified as such to arrange adjustments of their educational programs. These problems may be found in large numbers if there is an abundance of deprived and disadvantaged students in schools.

Unfortunately the home has not always satisfactorily or completely assumed its health role. In some instances this responsibility has been ignored or has not been recognized. Children continue to be sent to school with physical and emotional conditions that are considered to be unimportant or are unknown to parents. The school, therefore, has found it necessary to locate those boys and girls who are the health deviates. The procedures used to identify these children with health problems are called appraisals.

Health appraisals are part of the comprehensive health services program that should be found in school health programs (see Fig. 1-1). Health services also include health guidance and follow-up procedures, control of communicable disease, safety (with special reference to emergencies and first aid), nurses and other personnel, and evaluation. Chapters 5 to 7 and 14 provide detailed information.

PROBLEMS OF THE POOR

It was pointed out in Chapter 1 that deprived individuals generally have more health problems than those children and youth whose families are at higher socioeconomic levels. The American Academy of Pediatrics* has advocated that where school children do not receive adequate health care, school programs may need to provide screening, preventive, and some treatment services. In recent years federal and state funds have become available to help in this regard. In California, the Child Health and Disabilities Prevention Act of 1975 provided

for the early and periodic assessment of the health status of children and youth under 21 years of age. It specifically required children within 12 months before entering first grade to be given a health evaluation (screening) that consisted of: a health history; a brief physical examination; developmental assessment; eye and hearing tests; examination of teeth; and laboratory tests, including blood, tuberculosis, anemia, PKU (phenylketonuria), diabetes, urine, and sickle anemia. The evaluation must also include a check of the immunization record in order to bring up to date the following: DPT (diphtheria-

---

*School Health Committee: School health; a guide for health professionals, Evanston, Ill., 1977, American Academy of Pediatrics.

Timing and frequency of the routine school health services for pupils (1975-1976)*

Type of service	Kg.	1	2	3	4	5	6	7	8	9	10	11	12
Vision screening tests: at certain grades; all new pupils at other grades and referrals	☑	☑	☐	☑	☐	☑	☐	☑	☐	☐	☑	☐	☐
Hearing screening tests: at certain grades; all new pupils at other grades and referrals	☑	☑	☐	☑	☐	☐	☐	☐	☐	☐	☐	☐	☐
Dental education and/or inspections:													
a. at certain grades (except in a few schools) and some cleanings	☐	☐	☑	☑	☑	☑	☐	☑	☐	☐	☐	☐	☐
b. DMF surveys in high schools (about every 5 years)	☐	☐	☐	☐	☐	☐	☐	☐	☐	☑	☐	☐	☐
Weight and growth measurements: on all new and referred pupils (often done cooperatively with P.E. fitness program)	☑	☑	☑	☑	☑	☑	☑	☐	☐	☐	☐	☐	☐
Nurse interviews: with parents of new children	☑	←——————— (as indicated) ———————→											
Medical appraisals:													
a. all pupils who participate in varsity sports or ROTC who do not bring reports from private or clinic physicians	☐	☐	☐	☐	☐	☐	☐	☐	☐	☐	☑	☑	☑
b. pupils who participate in swimming classes when private or clinic physician appraisals are not obtained	☐	☐	☐	☐	☐	☐	☐	☑	☑	☑	☑	☑	☑
Medical and/or nursing appraisals:													
a. all pupils with suspected health or learning problems without current or complete reports from family or clinic physicians	☑	☑	☑	☑	☑	☑	☑	☑	☑	☑	☑	☑	☑
b. all pupils being considered for placement in special education	☑	☑	☑	☑	☑	☑	☑	☑	☑	☑	☑	☑	☑
Special services:													
a. mandatory tuberculin skin tests for those who have not had one within 9 months	☐	☐	☐	☐	☐	☐	☐	☑	☐	☐	☐	☐	☐
b. scoliosis screening	☐	☐	☐	☐	☐	☑	☑	☑	☐	☐	☐	☐	☐
c. inspections for nuisance diseases	←——————————— (as needed) ———————————→												
d. color vision rechecks	☐	☐	☐	☐	☐	☐	☐	☑	☐ ←—(new pupils)—→				

*From the Fifty-first Annual Report, 1975-1976, Denver Public Schools, Denver, Colo., Department of Health and Medical Services.

pertussis-tetanus), TOPV (Trivalent oral polio virus vaccine), MMR (measles, mumps, rubella), and TD (tetanus and diphtheria toxoids).

WHAT ARE HEALTH APPRAISALS?

Health appraisals refer to a series of procedures to assess or determine the health status of children through the use of teacher observations, screening tests, health histories or inventories, dental inspections, medical examinations, and psychologic tests. They are dependent on the cooperation of parents, teachers, physicians, dentists, health educators, nurses, and psychologists in the school program. The frequency of appraisals varies in school districts throughout the United States. The chart on p. 48 illustrates the types, grades, and times for the Denver Public Schools in Denver, Colorado.

A growing procedure in schools is to conduct preschool health appraisals, with or without the cooperation of the health department.

Appraisals exist for the following reasons:
1. To locate pupils needing medical or dental treatment
2. To locate pupils who are poorly adjusted and in need of special attention at school or treatment by a psychiatrist or child guidance clinic, for example, concerning behavior problems and emotional disturbances
3. To locate pupils who need modified educational programs, for example, those who are hard of hearing, partially sighted, blind, or mentally retarded
4. To locate pupils who need more thorough examinations than provided in school, for example, by means of x-ray examinations, laboratory examinations, or examinations by specialists
5. To inform school personnel and parents about the health status of children and to encourage parents to recognize and accept the responsibility for seeking necessary corrections
6. To help pupils with health problems make adjustments or compensations for their conditions in schools

7. To serve as learning experiences for children, teachers, and parents

A description of the nature of health appraisals together with the responsibilities of the teachers are discussed in the pages that follow. The degree to which the teacher participates differs in every school district and is dependent on the extent of the school program as well as on the availability of special school health personnel.

Three important points related to the teacher's role must be recognized:
1. Teachers, nurses, and nonmedically trained people should not attempt to make diagnoses. However, nurses are able to make preliminary diagnoses because of their training and experiences. Observations of runny noses, flushed faces, and elevations of temperatures do not permit untrained individuals to identify these conditions as colds, the flu, or other diseases. Signs and symptoms that are noted in young people should result in the referral of these children to the school personnel capable of making diagnoses or of determining necessary action.

2. Ordinarily schools and school personnel should not render medical care, and employees in general should not attempt to provide treatment services; this is the function of physicians, dentists, and other qualified specialists. Some school districts try to make provision for treatment services for needy children.

3. Health information about pupils should remain confidential. Teachers and others in schools who need this knowledge should have access to it.

WHAT ARE TEACHER OBSERVATIONS?

Teachers are in a strategic position to observe the appearance and behavior of children because they are with pupils for many hours each day and many weeks each year. They see children perform a variety of activities under different environmental circumstances. They are continually noting pupils with headaches, frequent respiratory infections, and recurrent earaches, or those suffering from overfatigue, skin infections,

Text continued on p. 56.

Table 4-1. Good health characteristics of children

Physical	Social-emotional	Work habits
Endurance: completes a task without undue fatigue	Enthusiastic	Attentive
Enjoys vigorous play	Objective interests: friends, hobbies, games, work, people	Carries a task through to completion
Alert, buoyant, pleasant	Curious: interested in things about him	Ability to concentrate
Looks refreshed in morning	Enters into activities	Persistent in work
Assumes good posture	Happy, cheerful, agreeable, friendly	Works independently
Posture expresses buoyancy, alertness, success, happiness	Refrains from quarreling	Orderly in work habits
Prompt, efficient muscular coordination	Confident: expects success, meets failure	Shows originality and initiative
Poise: freedom from unnecessary activity	Shares group responsibility	Creative
Muscles firm	Protects others' property	Takes responsibility
Hair: natural luster	Appreciation and understanding for others	Prompt in meeting appointments
Clear skin, clear bright eyes, clean, neat in appearance, inoffensive breath, wholesome appetite	Does things for the group, not for self alone	Responds quickly and cheerfully to directions
	Shows courage in meeting difficulties	Shares group responsibility
	Cooperative with peers	Cooperative with peers
	Adapts to new situations	
	Exercises control	

Table 4-2. Growth and development characteristics

Physical development	Characteristics	Health education implications
	5 to 7 years of age	
Growth is relatively slow: at age 7 may be 2 to 3 inches and 3 to 6 pounds yearly	Upon entering school may be a resumption of earlier tensional behavior; thumbsucking, nail biting, toilet lapses	Mental health: Wants to get along with agemates
Large muscle better developed than small ones; improving by age 7	Eager to learn, exuberant, restless; exaggerates, overactive, and susceptible to fatigue; dawdling may occur	Praise, warmth, and patience with independence and encouraging support from adults
Some postural defects may have been established by age of 6	Criticism difficult; thrives on encouragement	Some responsibilities without pressure of being required to make decisions or meet rigid standards
Hand-eye coordination is incomplete; 90% are right-handed; small muscle control difficult especially of fingers and hands	Attention span short but increasing; interested in activiity, not results, learns best through active participation	Help to make adjustments in playground; withdrawn child needs encouragement to find place in group
Eyeballs are still increasing in size; tendency toward farsightedness	Has difficulty making decisions	Provide sense of accomplishment for each child; engage in real tasks; needs freedom
Heart is in a period of rapid growth	Self-assertive; aggressive; wants to be first; becoming self-dependent; can take care of own toilet needs and dressing; likes to climb and jump; by 7 is apt to be talkative and prone to exaggeration; competition developing	Provide active participation in learning with concrete objects
Permanent teeth begin to appear; baby teeth begin to be lost		Exercise and safety: active, boisterous games for large muscles; stress safety
Susceptible to respiratory infections; childhood diseases (measles, mumps, chickenpox, etc.), rheumatic fever		
Lungs relatively small		

Table 4-2. Growth and development characteristics—cont'd

Physical development	Characteristics	Health education implications
Tires easily Teeth: 6-year molars appearing and loss of primary teeth	Interest of boys and girls diverging, less play together; gets along best in small groups Able to assume some responsibility concerning right and wrong and simple tasks; acts grown up at times Bright eyes, color in face, great vitality Enjoys rhythms, active play, fairy tales, comics, TV, myths, dramatic play and stories Moods fluctuate; quick resistance to bathing	Vision care: protect eyes Sleep and rest: need 11 or more hours of sleep and possibly daytime naps Dental health: emphasis on tooth care Disease control: development of personal hygiene; cover coughs, sneezes, fingers away from mouth, washing hands, and others

8 to 10 years of age

Growth still slow and steady; some children reach plateau preceding growth of preadolescence; differences in individual bone ossification may vary as much as 5 to 6 years; girls' growth spurts at about 10 years Small muscles developing; manipulative skill is increasing Poor posture may develop; presence may indicate attention; chronic infection, fatigue, orthopedic difficulties, emotional maladjustment, etc. Hand-eye coordination improved; hands ready for crafts Eyes ready for both nearsightedness and farsightedness; nearsightedness may develop during eighth year Incisors and lower bicuspids appear; often a period of dental neglect; orthodontia may be necessary Internal changes in glands and body structure taking place; wide range in beginning of sexual maturity; period of rapid growth comes earlier for girls, it lasts longer in boys: Boys: beginning puberty cycle 10 to 13 years; ends 14 to 18½ years Girls: appearance of menstruation 10 to 16 years; average 12 years Lungs, digestive and circulatory systems still developing	Wants to do well but loses interest if discouraged or pressured; sensitive to criticism Gangs strong and of one sex only, of short duration and changing membership; response to structured groups and activities Allegiance to peer group instead of adult in case of conflict; want a "best friend" Capable of prolonged interest; often makes plans and goes ahead on his or her own; increased attention span; realism replacing fantasy Enjoys conforming to rules of game, testing his or her skill against perfection; can be fairly responsible and dependable Gaining self-control; conscience becoming strong; awareness of self-energy Fairly good eater; may neglect vegetables Decisive, responsible, dependable, reasonable, strong sense of right and wrong; much arguing over fairness of games Is untidy, deliberately throws over table manners, handwashing, hair combing; protests parents' choice of new clothes; general coolness toward all adults Is prone to accidents Health usually good; has much energy Fond of sports and games, collections, comics, adventure stories Girls less noisy and less full of spontaneous energy than boys	Mental health: Self-concept; values Needs friends and group membership Training in skills without pressure Wise guidance and channeling of interests rather than domination or overcritical standards Praise, encouragement; warmth from adults Help gain self-confidence by excelling in one thing Definite responsibility; reasonable explanations; no talking down Exercise: Activities involving use of whole body; sports and games Posture development in need of attention Sleep and rest: 10 to 12 hours sleep Nutrition: balanced intake of foods Dental health: care of teeth reemphasis Disease control: handwashing, hair washing, food washing, etc. Safety: accident prevention Sex education: growth and developmental changes

Continued.

Table 4-2. Growth and development characteristics—cont'd

Physical development	Characteristics	Health education implications
	11 to 13 years of age	
A "resting period" followed by a period of rapid growth in height, then weight; usually starts somewhere between 9 and 13 years; girls usually taller and heavier at 11 years than boys	Wide range of individual differences and maturity level	Mental health:
		Self-image; success experiences
Rapid muscular growth; uneven growth of different parts of body; awkwardness prevalent; posture may be slovenly	Gangs or groups important; prestige is more important than adult approval; gang interest is changing to interest in one or two best friends (girls more than boys)	Warm affection, approval, no nagging or condemnation
		Increase opportunities for independence
	Loves parents but does not show it, cool toward adults	Relations with others
Secondary sex characteristics beginning to develop; may cause embarrassment; in girls hips and breast development; in boys voice changes	Strong sense of responsibility about matters he thinks are important	Sense of belonging and peer group relations
		Values development
	Girls mature earlier than boys; girls are taller, heavier	Individual health and emotional counseling
Heart developing; blood pressure may fall; more rest is needed	Strong interest in sex, much teasing and antagonism between boy and girl groups; sex consciousness may cause self-consciousness and shyness	Nutrition: adequate diet importance
		Rest and sleep: 9 to 11 hours sleep
Permanent dentition of 28 teeth is completed by 13 to 14 years	Child approaching adolescence often becomes hypercritical, changeable, rebellious, uncooperative; exhibits extremes of conduct from independence to childish dependence; may rebel against rules	Exercise: sports and games both individual and team
Resistance to infection may be low		Dental health: care of teeth
		Safety: accident prevention and first aid
	Interest in activities to earn money	Disease control: acne especially
	Reading differences in ability and tastes apparent	Sex education:
		Physical and social changes
	Ravenous but finicky appetite may develop	Boy-girl relations
		Venereal disease
	May be overanxious about his or her own health and normalcy	Reproduction
	Competition is keen; development of coordination and skills through games especially for boys	
	Awkwardness and laziness common because of rapid and uneven growth; may need rest	

Table 4-3. Signs and symptoms of health defects and illnesses*

Point of observation	Physical signs	Behavior	Complaints
General appearance and behavior	Excessive thinness; excessive overweight; very small or very large in body build for age; pallor; weary expression; poor posture; dark circles under or puffiness of eyes; unusual gait or limp; uncleanliness; lethargic and unresponsive; facial tic	Acts tired or apathetic; is easily irritated; makes frequent trips to toilet; has persistent nervous habits, such as muscular twitching or biting of nails or lips; is subject to spasms (fits), fainting spells, or frequent nosebleeds; gets short of breath after mild exertion and climbing stairs; lacks appetite; vomits frequently; has frequent accidents	Feels tired; does not want to play; has aches or pains; feels sick to stomach; feels dizzy
Hair and scalp	Stringy, lusterless hair; small bald spots; crusty sores on scalp; nits in hair	Scratches head frequently	Head itches
Ears	Discharge from ears; cotton in ear; tired, strained expression long before day is over; watchful, sometimes bewildered expression	Is persistently inattentive; asks to have questions repeated; habitually fails to respond when questioned; mispronounces common words; cocks one ear toward speaker; fails to follow directions	Has earache; has buzzing or ringing in ears; ears feel stuffy; hears noises in head
Eyes	Inflamed or watery eyes; frequent styes; redrimmed, encrusted, swollen lids; crossed eye; recurring styes; sensitivity to light	Holds book too close to, or too far from, eyes; squints at book or blackboard; persistently rubs or blinks eyes; reads poorly; attempts to brush away blur; tilts head to one side; shuts one eye; tends to reverse words or syllables; tends to lose place on page; shuts or covers one eye; unable to see distant things clearly	Headaches; dizziness; nausea; eyes ache, itch, smart, or feel scratchy; cannot see well (blurred or double vision); sensitivity to light
Mouth and teeth	Cavities in teeth; excessive stains; tartar at necks of teeth; malocclusion (uneven bite); irregular teeth; bleeding or inflamed gums; swollen jaw; sores in mouth; cracking of lips and corners of mouth	Acts depressed or resentful if many missing teeth or severe malocclusion subjects him or her to teasing or adverse comments from other children; this behavior is especially likely to occur in adolescence	Has toothache; mouth or gums feel sore
Nose and throat (upper respiratory tract)	Frequent or long-continued colds; persistent nasal discharge; persistent mouth breathing; enlarged glands in neck	Is frequently absent from school because of a cold; constantly clears throat or has frequent coughing or sneezing spells; is always sniffling or blowing nose; breathes persistently through mouth	Throat feels sore or scratchy; has difficulty in swallowing; nose feels stuffy or sore
Skin	Rashes or inflamed skin areas; scales and crusts; persistent sores, pimples, and blackheads on face; boils; hives; persistent warts; accidental injuries, such as cuts, scratches, bruises, burns, blisters; dry, red, rough skin	Is always scratching; is subject to skin irritations (hives, eczema, puzzling rashes, etc.), which suggest sensitivity to one or more substances (allergic manifestations); is easily bruised	Skin itches or burns; is concerned about pimples, blackheads, and other skin conditions that affect personal appearance

*What teachers see and Looking for health, 1969, New York, Metropolitan Life Insurance Co.

Table 4-4. Other signs and symptoms of health defects, illnesses, and problems

Condition	Signs and symptoms	
Allergy	Stuffy and runny nose, sneezing, persistent cough, swollen eyelids, and rash, itching, watery and burning eyes, paleness, mouth breathing	Tired and listless, recurrent headaches, recurrent gastrointestinal cramps, vomiting, diarrhea
Cancer	Leukemia: tires easily, irritable, pale (anemic), recurrent and serious infections, prolonged bleeding from injuries	Brain tumors: irritability, fatigability, decreased appetite and activity, intermittent headache
Contagious diseases of childhood	Chill or chilliness; fever (flushed face, lassitude, malaise); sore or scratchy throat; red, watery eyes; watery nasal discharge	Tight, dry cough; sneezing; headache, earache, or aching in back or legs; nausea or vomiting
Diabetes	Constant urination, abnormal thirst, unusual hunger	Rapid loss of weight, irritability, obvious weakness and fatigue, nausea and vomiting
Diabetic insulin reaction*	Excessive hunger, perspiration, pallor, headache, dizziness, nervousness/trembling, confusion, crying	Irritability, drowsiness, fatigue, blurred vision, poor coordination, abdominal pain or nausea
Drug misuse and abuse	Physical: possible odor on breath and clothes; mouth and nose irritations; red, watery eyes; fingers with burns from smoking; poor appetite and/or weight loss; distraction of time and sense of perception; needle marks and scars on body; appearance of intoxication; dryness of mouth and nose	Behavior: changes in attendance, discipline and academic performance; display of unusual degrees of activity and excitement; display of unusual inactivity—moodiness, depression; deterioration of physical appearance and concern for health habits; unpredictable outbreaks of temper and flare-ups
Heart	Pale, blue lips, short of breath on rest of exertion, undersized, deformed chest	Rapid pulse at rest, clubbed fingers, easily fatigued, undernourished, fainting after exertion or excitement
Lead poisoning	Fatigue, lethargy, stomach pains, constipation, vomiting, anemia, irritability	Temper tantrums, unsteady walking, insomnia, convulsions, poor appetite or paleness; may be no symptoms
Nutrition	General appearance: fatigue slouch or posture; round shoulders or flabby muscles; excessively thin with spindly legs; lack of or finicky appetite; fails to gain weight steadily; excessively fat or poor distribution of fat; strained and worried look; listless and inactive or high-strung and overactive; easily fatigues and possibly irritable and and difficult to manage Hair: dry, coarse, brittle, lacking luster, dull	Eyes: tiny red line (engorged capillaries) extending around or across the cornea and inward toward pupil; dark circles under eyes; inflammation and crusting of lids Teeth and gums: decayed teeth; swollen, bleeding, or spongy gums; or abnormal color Tongue: beefy red and magenta Mouth: scarring, fissuring, or sores on angles of lips Skin: small nodules (like gooseflesh) or scaly and rough Chest, knees, legs and feet: pigeon-breasted, knockkneed, bow-legged, flatfooted—abnormal bone growth

*Give sugar immediately in form of sugar, fruit juice, carbonated beverages, or candy.

Table 4-4. Other signs and symptoms of health defects, illnesses, and problems—cont'd

Condition	Signs and symptoms	
Posture	Head tilted to side when reading or listening Head tilted forward when sitting, standing or walking Feet pointed inward or outward; stands with weight on inner ankles (pronated); drags or scuffles feet	Shoulders not level: one higher, lower, or forward Round shoulders with protruding shoulder blades One hip higher or more prominent Knees pointed inward (knock-kneed), outward or hyperextended (bowlegs)
Rheumatic fever	Failure to gain weight, or loss in weight; pallor; irritability	Poor appetite, repeated colds and sore throats, unexplained nosebleeds, muscle or joint pains
Sickle cell anemia	Pains in arms and legs, swelling in joints, loss of appetite	Weakness, pain in abdomen, jaundice
Social-emotional maladjustment	Overtimidity: withdrawing, crying easily Overaggressiveness: bullying, quarreling, boisterousness; cruel behavior Excessive daydreaming: persistent inattentiveness Extreme sensitiveness to criticism: cries easily, temper tantrums Difficulty in reading or reciting Failure to advance in school at normal rate despite good physical health and adequate intellectual capacity Stuttering or other forms of speech difficulty Lying, stealing, cheating, truant Resistance to authority: constant complaints of unfairness, "picked on," may engage in vandalism	Excess boasting or showing off Poor sportsmanship Undue restlessness: hyperactivity, habit tics, stammering, nail biting Frequent accidents or near accidents Poor coordination Abnormal sex behavior Unhappy and depressed Gradual deterioration or marked sudden drop in educational achievement Lack of interest or motivation Withdrawal, shyness, inferiority feelings Intense ambition, especially if inconsistent with potential Inconsistent bladder or bowel control Constantly seeking attention or popularity
Suicide	Sudden shift in quality of work; excess use of drugs and alcohol; changes in early behavior and learning patterns; extreme fatigue; boredom; decreased appetite; inability to concentrate; truancy; gives away prized possessions	Open signs of mental illness—delusions, hallucinations; distress signals—"Notice me; I need help; you'll be sorry when I'm dead"
Tuberculosis	Persistent cough, spit blood, nervousness, lack of energy, easy fatigability, fever	Loss of weight, chest pain, rapid pulse, night sweats or afternoon fever, pallor, feeling of tiredness
Venereal diseases	Syphilis: within 10 to 90 days—small sore (chancre) at sight where germs entered body tissue 6 weeks to 6 months—rash on palms or soles of feet; falling hair; ugly sores on body, in mouth, under arms, between legs or toes	Gonorrhea: within 3 to 8 days males—burning sensation on urination, pus from urethra females—no pain, male signs may not appear until serious damage to bodily organs occurs

and emotional disturbances. They are capable of becoming skilled observers of the signs and symptoms of ill health. The constant attention that they give to observing boys and girls throughout the day often results in the identification of pupils who are in the early stages of communicable diseases or who are suffering from physical defects or emotional disturbances needing care. Prompt attention to symptomatic behavior greatly helps in the maintenance and improvement of the children's health.

Teachers must be especially observant of disadvantaged children and those living in poverty. These young people generally have more dental caries and higher incidence of heart disease, mental illness, tuberculosis, and other health problems than do their classmates of higher socioeconomic standings.

The responsibility of observing children for illness indications does not carry with it the responsibility of diagnosing specific conditions. Diagnosis is a matter that rests with individuals with special professional ability. However, the more detailed and accurate the teacher's noting of pertinent symptoms, the more valuable the information can be for those responsible for diagnosis. A comment such as "George does not seem to feel well today" gives the physician little specific aid; but a brief account of signs and symptoms, such as a runny nose, frequent fatigue, and constant cough, which led the teacher to believe that George was not feeling well, is likely to be much more helpful.

Health observations by the teacher (Tables 4-1 to 4-4) are now considered to be a continuous procedure that takes place daily and throughout the entire day. It is no longer the formal type of health inspection that occurred early in the morning and was relegated to a specified few minutes in the schedule. It is much more than the mere checking of the cleanliness of hands, hair, teeth, skin, and other parts of the body. The teacher must realize that pupils' health may change from minute to minute, or from hour to hour, and must constantly be on the alert for these

changes. These observations involve the mental and emotional status of pupils as well as their physical status. The foundation of all pupil health appraisal activities is the continual informed observation of students by teachers.

Recent studies* indicate that teacher observations together with the use of screening tests are potentially capable of identifying nearly all kinds of health problems that develop after the initial health examination.

Specific learning disabilities or perceptual problems

Teachers will also observe a variety of children's problems that have been identified by these synonyms: minimal brain damage, minimal cerebral function, minimal brain dysfunction, dyslexia, hyperkinesia, hyperkinetic impulsive disorders, hyperactivity, autism and developmental aphasia. These central nervous system disabilities are not clearly defined but generally refer to those pupils with near average, average, or above average general intelligence with learning or behavioral abnormalities ranging from mild to severe that are associated with subtle deviant functions of the central nervous system. They are characterized by difficulties in listening, thinking, talking, reading, writing, spelling, and arithmetic. They involve memory and control of attention, impulse, or motor function. There is a significant difference between children's achievement level and their functioning capabilities based on their mental abilities. These conditions are independent of errors of refraction, muscle imbalance, and imperfect binocular vision, including problems due primarily to hearing or motor handicaps, to mental retardation, to emotional disturbance, or to environmental disadvantage.

Learning disabilities may be found in 5% to 15% of the school population. It is estimated that ten million children suffer learn-

---

*Jenne, F. H.: Variations in nursing service characteristics and teachers' health observation practices, Journal of School Health **40:** May, 1970.

ing disabilities; five million are hyperactive according to B. F. Feingold.* Boys are affected ten times more often than girls. Feingold states that these disabilities may be genetic in origin or may be caused by toxemia, infection, drugs, and anoxia during delivery, and toxicants, infection, trauma, and drugs after birth. He claims that additives, especially artificial colors and flavors, which occur in 80% of all foods and beverages, and the salicylate radical (related but not identical to aspirin) are especially involved after birth.

Children with specific learning disabilities may exhibit the following behavior:

1. Hyperactivity—constantly moving, poor concentration, short attention span, talkativeness
2. Impulsiveness—easily distracted by stimuli; speaks out of turn
3. Variability and unpredictability—may cry or laugh easily; explosive irritability
4. Emotional instability—overreacts to trips, parties, and such activities; delay and failure may produce tears and temper tantrums; not accepted by peers; gullible and trusting; low tolerance for failure and frustration
5. Perseverance—continuous repetition of an action or response after a successful performance; may write a letter over and over, or talk incessantly about a subject for months
6. Poor sleep habits—easily awakened; hard to fall asleep
7. Muscle coordination—cannot function in sports; exceptionally clumsy; difficulty with buttoning, writing, speech, reading (dyslexia)

Diagnosis of students with perceptual problems is difficult and complex. It is a medical matter. It may involve a team of individuals including school personnel. The procedure involves obtaining a complete medical history, conducting a thorough physical examination, including a neurologic survey, as well as a psychiatric and psychologic examination and an electroencephalogram. There is question by some authorities regarding the use of the EEG because they claim so-called normal children may exhibit abnormal brain wave patterns.

Treatment for learning disabilities is not easily rendered. It may include helping students to recognize sensory information (perception), to improve memory, to understand oral and written language, to increase cognitive skills—conceptualizing rational, psychologic, and social factors. It may also include the use of such drugs as stimulants (Ritalin, Dexedrine, Mellaril), tranquilizers, sedatives, antidepressants, antihistamines, and anticonvulsants, which have been beneficial to a variety of children. If drugs are to be administered at school, the role of the teacher should be clearly defined.

Harlin* reports that in March, 1972, a report of a panel of experts regarding the management of the hyperkinetic child stated that certain disorders improved from the standpoint of alertness, learning, and social behavior when amphetamines were used. They found no evidence that such drugs, when properly administered, led to drug addiction in later life.

The American Academy of Pediatrics† believes that other methods of behavior modification at home should be tried before treatment with drugs is attempted. They do not advocate the use of tranquilizers for the learning disability syndrome per se except perhaps for grossly disturbed, hyperactive,

*Feingold, B. F.: The role of the school luncheon program in behavior and learning disabilities, Oversight Hearings on the School Lunch Programs, Hearings before the Subcommittee on Elementary, Secondary and Vocational Education, Committee on Education and Labor, House of Representatives, Washington, D.C., 1976, U.S. Government Printing Office.

*Harlin, V. K.: The hyperkinetic child, School Health Review 4: March/April, 1973.
†Committee on School Health: School health; a guide for health professionals, Evanston, Ill., 1977, American Academy of Pediatrics.

and prepsychotic children. Feingold* has observed 350 children whom while under his care he placed on diets that eliminated all foods with a natural salicylate radical and that contained artificial colors and flavors. He states that he has had a favorable response in the behavioral pattern and learning abilities of 30% to 50% of these children.

Control of communicable diseases

Although local health departments generally have the legal responsibility for the prevention and control of disease, teachers need to be concerned with the control of communicable diseases because of the hazards they present to the pupils attending school. A variety of microorganisms including bacteria, viruses, protozoa, and fungi, can enter the body, cause infectious disease, and, if they are transmissible from person to person, are considered to be communicable.

Teachers must be alert for symptoms (Tables 4-3 and 4-4) that will identify suspected disease conditions in pupils. They are expected to isolate those children discovered and send them to the nurse, principal, or appropriate school authority for possible exclusion from school. When such pupils return to school, teachers should be familiar with the readmission procedures to be certain that the pupils have sufficiently recovered from their communicability to permit their return.

Where nursing services are limited or nonexistent, it may be the teacher's responsibility to inform parents of the symptoms observed.

The essential features of health observations comprise:
1. The teacher's constant alertness to health matters

---

*Feingold, B. F.: The role of the school luncheon program in behavior and learning disabilities, Oversight Hearings on the School Lunch Programs, Hearings before the Subcommittee on Elementary, Secondary and Vocational Education, Committee on Education and Labor, House of Representatives, Washington, D.C., 1976, U.S. Government Printing Office.

2. The teacher's awareness of the characteristics of good physical and emotional health
3. The teacher's understanding of the growth and development characteristics of children
4. The teacher's knowledge of the signs and symptoms of health deviations

Tables 4-1 to 4-3 provide information that will enable teachers to understand better their role in health observations. Specific details regarding the more common communicable diseases may be found in Appendix A.

It is possible to prevent and control many diseases through immunizations for smallpox, diphtheria, whooping cough, tetanus, poliomyelitis, measles, mumps, and German measles. Some school districts make available these immunizations. (See Appendix B for state regulations.)

TEACHER-NURSE CONFERENCES

A common practice in elementary schools is for teachers and nurses to hold periodic meetings during the school year to share their observations and information about the health status of pupils. The frequency of these meetings and their exact nature vary in schools and school districts, but their significance and importance is widely recognized. In general, the following are the reasons for these conferences:
1. To discuss the nature of teacher observations
2. To provide understandings regarding known health problems, such as diabetes, epilepsy, and heart conditions, and to make provisions for individual pupil needs
3. To help teachers to know what action to take in emergencies to help pupils with known health problems, such as epilepsy and diabetes
4. To help teachers make environmental adjustments in their classrooms and in school, such as having children sit in the front of the room or having them participate in limited activities
5. To make decisions about referral cases to

parents for diagnosis, information, or other action

6. To help teachers with the techniques of discussing health problems with parents
7. To inform teachers about future examinations and screening tests

Teacher observations serve as supplementary measures to the various screening procedures and examinations that take place in schools. They help to identify pupils with health problems in the interval between medical examinations and to identify children with problems who need special examinations. In schools that do not conduct periodic medical and dental examinations, teacher observations combined with screening tests and health inventories or histories, together with teacher-nurse conferences, may have to be used in substitution.

WHAT ARE SCREENING TESTS?

Screening tests are those preliminary health evaluations used in schools to assess the health status of pupils. They may include vision, hearing, growth and development, tuberculosis, dental inspections, posture, nutrition, sickle cell anemia and others. They should be low in cost so they can be available to large numbers of students. They are likely to be administered by teachers, nurses, technologists, and other school personnel. They serve as rough measuring devices that supplement and complement teacher observations as well as other procedures used to determine the health of pupils. If children are found to be in need, they should be referred to health specialists for diagnostic tests.

State laws widely differ in regard to requirements and frequency for these tests, but many include specific provisions for periodic screening of vision and hearing.

Vision

Vision testing usually concerns itself with problems of central visual acuity, direct vision of near and far objects, or the ability of the eye to perceive the shape and form of objects in the direct line of vision. However, constant alertness for signs of eye diseases

and other abnormalities must also be maintained. Children with acuity defects are not able to perceive and discriminate the details of objects or printed symbols. Thus, they are likely to encounter learning difficulties.

School vision screening usually attempts to reveal the following eye problems:

1. Errors of refraction—eye defects in which images are focused improperly on the retina.
   a. Hyperopia—farsightedness; light rays focus behind the retina, common in those under 10 to 12 years and usually corrects itself as the eye matures
   b. Myopia—nearsightedness; light rays focus in front of the retina
   c. Astigmatism—irregular curvature of the cornea or lens
2. Strabismus—cross-eyes caused by muscle imbalance; the muscles of the two eyes do not work in coordination, resulting in failure of the alignment of the eyes; it is estimated that 1.5% of children are so afflicted; the afflicted eye may not be used and may bring about deterioration of visual acuity, a condition known as amblyopia, which can usually be prevented if treated early; some schools are advising preschool examinations, and others are trying to identify children in Head Start programs.
3. Color blindness—inability to perceive colors; this condition may be congenital or acquired, with the congenital form being more prevalent; congenital defects may be either total or partial; total color blindness is rare, and when it occurs, all colors appear as grays; the partial type is most common and is primarily inherited through the mother who carries the recessive gene and is generally not affected; red and green colors are usually confused in most cases, but blue-yellow defects also occur; acquired defects of color may often develop in the course of ocular, mainly retinal, disease; approximately 3.8%* of children 6 to 11 years of age have

---

*U.S. Department of Health, Education, and Welfare, Public Health Service, National Center for Health Statistics: Color vision deficiencies in children, United States, Washington, D.C., 1972, U.S. Government Printing Office.

color vision deficiencies; by sex, 6.95% of boys and 0.53% of girls are affected; the problem among white boys is about twice as great as among black boys.

The minimum recommended vision screening program varies in schools throughout the United States. The National Society for the Prevention of Blindness believes an annual test for visual acuity is ideal in lieu of a professional eye examination. In California the program that will identify pupils with visual acuity deviations includes the following:

1. An examination by an eye or vision specialist (ophthalmologist or optometrist) before a child enters school to discover muscle imbalance, marked astigmatism, hyperopia, and amblyopia—a condition appearing in the very young child and rarely appearing later in life
2. The Snellen test for nearsightedness administered early in the school year to every child in kindergarten or first grade and to each pupil in any other grade who is enrolled for the first time in a school, and repeated in grades 3, 5, and 7
3. Systematic observation by teachers of the appearance, behavior, and complaints of pupils
4. Systematic investigation when a pupil's school performance shows evidence of the existence of a vision problem
5. Administration of a test for color vision preferably in early grades but no later than sixth grade to male students

Numerous other instruments, devices, and procedures, with varied opinions regarding their value, are available for vision screening, including the Maddox rod test (muscle imbalance), the telebinocular (a stereoscopic instrument to measure muscle imbalance, visual acuity, and color vision), the Ortho-Rater (similar to telebinocular), the Titmus vision tester (near- and far-sightedness), and the Massachusetts vision kit (visual acuity plus sphere and Maddox rod test and muscle imbalance). They all use some of the procedures mentioned in the California program and are more complex in nature. The modified clinic technique (MCT) is a procedure for testing vision that was used in the Orinda,

California, Vision Study. It is a technique administered by optometrists or ophthalmologists to all first graders and new children in school whereby refractive error is measured by skiametry (use of a retinoscope) and includes a cover test and inspection for organic problems. The Snellen test and teachers' observations are then used for additional periodic screenings. The Orinda study revealed that children needing eye attention are not missed, or underreferred, in schools where the modified clinic technique is used.

Preschool vision screening is now being recommended as an appropriate procedure. Such defects as cross-eye and amblyopia or so-called lazy eye can lead to unnecessary loss of vision in the affected eye if not detected or treated before the age of 6 years.

Because of the constant changing of children's eyes during their growth and development, it is recommended that vision be screened annually. The question of who does the screening differs in schools and school districts. Common practice indicates that teachers, nurses, technicians and volunteers are assigned to perform this service. Some state laws require teachers to give the tests. Reasons often advanced for teachers doing the vision testing are the following:

1. There is a greater possibility of every child being tested annually.
2. They understand better the children with vision problems in their classes.
3. They become more sensitive to and concerned with opportunities for continually observing children for vision deviations.
4. They can make the vision screening program a part of the health instruction program.

Snellen test. The Snellen test is designed to discover those children with myopia, although other difficulties may also be found. It has been widely used in schools because it is simple, economical, and practical. It has been considered by the National Society for the Prevention of Blindness as well as other authoritative groups as the best single measurement for vision screening.

The test makes use of a chart that has square-shaped letters or symbols resembling the letter E (Fig. 4-1). These are in specified sizes and in printed rows. The symbol at the top line of the chart is of such a size that a person with normal vision is able to see it from a distance of 200 feet, whereas the person with a vision problem can view it only from 20 feet. In each succeeding row, from the top downward, the size of the symbols is reduced to a point that a person with normal vision can see them at distances of 100, 70, 50, 30, and 20 feet, respectively.

To determine visual acuity, the student stands at a distance of 20 feet from the chart and with one eye covered reads the smallest letter that can be seen. The pupil's acuity is recorded by stating the distance at which the test has been completed and the line the student reads. These numbers are recorded as

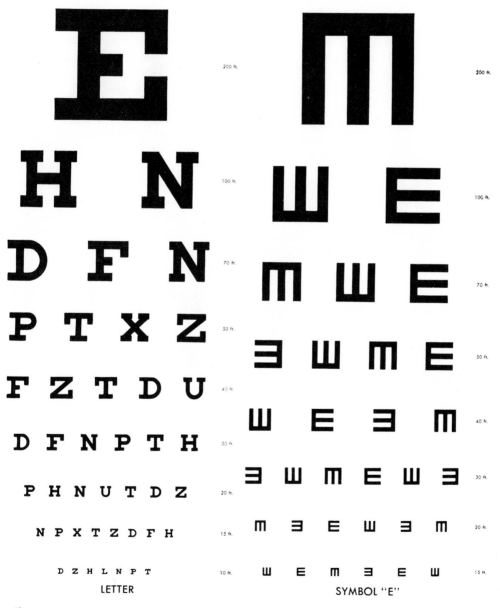

Fig. 4-1. Snellen charts. (Courtesy National Society for the Prevention of Blindness, New York, N.Y.)

fractions: 20/20, 20/40, 20/70. They are not actually fractions, but represent a simple method of reporting facts. Thus an acuity of 20/70 means that the student was tested at 20 feet and could read only the letters on line 70. The vision of each eye is tested separately.

Criteria for recommending pupils for a retest may be the following:

1. 12 years and under—20/40 in one or both eyes
2. Over 12 years—miss one symbol on line 30 with one or both eyes
3. Pupils with unequal vision between both eyes such as 20/20 in one and 20/40 in the other

After being retested, children for whom the second findings are the same as those recorded after the first test and concerning whom the teacher's observations indicate signs of abnormality are referred to examination to a professionally qualified person.

Plus sphere lens. The plus sphere lens is used to detect pupils with hyperopia. The test is administered by having such children wear a pair of glasses with convex (hyperopic) lenses of specified strength (+2.25 diopters* for the first three grades and +1.75 diopters from fourth grade on) and requiring them to read the 20-foot line of the Snellen chart. Each eye is tested separately. If they read the line, they have failed the test. The convex lens blurs the vision of the children with no refractive error and makes correction for the hyperopic youngsters enabling them to read the chart. Pupils who fail the test should be retested. If the results are the same and there are other signs noted through teacher observations, these children should be referred for professional diagnosis. The plus sphere test should be given only to those pupils not wearing glasses and who satisfactorily perform the Snellen test.

Cover test. There is no satisfactory screening procedure for muscle imbalance. However, a rough, and not very accurate, method is the cover test. It is a simple way to detect

---

*Diopter, unit of measurement of strength or refractive power of lenses.

latent strabismus (crossed eye not readily noticed). In some children this condition reveals itself only when they are very tired or under emotional stress. Latent strabismus may manifest itself in only one eye, or it may alternate between the eyes.

The cover test determines whether eye alignment is maintained when one eye is covered while the other is fixed on an object. The alignment of each eye should be determined for both distant and near points.

The procedure for testing should be as follows:

1. Have the pupil look at a small light or object 20 feet away.
2. Place a cover card in front of one of the pupil's eyes in a manner so that the light or object cannot be seen with that eye. Watch to see if the alignment of the covered eye is maintained; note whether the eye turns in, out, up, or down or holds its fixed position.
3. After a few seconds, move the cover card to the other eye. The previously covered eye is watched for a shift in the direction of its fixation.
4. Repeat the test, having the pupil look at a small light or object 8 to 10 inches in front of the nose. If the muscle balance of the eye is essentially normal, there should be no marked change in its fixation upon covering or when the cover is removed.

Pupils who show marked deviation from normal should be retested, and if the same results are discovered, they should be referred for professional diagnosis.

Color vision test. The color vision test is a procedure to determine whether a person is color blind, or unable to discriminate between certain colors, usually red and green and sometimes blue and yellow. Two satisfactory tests for school use are the Hardy-Rand-Ritter test and the Ishihara test.

Color blindness is inherited and cannot be corrected. Adjustments to the abnormality are important, and students should be aware of this limitation, especially when making vocational choices, when learning to drive automobiles or when crossing streets. It is desirable to test young people before they enter junior high school.

Hearing

The procedure generally used to test the hearing of children is the puretone audiometer. It requires technical training to administer and interpret.

The American Academy of Pediatrics recommends that hearing should be tested annually. This may be too costly for many school districts or may be impossible because of logistical problems. The 1960 National Conference of Identification Audiometry advocated an adequate program in the early school years with annual testing in kindergarten and first, second, and third grades. It further suggested that less frequent testing could be planned in subsequent school years, but that there should not be more than a 3-year interval after the fourth grade.

Puretone audiometer. The puretone audiometer (Fig. 4-2) is an individual testing device that measures the ability to hear sounds of varying frequencies* at different intensities of sound called decibels.†

A procedure known as the sweep-check test method (may be administered on an individual or group basis) has been used in schools to speed up the hearing screening process. Testing each ear separately, the intensity dial is set at 10 decibels; and the tone dial is changed rather quickly through the 1,000, 2,000, 4,000, and 6,000 frequencies and reset at 20 decibels for 4,000 frequencies. The extremely low and high tones are omitted. Some sweep-check methods involve the 500, 1,000, 2,000, and 4,000 frequencies at 25 decibels. It is estimated that from 5% to 10% of the students will fail to pass this test. Those students who fail to hear one tone or more in either ear in this sweep

---

*Frequencies, qualities of sound caused by the number of vibrations per second of an object resulting in high and low tones, for example, strings on a piano.
†Decibels, units of sound intensity.

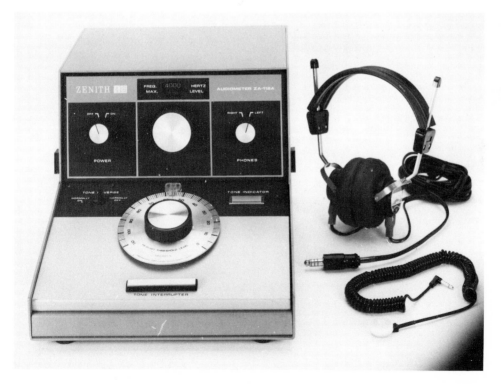

Fig. 4-2. Puretone audiometer. (Courtesy Zenetron, Inc., Chicago, Ill.)

DENVER PUBLIC SCHOOLS   **AUDIOGRAM**   DIVISION OF HEALTH SERVICES

Name_____ Age_____ Grade _____ School_____

Address_____ Room No._____ Audiometrist_____ Date_____

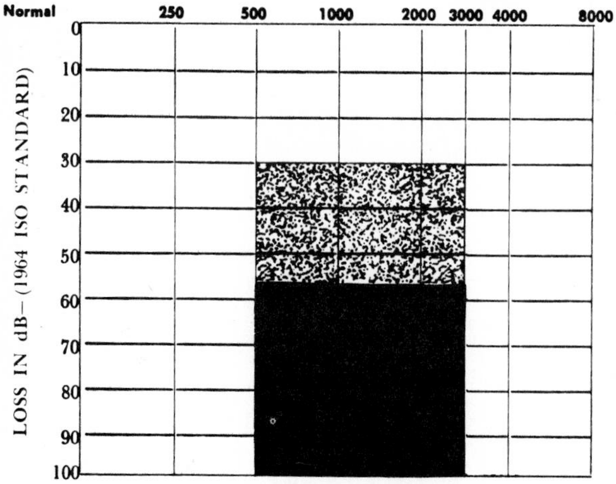

Normal   250   500   1000   2000 3000 4000   8000

LOSS IN dB—(1964 ISO STANDARD)

0 10 20 30 40 50 60 70 80 90 100

HEARING LOSS

		DECIBELS	WEBER TEST
RIGHT	Air		Lateralized
	Bone		R
LEFT	Air		L
	Bone		M

TEST CONDITIONS

Reliability_____

Has cold today_____

Follow-up_____

(See other side for code.)

Key:	Air	Air Masked	Bone	Bone Masked
Right (red)	O	⚛	>	▷
Left (blue)	X	X̄	<	◁

FORM 941   DSP   12-70-100 PADS   J-901-64473

CODE: 1. RETEST AT CENTRAL OFFICE.
      2A "HOME REPORT"—*To recommend medical care.*
      2B "HOME REPORT"—*With no medical care recommended at present.*
      3. RECHECK NEXT YEAR.
      4. STATIONARY CONDITION—NO RECHECK NEEDED.

ADDITIONAL INFORMATION ON PUPIL

Frequent sore throats_____ Earaches_____ Drainage_____

Comments:
Special seating, etc._____

General_____

_____

_____

_____

Medical information after referral:_____

_____

_____

_____

Fig. 4-3. Audiogram. (Courtesy Denver Public Schools, Denver, Colo.)

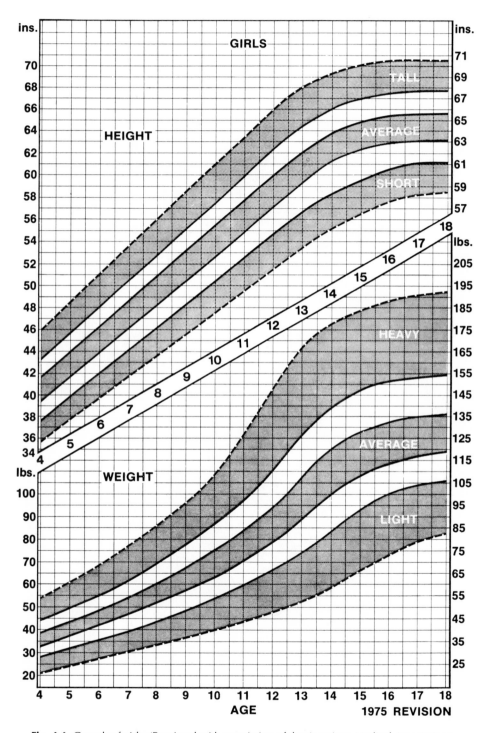

Fig. 4-4. Growth of girls. (Reprinted with permission of the American Medical Association.)

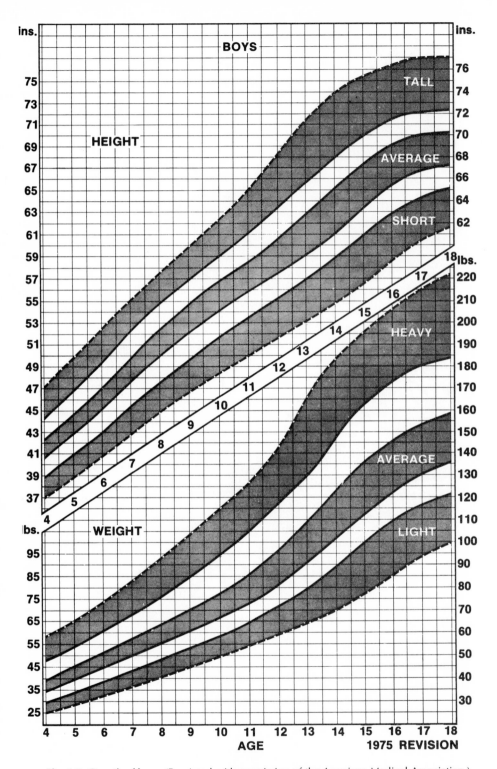

Fig. 4-5. Growth of boys. (Reprinted with permission of the American Medical Association.)

method should be given a threshold test. In this test, pupils listen to all the intensities of sound of each frequency, with the results plotted on audiograms (Fig. 4-3). The findings are then interpreted by technologists administering the test and decisions made whether to refer these children for specialized examinations. The criteria for referral generally include hearing losses of 20 decibels or more at any two frequencies in either ear, or a loss of 30 decibels or more at any single frequency in either ear. The degrees of hearing disability may be categorized as mild, moderate, moderately severe, and severe.

Audiometers are usually calibrated in round-numbered frequencies such as 125, 250, 500, 1,000, 2,000, on up to 8,000, the range of sounds that are normally heard by human beings. The machines are also calibrated by sound intensities with the step intervals being from 5 or 10 decibels to a maximum of 100 decibels.

Growth and development

Periodic measurements of the heights and weights of children will aid in understanding the growth and development of boys and girls. However, Eisner* states that routine growth measurements have not proved their general usefulness in health service programs and are not of sufficient educational value to justify a large investment of nurse time. Mere observations of weight and height increases, or the failure of children to gain weight, may not in themselves be of much significance in the growth process. Childrens' growth patterns are individual, and unless an instrument is used to show this, school personnel may be led to erroneous conclusions about overweight, underweight, or abnormal growth conditions. Weighing and measuring can be valuable in the appraisal process if the information is recorded and plotted on growth charts for interpretation, as illustrated in the height-weight records shown in Figs. 4-4 and 4-5.

The taking of heights and weights should be done three times yearly—at the beginning, middle, and end of the school year. It is important that measurements be accurately taken and recorded.

Tuberculosis

Tuberculin testing in elementary schools has been on the increase since 1963 when the Surgeon General's Task Force of the U.S. Public Health Service advocated that the identification of positive reactors among school children would be a good procedure for finding the active cases in society who had infected the pupils. A fluid in which tubercle bacilli have been grown, or the proteins of the tubercle bacilli extracted from it called tuberculin, is injected between the layers of the skin (the Mantoux test) or into the skin through multiple punctures (the tine, Heaf, or Sterneëdle test), or gauze moistened with tuberculin is fastened to the skin with adhesive tape (the patch test). The patch test is no longer recommended by the American Academy of Pediatrics. If the test is positive, a reaction, an inflamed or red area, appears in about 48 hours on the skin where the test was made.

A positive reaction to the test (inflammation, redness) does not necessarily mean that a person has active tuberculosis. It is an indication that the person has tubercle bacilli within his or her body and there has been an allergic reaction to these germs. In areas of high socioeconomic conditions less than 2% of positive reactors may be found among elementary children, whereas in low socioeconomic areas this percentage may be as high as 10%. Positive reactors to tuberculin tests should receive thorough medical examinations, including chest x-ray films, to determine whether active tuberculosis exists.

The American Lung Association* recommends that tuberculin testing should be concentrated in areas where the prevalence of infection is constantly high over a period of time. Therefore, annual testing of school en-

---

*Eisner, V., Oglesby, A., and Peck, E. B.: Health assessment of school children, VI. height and weight, Journal of School Health **42:** March, 1972.

*Your patient's risk of tuberculosis, 1975, New York, American Lung Association.

trants and young adolescents should be stressed in those schools where the reactor rate is 1% or more and should take place in other schools on a selective basis only. The American Academy of Pediatrics* agrees with this procedure and adds that students through ninth grade should be tested at 3-year intervals.

Dental inspections

Dental inspections refer to procedures generally performed by dentists or dental hygienists using mouth mirrors and explorers to locate decayed teeth, as well as to check for diseases of tissues surrounding the teeth and for malocclusion. These inspections are not complete examinations since they do not include x-ray examinations.

Ideally, children should visit their family dentists twice yearly for appraisal and necessary treatment. There is evidence to indicate only 20% of the population is following this practice.

Opinions differ regarding whether periodic dental inspections should be conducted in schools. Several reasons causing this dilemma include the following:

1. Dental decay is the most common defect found in school-age children, and there is little need to locate problem cases.
2. Increased pressure on parents by the schools to obtain corrections may make it impossible for dentists to provide the needed services. The schools would be criticized for not being aware of this difficulty.
3. Many school districts do not employ dentists or dental hygienists.
4. There is an inadequate supply of dentists and dental hygienists as well as poor geographic distribution of these specialists.

Dental inspections in schools vary widely as to their inclusion and frequency. In Pennsylvania, dental examinations by a dentist must be conducted by schools on the original entry of children as well as in the

third and seventh grades. In elementary schools, however, substitution is permitted by service from dental hygienists provided it includes a screening process, prophylactic care, and an educational program. In Denver, all pupils are inspected annually by dental hygienists.

Sickle cell disease

Sickle cell disease is a disorder of red blood cells caused by abnormal hemoglobin and their ability to carry oxygen. The normal red blood cells that usually appear disc shaped are crescent or sickle shaped. The condition is found among the black population as well as to a lesser degree in individuals with Mediterranean ancestry (Greece, Italy), in Caribbean islanders, and in people in South and Central America. The sickle cell trait is a genetic factor estimated to be found in 10% of the black population, whereas the disease itself, sickle cell anemia, is found in approximately 1 in 400 to 500 blacks. The condition results in the swelling of joints, pains in the abdomen, legs, and arms, and fatigue. The anemia cannot be cured, but the "crisis" situation when cells are deprived of oxygen can be treated. The crisis condition can be prevented or ameliorated. One valid procedure used to screen for this condition among junior and senior high school students is to draw venous blood and test it by direct hemoglobin electrophoresis to determine if the blood cells differ from normal ones.

Diabetes

Diabetes is not an infectious disease. It can be detected by urine testing to determine the level of sugar in the blood. The condition results from failure of the pancreas to make a sufficient amount of insulin. Without insulin food cannot be used properly. Diabetes currently cannot be cured but can be controlled by daily injections of insulin and a prescribed food plan. Afflicted children can participate in all school activities but should be carefully observed in class. Physical education should not be scheduled just before lunch, nor should a child be assigned a late lunch period. These young people may

---

*Committee on School Health, School Health: A guide for health professionals, Evanston, Ill., 1977, American Academy of Pediatrics.

need midmorning or midafternoon snacks. Teachers should have sugar readily available in the event of insulin shock.

Epilepsy

Epilepsy is a disruption of the electrical impulses to the brain that causes nerves to send out erratic impulses through the body resulting in a seizure, or sudden onset of symptoms, such as convulsions. It occurs in approximately 1 child in 50, with 75% of the cases beginning before the twenty-first birthday. Four out of five seizures, where known, can be controlled with medication; 50% can be totally controlled, and 30% partially. Teachers should be aware that excessive fatigue, overexposure to heat or sunlight, and situations that cause emotional disturbances can affect the seizure threshold in children and increase the incidence of attacks. There are three types of epilepsy:

1. *Grand mal (major seizure)*—the body shakes violently; the person may cry out and fall to the ground, thrashing about; the child may suffer temporary loss of consciousness.
2. *Petit mal*—this results in a simple staring spell that lasts only a few seconds; it may go unrecognized with the belief the child is "daydreaming" or "inattentive." The child may suddenly appear immobilized, the eyes may have a vacant look, and the condition may reoccur several times during the day. It is found principally in children 4 to 12 years of age and is less common than grand mal.
3. *Psychomotor*—the brain cells affected are those that govern repetitive behavior; the person may engage in purposeless, or inappropriate, behavior lasting 1 or 2 minutes and will probably remember nothing afterward. It is manifested by abrupt changes in consciousness, illusions, hallucinations, and dreamlike states, as well as loss of speech, including incorrect and inappropriate loss of words.

Other screening procedures

A variety of additional types of screening appraisals such as posture, nutrition, and speech occur in schools. Their frequency and extent show wide variation throughout the United States.

WHAT ARE HEALTH HISTORIES AND INVENTORIES?

Histories and inventories (Fig. 4-6) are informational accounts of the health practices and behavior of children that take the form of written questionnaires or checklists. They are frequently neglected, yet they are one of the most important parts of periodic health appraisals. The basic content should include information about major past health problems (physical and emotional) and their treatment, an orderly review of body systems, information about current and past special problems of other members of the family, and information about the student's academic achievement and school adjustments. This information provides background data about the health of children not usually revealed by other procedures that are useful in the health appraisals of pupils. The teacher needs to know that a child with diabetes is taking insulin. A periodic health examination may not reveal that a student has asthma or occasional epileptic attacks. These inventories serve for better understanding of the health status of boys and girls and may be particularly useful when school medical examinations are conducted. The forms may be sent to parents of young children for completion or may be finished at school when the child is brought in for enrollment. The data obtained become a part of the child's health record.

WHAT ARE MEDICAL EXAMINATIONS?

Medical, health or physical, examinations refer to those appraisals completed by physicians who are qualified to make diagnoses and to render treatment. Accurate evaluations of health require medical examinations.

Because of the shortage of school health physicians (estimated less than 500 full-time in U.S.) and their limited availability to schools, a growing number of *school nurse practitioners* are being prepared to perform health examinations and to provide expanded

HEALTH INVENTORY FOR ELEMENTARY PUPILS

Name_____ Grade_____ Teacher_____ School_____

To Parents: Please fill out and return this form tomorrow. This information is used in the school program to promote and protect the health of students.

I.   Immunization History: Give month and year completing immunizations for:

Measles vaccination (Rubeola)_____ Had Disease _____
                                          YEAR   YEAR

Polio initial series_____ Booster _____
                             NUMBER – YEAR   MONTH AND YEAR

DPT (diphtheria, pertussis and tetanus) Series_____ Booster _____
                                                    YEAR   MONTH AND YEAR

Tetanus (Latest) _____
                                                          YEAR

Smallpox vaccination (Latest) _____
                                                                  YEAR

Mumps vaccination_____ Had Disease _____
                                   YEAR   YEAR

German Measles (3 day-Rubella)_____ Had Disease _____
                                            YEAR   YEAR

Date of last tuberculin skin test_____ Positive _____ Negative (OK)_____

Has he/she had a chest x-ray?_____ BCG vaccine? _____
                                  MONTH AND YEAR   YEAR

II.   History of Illness: Give age

____ Anemia   ____ Diabetes   ____ Heart Disease   ____ Rheumatic fever

____ Asthma   ____ German Measles   ____ Hernia (Rupture)   ____ Skin Problems

____ Chicken Pox   ____ Hay fever   ____ Measles   ____ Tuberculosis

____ Convulsions   ____ Hearing Problem   ____ Mumps   ____ Vision Problem

Surgery_____ Injury_____

Any other serious illness?_____

PLEASE COMPLETE OTHER SIDE
(Front)

Fig. 4-6. Informational account of the health practices and behavior of children in the form of a questionnaire. (From Bryan, Doris S.: School nursing in transition, St. Louis, 1973, The C. V. Mosby Co.)

III. History of Symptoms: Give age

___ Frequent colds or   ___Frequent use of toilet   ___ Angers easily
___ sore throats   ___Frequent stomach ache   ___ Worries a great deal
___ Nosebleeds   ___Toothaches   ___ Many fears
___ Persistent cough   ___Frequent pains in legs   ___ Nervousness
___Running ear   ___ Bedwetting   ___Tires easily
___ Frequent headache

IV. Medical and Dental Care:

Name of child's doctor or clinic _____

MEDICAL RECORD NO.

_____
ADDRESS

Date of most recent visit_____ Reason for visit _____

_____

Name of child's dentist or dental clinic _____

ADDRESS

Date of last visit_____

Was all necessary dental work completed? _____   _____
                                      YES   NO

V. Are there any other health problems or family matters which you think would be helpful for the school to know?_____

_____

_____

_____

_____

_____

_____
PARENT-S SIGNATURE

_____   _____
DATE   HOME TELEPHONE

13-0150-09 20M771-3

(Back)

Fig. 4-6, cont'd. For legend see opposite page.

and improved health care to children. These individuals are school nurses who have completed a special education and training program under the direction of the local medical society or provided by a local medical center at a university. Such preparation may include taking and evaluating medical health history; performing a thorough physical examination including the use of the stethoscope and otoscope; performing a variety of specialized clinical and laboratory tests and procedures, such as urinalysis, throat cultures, and hematocrits; and identifying and assessing factors leading to a variety of behavioral, learning, and perceptual disorders. These practitioners work closely with school personnel, school physicians, health personnel, and physicians in private practice. Nurses prepared can be especially useful in ghetto schools and school districts, where health problems are numerous.

In schools these examinations may be classified as periodic and referral types. The periodic examinations are those conducted at intervals on apparently normal or healthy children. Referrals are those examinations given to pupils who have been sent to physicians because of symptoms of abnormality noted by school personnel.

The health examination usually includes the followincg conditions and parts of the body.

Nutrition
Skin and hair
Head and neck
Lungs
Muscle tone
Nose, throat, and tonsils
Feet
Eyes
Genitalia
Heart
Nervous system
Posture
Thyroid gland
Teeth and gums
Bones and joints
Ears
Pulse resting and after exercise
Blood pressure
Abdomen
Lymph nodes
Inguinal and umbilical region for hernia

Although these are not frequently done in schools, examinations should also include urinalysis, blood work, and other laboratory tests.

Results from the various screening tests, teacher observations, nurse opinions, health histories, and other data aid physicians in making accurate diagnoses when conducting examinations. The practice of having parents present makes for better communication and greater possibility of obtaining necessary corrections.

Common practice in schools indicates that examinations are being completed by school physicians as well as family physicians and more recently by nurse practitioners. There is a trend for schools to encourage parents to have examinations completed by personal doctors. In some districts these outside specialists have performed from 50% to 75% of all evaluations. This indicates that the home is capable of assuming this responsibility. If all schools were to achieve these results, it still would be necessary to conduct examinations for needy and ghetto children, as well as for those pupils whose families fail to have them completed.

In ghetto areas where poverty exists, children generally receive few or no health appraisals or other services. Yet most of the health problems in children are found among the deprived, the disadvantaged, and the poor. In one New York City elementary school in Harlem, a survey revealed that positive tine tests for tuberculosis were three times the national average for the same age children. Health services will need to be provided by the schools, in schools by community resources, or in the community itself. In a deprived area in Washington, D.C., a full-time school physician was assigned to a neighborhood health center to identify students with health problems, to provide immediate treatment, and to attempt to get 100% referrals and follow-up action. Where physicians are not available, school nurse practitioners may need to be trained and readied to work closely with the resources found in the community.

Several reasons supporting family physicians' examinations are the following:

1. The physician perhaps knows the patient for longer periods of time and has better understandings of the background factors in the life of the child.
2. The examinations will be more complete with the probability that laboratory analyses will be included in the procedure—urinalysis, blood tests, and others.
3. Parents are more likely to be present, and better guidance can occur.
4. The primary responsibility for the health of children rests with the home.
5. There will probably be better continuity of care from childhood to adolescence.

Some of the advantages of school physicians' examinations are the following:

1. The type of examination can be suited to meet the school needs.
2. The examination can be adapted to provide an educational experience for both parents and children.
3. A large number of pupils might be examined.
4. School facilities may be more complete than those of personal physicians.

Yearly health examinations of all children in schools is now being questioned as an advisable practice. The lack of sufficient physician services, the difficulty in performing quality examinations, the cost, the ineffectiveness of the procedure for case-finding, and the consideration that this may be an unwise expenditure of money and professional time are some of the reasons advanced for the present attitude. There is evidence to indicate that routine yearly examinations in schools may not be advisable or necessary in the first through fourth grades. Studies show that examinations performed regularly on entrance to school by school physicians do not reveal much new information about the health status of children that could not be obtained by other less time-consuming and expensive methods except in the areas of dental, vision, and hearing testing.

The shortage of physicians' services and especially of pediatric cardiologists in schools has led to the development of a new procedure to help in detection of unrecognized heart disease (incidence about 10 per 1,000) among school children through mass screening programs using an electronic heart-sound screening device. A small transistorized computer, the PhonoCardioScan (PCS), has been designed to scan heart sounds and to differentiate between the normal and the abnormal sounds and murmurs. This instrument, which can give immediate visual readouts, can be operated by a technologist, and the average screening takes 2 or 3 minutes per child.

Although the frequency still needs evaluation, it is now recommended that children receive a minimum of three periodic health examinations during their school years; one at entrance to school, one at the beginning of adolescence, and one shortly before leaving school. The two examinations during the elementary grades should be supplemented by well-planned screening procedures and teachers' observations. Fewer examinations but of good quality, with time for instruction and counseling, are preferred to frequent and incomplete coverage. Referral examinations should also be conducted for those students having special health problems. The American Academy of Pediatrics gives priority to those children of high risk, low socioeconomic status, poor school performance, with existing handicaps, who are frequently absent, or are disciplinary problems.

The American School Health Association* passed a resolution that medical examinations should be given to pupils at or near enrollment into school and thereafter when health problems arise that indicate that medical evaluations of children are warranted. They added that periodic medical appraisals at appropriate grade levels are of value but are less important than those conducted at entrance to school or completed to meet an apparent need, a referral assessment.

---

*American School Health Association resolutions for the year 1972, Journal of School Health **43:** Feb., 1973.

The teacher's functions in health examinations may be considered as being fourfold in nature:

1. To help encourage children to obtain these examinations when advisable
2. To help reduce fears or anxieties that students may develop
3. To cooperate with nurses and others in getting children prepared for the examinations
4. To use the opportunities for health education

WHAT ARE PSYCHOLOGIC EXAMINATIONS AND TESTS?

Psychologic examinations and tests include a variety of procedures to test personality, behavior, and social acceptance of pupils as well as intelligence, achievements, and aptitudes. They are usually administered by psychologists and psychometrists who are members of a child guidance or pupil personnel services program. School districts occasionally employ consulting psychiatrists to help with emotionally disturbed students. Mental health specialists and mental health counselors are beginning to be trained and used in some schools. The findings from these appraisals, together with teacher observations, help determine the necessary action. Pupils with suspected emotional difficulties who are located through these evaluations may need to be referred for medical or psychiatric consultation. In California, upon a report of the school principal that a pupil shows evidence of impaired mental health and that a mental examination is desirable, the governing body of any school district may, with the written consent of the pupil's parent or guardian, provide for the mental examination of said pupil. The American Academy of Pediatrics states that children with emotional problems are difficult to identify. They claim that the management of children with emotional problems is the most common unmet health need of school children.

Teacher feelings, emotions, and expressions affect pupil emotions. Teacher attitudes are reflected in the attitudes of pupils. The teacher who is kind but firm, sympathetic but exacting, and friendly but reserved exerts a beneficial influence on emotional health. The nagging, scolding, domineering, sarcastic, or emotionally unstable teacher may lead to serious emotional difficulties in pupils.

WHAT ARE HEALTH RECORDS?

Health records (Fig. 4-7) refer to those materials that contain all pertinent data about the health status of pupils. Cumulative records should be maintained for all pupils in school and not merely for those with known health problems. They should be accessible to those persons who need to use them and should follow students from grade to grade, from school to school, and from school district to school district.

There is no common type of health record used in schools. However, records information should be kept confidential and should not be available without permission of school health personnel. Parents or guardians should have access to their contents.

Records usually contain the following information:

1. Teacher observations
2. Screening tests results
3. Findings of medical, dental, and psychologic examinations
4. Notes on health counseling and follow-up procedures

Despite the amount of information found in health records, they are not used with any degree of consistency by teachers and others. This is probably because of any, or all, of the following reasons: (1) there is no central, master file on every student, and retrieval of information is difficult; (2) it takes a great deal of time to transcribe the data by hand; (3) information is frequently lost or misinterpreted, and records may be incomplete; (4) little anecdotal information can be included; (5) if a record is lost, a completely new one must be reconstructed; and (6) an adequate study of the total student population is virtually impossible.

A new approach to records is the Problem Oriented Medical Record (POMR) that was

DENVER PUBLIC SCHOOLS • DEPARTMENT OF HEALTH SERVICE

HEALTH RECORD

ROOM												
YEAR												
GRADE AGE												
HEIGHT												
WEIGHT (follow up)												
WEIGHT (Spring)												
VISION— With Glasses R. / L.												
VISION— Without Glasses R. / L.												
HEARING, R.												
HEARING, L.												
TEETH												

NURSES SUMMARY OF **PERMANENT** DATA.

NAME

BIRTH DATE   FATHER'S NAME   MOTHER'S NAME

ADDRESS 1.	5.	9.
2.	6.	10.
3.	7.	11.
4.	8.	12.
SCHOOL 1.	5.	9.
2.	6.	10.
3.	7.	11.
4.	8.	12.

NAME AND **BIRTH YEAR** OF OTHER CHILDREN IN FAMILY

1.	4.	7.
2.	5.	8.
3.	6.	9.

RECORD OF PREVIOUS HEALTH (date)

1. Allergies	6. Diphtheria	11. Kidney trouble	16. Polio
2. Bed Wetting	7. Encephalitis	12. Measles, Regular	17. Rheumatic fever
3. Chorea	8. Fractures	13. Mumps	18. Scarlet fever
4. Convulsions	9. German measles	14. Operations	19. Whooping cough
5. Diabetes	10. Infectious Hepatitis	15. Pneumonia	20. Other health problems

MEDICAL RECORD   (FOR DESCRIPTIVE **REMARKS** USE A SECOND SHEET.)

CODE

MONTH AND YEAR OF EXAM.						O = satisfactory; Numbers (1-10) = type or degree of defect	Date and Use Pencil for COMMENTS
PARENT PRESENT						I. 1. Little or no milk 2. No breakfast 3. Unsatisfactory sleep 4. Excess piecing between meals 5. Habitual use of tea and coffee 6. Sleeps with mouth open or snores 7. Excessive outside activities 8. Nail biting 9. Poor social adjustment 10. Exposure to tuberculosis	
I. HISTORY							
II. HEALTH						II. 1. Poor 2. Frequent colds 3. Stomach trouble 4. Headache 5. Constipation 6. Earaches	
III. EYES						III. 1. Blepharitis 2. Conjunctivitis 3. Trachoma 4. Strabismus 5. Eye strain	
IV. EARS						IV. Membranes R / L 1. Retraction 2. Wax 3. Discharging 4. Perforated 5. Scarring	
V. NOSE						V. 1. Nasal obstruction 2. Mouth breather 3. Deflected septum 4. Nasal allergy	
VI. THROAT						VI. Tonsils 1. Injected 2. Tag 3. Enlarged 4. Infected 5. Arched palate 6. Removed	
VII. LYMPH GLANDS						VII. 1. Cervical 2. Axillary 3. Inguinal	
VIII. THYROID						VIII. 1. 2. 3. Englargement 4. With symptoms	
IX. SKIN						IX. 1. Acne 2. Athletes foot 3. Eczema 4. Pallor 5. Ringworm 6. Scars 7. Warts 8. Moles	
X. CHEST						X. 1. Flat 2. Funnel 3. Pigeon 4. Deformed	
XI. NUTRITION						XI. 1. Fair 2. Poor 3. Serious 4. Obese	
XII. ORTHOPEDIC						XII. 1. Spine A. Kyphosis B. Functional scoliosis C. Structural scoliosis D. Lordosis 2. Prominent shoulders 3. Fatigue posture 4. Pronated feet 5. Flat feet 6. Muscle astrophy 7. Flabby muscles	
HEART XIII. ENL.						XIII. A. Systolic 1. Apex 2. Pul. I—Innocent	
HEART XIV. MURMUR						XIV. B. Diastolic 3. Aortic O—Organic 4. L. Sternal border	
XV. LUNGS						XV. 1. Asthma 2. Rales	
XVI. ABDOMEN						XVI. 1. Hernia A. Inguinal i. indirect d. Direct B. Umbilical 2. Pot-bellied 3. Post-operative scar	
XVII. GENITO URINARY						XVII. 1. Phimosis 2. Undescended testicle 3. Underdeveloped 4. Varicocele 5. Hydrocele 6. Circumcision	
XVIII. NERVOUS SYS.						XVIII. 1. Chorea 2. Speech defect 3. Hyperkinetic	
EXAMINED BY							

Fig. 4-7. From Department of Health and Medical Services, Fifty-First Annual Report, 1975-1976, Denver, Colo., 1976, Denver Public Schools.

SCHOOL HEALTH RECORD

Name _____ Smith, Mary _____

Problem list

Entry Date	Problem	Inactive
11-15-75	1. Stomachache	11-18-75
1-8-76	2. Leg injury	2-20-76 normal activity
2-4-76	3. Weight problem	5-28-76 12-pound loss

Date/time	Progress notes*	Signature
11-15-75 9:05 A.M.	1. Stomachache S: "My stomach hurts here." O: Points to lower right abdominal area; T 101° F., diarrhea x3 yesterday, x2 today. A: Gastrointestinal infection? appendicitis? P: Contact parent, send home, advise MD check if symptoms continue.	W. Jones
1-8-76 1:25 P.M.	2. Leg injury S: "I can't walk on it, it hurts to move it. I was running down the stairs and tripped and fell on my right leg." O: Swelling of right ankle, unable to place weight on foot without pain. A: Sprained/fractured ankle? P: Contact parent, advise MD check.	W. Jones
2-4-76 1:30 P.M.	3. Weight problem S: Home Ec. teacher (Mrs. Jones) referred student for weight/diet counseling. Student: "I don't think I'm really fat." O: 5 feet 4 inches 140 pounds = ±15 pounds above recommended height/weight (mod. heavy). A: Student not in agreement with need for weight loss/diet control. P: Personal and diet counseling.	W. Jones

*S = subjective; O = objective; A = assessment; P = plan.

Fig. 4-8. Adapted from Oda, D. S., and Quick, M. J.: Journal of School Health **47**:212-215, April, 1977.

introduced by the Darien Public Schools in Connecticut.* It is organized to acquire such basic data as history, physical exams, and laboratory. In addition it precisely defined student problems and provides monitoring of these problems through the use of progress notes. Oda and Quick (Fig. 4-8) illustrate one version that they believe provides simplicity, clarity, and uniformity of data.

Recently in New York an attempt has been made to put the data collected on computer cards so the facts can be more easily stored and more readily accessible. In Ontario, Canada, it was reported by Stennett† that a computerized system operative in a large school system (over 10,000 students) and called an Electronic Data-Processing (EDP) oriented record system appears to be successful. The American Academy of Pediatrics stated that computers may be helpful in large school systems to compile statistics, but they may not represent the most cost effective way to maintain and analyze school health records.

Teachers can better understand the health status of students by reviewing these health forms at the beginning of the semester as well as at other times. They may be expected to make notations of observations and other essential information about the health of children in their classes on these cards.

IDENTIFICATION OF DRUG USERS AND ABUSERS

The importance of the drug problem in society necessitates special consideration to this matter. In ghetto areas especially, some children are misusing and abusing drugs at very early ages. The evidence indicates that a large percentage of fourth graders have tasted alcoholic beverages. There is no question that individuals at all ages are using drugs for a variety of reasons and in a variety of ways.

To identify students who are misusing and abusing drugs may involve any, or all, of the following:

1. Awareness of observable signs and symptoms; general observations may be found by referring to Table 4-4. Telltale evidence such as syringes, pills, solvents, special cigarette papers, and other items found in student possession and around school are additional clues. Blum claims that potential users are behavioral problems at school, have mild conduct disorders, and lack self-confidence.

2. Taking prescribed medicines at school; students who have been recognized by nurses, parents, and others may be taking and using drugs while attending school for the control of such conditions as diabetes, epilepsy, and hyperkinesia as well as for other health problems.

3. Peer identification; friends may wish to help friends and thereby be willing to reveal information about drug use.

4. Self-identification; young people who discover their memory is failing, have problems of increased concentration, difficulty in speech, exaggerated feelings of self-confidence, or feelings of futility of life, may seek out assistance.

5. Clinical tests; urine testing for users of heroin, amphetamines, and barbiturates is a useful procedure that has received some notoriety because of its use by the military. There is question whether such a procedure should be used in schools.

THE TEACHER AND APPRAISALS

A review of the various procedures for assessing the health of pupils makes it evident that the teacher plays an important role in appraisals. The teacher should do the following:

1. Observe children for signs and symptoms of health deviations and know the referral procedures to follow
2. Be familiar with a variety of screening tests
3. Understand the meaning and importance of medical and psychologic examinations, dental inspections, and other assessment procedures
4. Know the importance of health records in

---

*Boone, S. F.: A new approach to school health records, Journal of School Health **44**:156-158, March, 1974.
†Stennett, R. G., Cram, D. M., Gibson, D., and Dukacz, K.: Exploring the possibilities of computerized student health records, Journal of School Health **41**: Feb., 1971.

helping to better understand pupils and realize that he or she may have to make notations on these records

5. Occasionally be prepared to discuss student health problems with parents

The teacher should also realize that health appraisals offer numerous opportunities for health education:

1. Teaching about care of the eyes and ears is appropriate when pupils are taking vision and hearing tests.
2. The importance and need for health examinations or dental inspections can have its greatest impact when the instruction period coincides with the examinations or the inspections.
3. The control of communicable diseases should be discussed when tuberculin tests are being administered.
4. Understandings about growth and development can be achieved more easily by relating this process to the periodic taking of heights and weights.

It should be apparent that the more the teacher knows about the health status of pupils the better qualified that teacher will be to understand them, to make necessary classroom and school adjustments, to provide functional health teaching, and to increase the effectiveness of the total educational program.

QUESTIONS FOR DISCUSSION

1. Why must schools be concerned with the health status of students?
2. What is the meaning of the term "health appraisals"?
3. What are the purposes of health appraisals?
4. What is the role of the teacher when observing the health status of children?
5. What are the growth and developmental characteristics of children who are 5 to 7, 8 to 10, and 11 to 13 years of age, and what are their health education implications?
6. What are some of the signs and symptoms of pupils' health problems that teachers can observe?
7. What are the characteristics of a healthy child?
8. What is the meaning of the term "learning disabilities," how can a teacher identify such conditions, and what can be done to help children with these problems?
9. What are several of the communicable diseases that

children may bring to school, and how may teachers recognize them?
10. Why are teacher-nurse conferences necessary and important?
11. What are the general categories of health screening tests used in schools, and why are they necessary?
12. What types of vision screening tests may be used in schools?
13. How is hearing tested, and who does it in schools?
14. What are the values, problems, and frequency of periodic height and weight measurements?
15. What is meant by tuberculin testing, and under what conditions should it be completed in schools?
16. What are dental inspections, and why are they valuable?
17. What is sickle cell disease, what are its signs and symptoms, and how can it be clinically identified?
18. What is diabetes, how can it clinically be identified, and what can schools and teachers do to help such children?
19. Who should administer medical examinations to pupils, and why should they take place?
20. How frequently and why should pupil medical examinations be conducted?
21. What are psychologic examinations and tests, and what can schools and teachers do to help problem children discovered?
22. What is the meaning of the term "nurse practitioners," and how may they help ghetto children with health problems?
23. What behavior may be exhibited by hyperkinetic children, and what understandings are needed by teachers of these students?
24. How can teachers identify drug users and abusers?
25. What is the role of the teacher in health appraisals?

SUGGESTED CLASS ACTIVITIES

1. Discuss the responsibility of the home and the school for the health of pupils.
2. Discuss the nature and extent of health appraisals used in schools.
3. Show color slides and pictures of children with symptoms of health deviations.
4. Have a panel discussion on the good health characteristics of children.
5. Have committee reports on the growth and development characteristics of children.
6. Have a pediatrician or a school physician discuss common childhood diseases of significance to schools.
7. Discuss state and local legal provisions relating to health appraisals.
8. Have a school nurse discuss teacher-nurse conferences, teacher observations, health inventories, and health records.
9. Demonstrate vision screening and hearing tests used in schools.

10. Discuss the use and importance of health records in schools.
11. Discuss the value and importance of height-weight charts in appraisals.
12. Have a demonstration of the tuberculin testing procedure.
13. Have a dentist or a dental hygienist discuss dental inspections and examinations.
14. Survey schools to determine the frequency of vision and hearing testing and health examinations.
15. Prepare reports on psychologic examinations and tests.
16. Have a physician discuss and demonstrate the procedures used in health examinations.
17. Discuss the role of the teacher in appraisals.
18. Have students give the Snellen test.
19. Plan field trips to meet and talk with drug misusers and abusers; to VD clinic in community.
20. Invite "nurse practitioner" to discuss responsibilities and problems.
21. Prepare reports on the extent of health problems and health services available to ghetto children in school and discuss possible solutions.
22. Prepare a self-test for use in class discussion that contains questions relating signs and symptoms of health problems to specific conditions.

REFERENCES

American Association for Health, Physical Education, and Recreation: School health practices in the United States, Washington, D.C., 1961, The Association.

American Medical Association: Reports of Third, Fourth, Fifth, Seventh, and Eighth National Conferences on Physicians and Schools, Chicago, 1952-1961, The Association.

Anderson, C. L., and Creswell, W. H., Jr.: School health practice, ed. 6, St. Louis, 1976, The C. V. Mosby Co.

Blum, H. L., Peters, H. B., and Bettman, J. W.: Vision screening for elementary schools; the Orinda study, Berkeley, Calif., 1959, University of California Press.

Blum, R. H., and others: Horatio Alger's children, San Francisco, 1972, Jossey-Bass, Inc., Publishers.

California State Department of Education: A guide to vision screening in California public schools, Sacramento, Calif., 1964, State Printing Office.

California State Department of Public Health: Hearing testing of school children and guide for hearing conservation programs, Berkeley, Calif., 1962, State Printing Office.

Committee on School Health of the American Academy of Pediatrics: School health; a guide for health professionals, Evanston, Ill., 1977, The Academy.

Conrad, P.: Identifying hyperactive children, Lexington, Mass., 1976, Lexington Books.

Cornacchia, H. J., Smith, D. E., and Bentel, D. J.: Drugs in the classroom; a conceptual model for school programs, ed. 2, St. Louis, 1978, The C. V. Mosby Co.

Department of Health and Medical Services: Fifty-first annual report, 1975-1976, Denver, Colo., 1976, Denver Public Schools.

Dennison, D., and Fenimore, J. A.: A heartsounding screening program for elementary children, Journal of School Health **41:** Sept., 1971.

Dodge, P. R.: Neurological disorders of school-age children, Journal of School Health **46:** June, 1976.

Does your state have a free lead testing program for children? Journal of School Health **46:** June, 1976.

Feingold, B. F.: The role of the school luncheon program in behavior and learning disabilities, Oversight Hearings on the School Lunch Programs, Hearings of the Subcommittee on Elementary, Secondary and Vocational Education, Committee on Education and Labor, House of Representatives, Washington, D.C., 1976, U.S. Government Printing Office.

Gearheart, B. R., and Weishahn, M. W.: The handicapped child in the regular classroom, St. Louis, 1976, The C. V. Mosby Co.

Jenkins, G., Shacter, H. S., and Bauer, W. W.: These are your children, ed. 4, Glenview, Ill., 1975, Scott, Foresman & Co.

Jenne, F. H., and Greene, W. H.: Turner's school health and health education, ed. 7, St. Louis, 1976, The C. V. Mosby Co.

Joint Committee on Health Problems: Health appraisals of school children, ed. 4, Washington, D.C., 1969, National Education Association and the American Medical Association.

Joint Study Committee of the American School Health Association and the National Society for the Prevention of Blindness: Teaching about vision, ed. 2, New York, 1972, National Society for the Prevention of Blindness.

Knotts, G. R., editor: Guidelines for the school nurse in the school health program, Kent, Ohio, 1974, American School Health Association.

Mayshark, C., Shaw, D. D., and Best, W. H.: Administration of school health program, ed. 2, St. Louis, 1977, The C. V. Mosby Co.

MacDonough, G. P.: School health, 1977, Journal of School Health **47:** Sept., 1977.

Montgomery, T. A.: Health appraisal of school children in a rural area, California's Health, Dec. 15, 1960.

Moriarity, M. J., and Irwin, L. W.: A study of the relationship of certain physical and emotional factors to habitual poor posture among school children, Research Quarterly, May, 1952.

National Committee on School Health, Policies: Suggested school health policies, ed. 4, Washington, D.C., 1966, National Education Association and the American Medical Association.

National Conference on Identification Audiometry, Journal of Speech and Hearing Disorders, Monograph 9, Sept., 1961.

National Medical Foundation for Eye Care: Identification of school children requiring eye care, No. 7, New York, 1959, The Foundation.

National Society for the Prevention of Blindness: A guide for eye inspection and testing visual acuity of school age children, New York, 1975, The Society.

National Society for the Prevention of Blindness: Vision screening in schools, New York, revised, 1972, The Society.

Rapaport, H. G., and Flint, S. H.: Allergy in the schools, Journal of School Health **44:** May, 1974.

Ratchick, I.: Evaluation of health services for disadvantaged children under Title 1, elementary and secondary act, Journal of School Health **38:** March, 1968.

Ross, D. M., and Ross, S. A.: Hyperactivity; research theory, and action, New York, 1976, John Wiley & Sons, Inc.

Schneeweis, S. M.: The computer in school health services, Journal of School Health **40:** March, 1970.

Schneeweiss, S. M., and Locke, A.: New horizons in school health services; the computer, Journal of School Health **37:** Sept., 1967.

Smith, E. S.: New electronics device zips through mass heart screenings for children with good reliability, California's Health, March 15, 1969.

Starling, K. A., and Shepard, D. A.: Symptoms and signs of cancer in the school-age child, Journal of School Health **47:** March, 1977.

Walker, J. E.: What the school health team should know about sickle cell anemia, Journal of School Health **45:** March, 1975.

What teachers see, and Looking for health, New York, 1969, Metropolitan Life Insurance Co.

Welner, N. M.: Health care for inner-city school children, Journal of School Health **38:** June, 1968.

Wheatley, G. M., and Hallock, G. T.: Health observation of school children, ed. 3, New York, 1965, McGraw-Hill Book Co.

Wilson, C. C., editor: School health services, Washington, D.C., 1964, National Education Association and the American Medical Association.

Yankaur, A., Lawrence, R. A., and Ballou, L.: A study of periodic school medical examinations, American Journal of Public Health **47:** Nov., 1957.

Zoleynski, S. J., and McKee, J. M.: The development of a student mental health record, Journal of School Health **32:** June, 1962.

5 Health guidance

The school, having identified children with health problems such as vision and hearing difficulties, undernourishment, malnutrition, overfeeding, dental decay, emotional disturbances, skin infections, and heart disease, using the variety of health appraisals referred to in the previous chapter, is faced with deciding what to do for or about these pupils. Since good health is vital to effective learning, the school must decide whether to assist in the attempt to improve students' levels of wellness. It should be evident that unless attention is given to the conditions discovered among the young people, they will not be able to profit to the greatest extent possible from the educational program. Schools therefore have assumed the responsibility of trying to help students and parents. The procedures used have been considered to be part of the school health services program and are called follow-up procedures, which include guidance and counseling, use of community health resources, and adjustment of the school program. The emphasis in this chapter is on the guidance and counseling aspects.

WHAT IS HEALTH GUIDANCE?

Health guidance in schools is a broad term that refers to a variety of processes involving the interaction of school personnel, students, and parents that aid in the discovery, understanding, and resolution of health matters through self-effort and self-direction. It includes those activities in which individuals participate voluntarily in incidental, individual, or small-group counseling or in "rap" sessions in order to obtain information regarding health concerns or to seek solutions to health problems. The general aim of health guidance is to enable pupils to acquire the highest levels of wellness in accordance with their individual needs. Guidance plays an important role in *primary prevention* (before a condition arises) and in *secondary prevention* (after a condition has been discovered).

Health guidance involves the use of health appraisals and health records; more specifically it involves counseling to provide information and aid in regard to health problems, immunizations, reports of health examinations, program adjustments, identification of community health resources, relations between pupils and parents with medical, dental, and other health specialists, and numerous other matters. Its objective is not to give advice but to encourage, motivate, and help individuals achieve good health through their own efforts. It is purposeful action and organized effort directed toward intelligent decision making regarding corrections, care, service, treatment, and assistance. It is educational in nature.

Opportunities for health guidance exist in the *formal school health education program.* However, they are not discussed in this chapter. The procedures used in the formal program may be considered to be group guidance methods. Pupils requests for informal assistance frequently arise from the formal program. Chapters 9 to 12 on organizing, learning, and teaching techniques provide numerous suggestions for helping students in the classroom in a group or formal setting.

The educational procedures used in guidance are frequently referred to as *health counseling*. This is the direct contact between students or parents and counselors (nurses, teachers, physicians, and others) on a face-to-face basis, with discussion focusing on information and understanding that will assist in making wise choices about courses of action. This process may be identified as the *informal phase of the health education program.*

Informal health education

Informal health education must receive greater emphasis in schools if educational programs are to adequately meet the differing health needs of children and youth. It is a phase of the school health education program that has been neglected and has generally been thought to be the responsibility of the nurse. Although the nurse is an important contact person, the nurse's presence in school is frequently limited. Also, there are others who can provide assistance. A number of students require special, individual attention that cannot be obtained from a formal health education program. These young people need and often desire someone, some group, or some way in schools to be able to discuss concerns and interests about sex, drugs, personality development, stress and pressure, self-care, parent problems, and other health matters. The school nurse, a teacher, a counselor, the school psychologist, or someone who will be a good listener and has empathy for student concerns might serve. Informal health education needs to be recognized and established in schools. It would be helpful in secondary prevention of health problems and also could serve a useful purpose in primary prevention.

Informal education is learning that takes place without structure and without much planning. It may occur in the classroom, in the nurse's office, or in other school locations. It may take place outside the school, in the home, watching TV, talking with a parent, friend, or neighbor, while reading a magazine or newspaper, or anywhere else. It usually occurs on a one-to-one basis or in small groups. It is a communication procedure that provides information, counseling, and guidance that is nondirective and nonthreatening to students and is voluntary in terms of participation.

Implementation of informal health education may occur in a variety of ways. Several illustrations are provided. A student may ask a teacher a question about health or regarding the action to be taken because of the sudden appearance of a skin rash. A pupil visits the nurse for information and guidance in terms of excess weight, a severe cold, pregnancy, or fear of one or more aggressive students. The nurse, counselor, or other person encourages children and youth to make visitations to discuss health problems or concerns whenever they are free, at the noon hour, or in after-school rap sessions. The school newspaper prints articles on student health problems written by students. The nurse makes pamphlets and publications available to students. Special voluntary educational programs on drugs, venereal disease, teenage pregnancies, and emotional problems may be held as needs arise.

What are the purposes of health guidance?

Health guidance seeks to achieve the following:
1. To provide information and interpretation about pupils' health status, concerns, or problems
2. To provide understandings to parents of the nature of the health conditions that exist in their children and to encourage needed care
3. To promote pupils' acceptance of the responsibility for the promotion and preservation of their health
4. To motivate parents and pupils to seek care and treatment when needed for existing health conditions and to accept modifications in the school program where desirable
5. To encourage and promote where necessary the establishment or expansion of school and community health service and facilities especially for needy children and families
6. To encourage pupils and parents to use available medical, dental, and other health resources to the best advantage
7. To contribute to the health education of pupils and parents
8. To assist in the adaptation of school programs to the individual needs and abilities of students with health problems; to keep teachers informed

9. To inform teachers of pupils' health problems and concerns and to identify responsibilities

What are the general problems for which children need health guidance?

Children's health problems requiring guidance may be categorized in the following manner:

In some situations *more detailed examination* of the child is needed to establish a diagnosis. Observations of signs and symptoms might necessitate a chest x-ray for tuberculosis or a tuberculin test, special tests for a heart murmur, a blood count for anemia, a urinalysis for diabetes, a medical examination when chronic fatigue, overweight, frequent colds, and blackouts are noted, or a dental examination for decay or periodontal disease.

There are some conditions for which the child needs *treatment services,* such as undernourishment, malnutrition, overfeeding, epilepsy, dental decay, vision and hearing difficulties, skin infections, diseased tonsils, or allergies.

There are conditions that need *home care improvement.* These may include the need for breakfast or help with balanced lunches, cleanliness, dental care, proper clothing, or better sleeping facilities.

Problems of emotional and social adjustment may make *special counseling* mandatory. Opportunities to talk with understanding people may be most helpful to students. Teachers who have success communicating with pupils may be able to assist them with their problems regarding the abuse and use of drugs. It also may be necessary to interpret the emotional problem to parents to encourage their seeking additional help. These problems frequently are difficult and delicate to present to parents.

For some problems, *assistance regarding health practices and behavior* is advisable. This might call for individual discussion with students regarding covering noses and mouths when coughing and sneezing, the importance of washing the hands before eating and after using the lavatory, the misusing and abusing of drugs, using the drinking fountains properly, remaining at home when ill, eating of breakfast, and what to do about venereal disease. Some of these matters may also involve parental communications and should be handled discreetly.

ORGANIZATION AND ADMINISTRATION OF SCHOOL HEALTH GUIDANCE PROGRAMS

Although practically all schools provide some health guidance, in most cases it is done on an incidental basis. Schools in general do not have well-organized and well-developed health guidance programs, as identified in this chapter. In elementary schools the nurse is usually the key person in the counseling programs. Where health guidance does exist on an organized basis, it has been found that best results accrue when the program is carried out cooperatively; all departments and personnel of a school concerned with any phase of mental, emotional, and physical health of children should cooperate and participate in the formulation of health guidance policies. Objectives and responsibilities need clear definition.

Organized health guidance programs may be considered a relatively new development, therefore it may be well to consider some of the fundamental factors that are basic to sound organization. In this respect, it seems essential that recognition be given to such factors as (1) desirable principles of operation, (2) role of the counselor, (3) responsibilities of various school personnel, and (4) techniques for counseling.

Desirable principles of operation

As in other functions of the school, health guidance should be based on certain fundamental principles for effective operation. The following generalized list may serve as a guide for the establishment of such principles in local school situations:
1. The health guidance complements and supplements the total educational program within the school.

2. The health program should be such that it serves individual pupil needs.
3. The health guidance program should have the wholehearted support of the school administrators.
4. School staff members responsible for health guidance programs should be knowledgeable about community agencies and specialists available for referral purposes.
5. The health guidance program should communicate to parents, teachers, and others the objectives of the services.
6. Some means of in-service training in health guidance should be provided for teachers, administrators, and other members of the school personnel whenever necessary or advisable.
7. There should be full cooperation and coordination of all school departments concerned with the health of pupils.
8. The purposes and scope of each school department concerned with child health should be clearly defined to assure the most efficient service to pupils.
9. Responsibility for leadership in the health guidance program should be centered in individuals who possess, insofar as possible, interest, ability, and preparation for such service.
10. The responsibilities of all persons concerned with the program should be clearly defined and designated.
11. The best possible procedures for effective school and community coordination in health guidance should be provided.
12. The health guidance program should be subjected to constant and continuous evaluation so that constructive improvements may be effected.
13. All health guidance personnel should be encouraged to keep abreast of the latest research and changing conditions as they relate to their specific health area.

Role of the counselor

The counselor is involved in human relations and should be competent to interpret to pupils and parents and to encourage and motivate them to action. Since parents have the primary responsibility for the health of their children, schools should not try to tell them how they should be raised. Schools should attempt to acquaint parents with the health conditions of pupils that require attention, to interpret the importance of care especially as it relates to learning, and to inform parents regarding the nature of community health services and the necessary adjustments of the school program.

School personnel must be familiar with blacks, Indians, Mexican Americans, and those of other ethnic backgrounds. They should understand the cultural heritage and customs and be conversant with the languages for effective communication.

The responsibility for counseling involves a variety of school people including teachers, nurses, physicians, psychologists, principals, counselors, and students.

Responsibilities of various school personnel

One of the principles previously mentioned suggested that the responsibilities of all concerned with the health of pupils should be clearly defined and designated. This statement should perhaps be amplified to the extent that *every* person in the school system should accept responsibility for the health guidance of the school population. In other words, every person associated with the school should have the physical, emotional, mental, and social well-being of pupils as a major concern. The fact that pupils' academic and nonacademic interests relate to their physical and mental health cannot be overstressed. For example, the child who is fatigued, hungry, or unable to understand why people do not want the pupil around may have a learning problem.

Although all school personnel rightfully should take an interest in health guidance of pupils, the extent of responsibilities naturally must vary. Someone should be available in schools with whom students are able to communicate when necessary about health matters, but especially regarding venereal disease, drugs, human sexuality, pregnancies, and home and school problems. This might be the nurse or a teacher or some other knowledgeable, capable individual. The following discussion indicates some of the more or less specific responsibilities of various members of the school health personnel depending somewhat on the size and existing conditions within the individual school system.

School administrators and officers. The responsibilities of the school board member, superintendent, and principal of the school within the community center around the leadership necessary to carry out a successful health guidance program. These groups actually have the final vote of approval as far as the budgetary needs, the acquisition of new equipment, and the hiring of personnel. It should be strongly emphasized that these kinds of service will entail a cooperative kind of leadership in which the administrator plans with his staff on matters pertaining to the broad scope of the program. It is obvious that continued pooling of the competencies of mental health professionals and educators will be needed to achieve the related goals of better mental health and effective learning for more school children.

School administrators need to have adequate knowledge of the objectives of the program, because they are usually the liaison persons between the school and the community and are expected to interpret the objectives. In addition, administrators should also initiate plans for the coordination of school and community relationships and strive to maintain the highest standards for total school health. They may also need to initiate community action to help with the provision of comprehensive health care services, especially for children in the ghetto areas.

Health service personnel. One of the main responsibilities of the school physician, school nurse, school dentist, and others in health service is concerned with helping youths who evidence health needs. Frequent follow-up is necessary. For example, certain pertinent information derived from examinations by the school physician can be relayed to teachers and guidance counselors through the proper channels. More and more use is being made of the case study method whereby those people directly working with a child meet and discuss their findings. The various reports add to the separate impressions, and the goal of assisting in the development of the whole child is more fully realized. In other cases in which either the school nurse or school social worker serves as a direct link between the home and school, she is in a desirable position to refer to guidance counselors and teachers information that may reveal physical, mental, and emotional health problems arising out of home situations.

School nurse. The work of the school nurse continues to grow in importance in the school health program. The committee on School Health Service of the World Health Organization states that nurses, like physicians, have a different type of task when they work within the framework of the school, for it is not the clinical situation to which they have been accustomed in their hospital experiences. It is a new kind of experience, one with children to whom these nurses must bring warmth, acceptance, and understanding. To the teacher the nurse must be a source of information and guidance. To the parent the nurse must be a friendly counselor, cognizant of community resources, sympathetic with family problems, and an interpreter par excellence of the child's needs as revealed by medical examination and school behavior.

Although the responsibilities and duties of school nurses are numerous and varied, special emphasis should be placed on their part in health guidance. The following list summarizes some of the ways the school nurse contributes to the health guidance program:

1. Keeping individual health records up to date for general use and for specific use when health counseling is indicated
2. Assisting with examinations and inspections that may reveal a need for guidance and counseling
3. Interpreting the results of health appraisals to pupils, teachers, and parents
4. Providing information and direction con-

cerning community resources available for the care of physical, mental, and emotional problems of children

5. Assisting in motivating pupils to develop and maintain optimum health
6. Helping children to find solutions to their personal problems, particularly those involving or likely to involve physical, mental, and emotional health
7. Assisting in the identification of pupils needing modified education programs
8. Counseling pupils with health problems
9. Counseling parents concerning the health problems of children
10. Serving as a liaison between home, school, and community organizations and agencies
11. Providing care in emergencies and accidents
12. Participating in formal and informal health education

The role of the school nurse is changing and Oda has identified the expanding duties that include*:

1. Greater stress on health education, counseling and consultation
2. Emergence as a school nurse practitioner in which special training is providing competency to conduct in-depth assessment of physical, psychomedical, and psychoeducational behavior and learning disorders of children (see Chapter 4)
3. Involvement in the development, implementation, and evaluation of health care plans and programs
4. Utilization of increased technologic health assessment skills

The number of nurses found in schools varies because standards are not uniform or consistent throughout the United States. New York advocates that there be one nurse for each 600 to 700 pupils, whereas California recommends that the ratio be one nurse for 1,000 to 1,400 students. Common practices differ widely. Many schools have no services while in others nurses are limited to one-half day weekly.

*Oda, D. S.: Increasing role effectiveness of school nurses, American Journal of Public Health **64:** June, 1974.

Health coordinator. The person assuming the responsibilities of school health coordinator should direct, supervise, and coordinate all activities concerning the health of students. In other words, the success or failure of health guidance programs may depend upon the extent to which proper use of information is made. For example, many schools have an excellent program of health appraisal, yet they do not have adequate organization, ways, or means of following up the findings of the appraisals. The school health coordinator should fill any gaps that may exist by coordinating all information that might be used to guide the pupil in matters that concern his health.

Another important function of the school health coordinator is that of conducting needed research. All too often records are kept and up-to-date entries made so that the pupils' growth and development are charted, with little if any attempt made to utilize these data for study purposes. The analysis of records could certainly aid in pointing out trends, changes in physical, social, and emotional patterns of both boys and girls, and the limitations of the school's health program, to name a few.

Unfortunately, health coordinators per se are not frequently employed in school districts. Where they are found, these individuals may be nurses, physicians, health educators, or others.

Guidance personnel. Guidance directors, psychometrists, and other guidance personnel have the responsibility of helping pupils in their efforts to handle their health problems. If counselors and others expect to have pupils referred to them for individual help, then a knowledge of the objectives of the health guidance program is essential. They should have not only sufficient background in the psychodynamics of behavior, but also understanding of health education in that most of the problems found among children involve, either directly or indirectly, physical, mental, social, and emotional health. They may also contribute to the health guidance program by offering in-service education to teachers and other school personnel with respect to the counseling methods that would be more effective with those pupils needing counseling and guidance.

Because guidance personnel are generally involved in a helping relationship, children, parents, teachers, and others often share with them various types of personal concerns, some of which may relate to the school environment. It is possible, without breaking confidence, for the guidance personnel to assist in calling attention to health problems that are not being cared for or even detected.

School psychologist. In school systems in which the services of a psychologist are available, many contributions can be made to the health guidance program by the person serving in this capacity. At the present time one of the major functions of the school psychologist is more nearly that of a psychometrist who administers group and individual psychologic tests. In addition to this primary function, many school psychologists confer with parents and teachers about individual pupils with problems that particularly concern emotional health. The school psychologist should be in close contact with the school administrators, school physician, school nurse, school social worker, teachers, and family physicians and psychiatrists who may be in a position to act on his or her recommendations regarding children who are in need of adjustment to problems that concern their health. Although most school personnel have taken course work in the area of the behavioral sciences, the school psychologist can be most helpful in aiding in the understanding of unusual behavioral patterns. Often the school psychologist will administer various types of tests and submit a report of these findings for the school to keep on record. Since these reports are more often than not psychologically descriptive, care must be taken in their use and circulation.

Elementary school teachers. Classroom teachers are actually the hub in a successful health guidance program at the elementary school level. As mentioned previously, in the majority of cases elementary school teachers are in a position to observe pupils day by day. It becomes their responsibility to detect physical, social, and emotional behavior patterns that are unusual and refer them to the nurses, physicians, and administrators. Elementary teachers probably are the most important people, outside of the family, in providing for the cultivation of health attitudes and values through the health instruction program. The student will seek out the teacher for information if communication has been established in incidental and informal settings.

Special teachers. Teachers dealing with special groups, as in rehabilitation, special education, and the various special subjects, such as physical education, home economics, and health education, very definitely have considerable responsibility in all matters of pupil health, including health guidance since they ordinarily come in closer contact with situations that deal with health status. For instance, the physical education teacher has an opportunity to watch the organic development of pupils as well as peer acceptance of the group members. Whether physical educators are aware of their responsibility for health guidance has been questioned, but it is the feeling that physical development should not be their only concern.

Drug counselor. A person known as a drug counselor is beginning to be available to students in the upper elementary and junior and senior high schools. Responsibilities may include establishment of communication with drug users, misusers, and abusers; student and parent guidance; liaison with community resources including the police and courts; and the preparation of policies and procedures. This individual should be one who is approachable by students, is readily available and accessible, is willing to talk and not to preach, is honest and trustful in approach, is willing to discuss any topic of interest to pupils, and is knowledgeable about the drug scene.

Students. There have been a variety of attempts by schools to use student peers in an attempt to help pupils with drug problems. Upper elementary school youths have made formal presentations to sixth graders and other students in their own schools. They have also been available for indirect, informal individual and group meetings. Students who are familiar with drugs have been able on occasions to establish rapport with drug misusers and abusers. The value of such activities has not been clearly defined, but indications reveal they create interest and enthusiasm on the part of both the participants and the performers. The use of students in a variety of health counseling situations should receive greater consideration and experimentation in schools.

Techniques for counseling

The specific procedures for communicating with students and parents include informal and formal talks, notes home, home and school visits with parents, and telephone calls.

When counseling parents or students, or both, the following suggestions should receive consideration:

1. Try to develop rapport and thereby improve the effectiveness of the communication. Attempt to be friendly and nonofficious in approach. Demonstrate sincerity in wanting to be helpful. Create the feeling that information and aid, if desired, is the intent of the meeting. Refrain from telling the parent or student what action to take; hopefully a request for help will be forthcoming. Be tuned in on expressions and language indigenous to inner-city children. Be familiar with differences in values and cultural conflicts without becoming judgmental. Permit cultural identification to emerge in the development of a source of pride.

2. Help parents and pupils to analyze or recognize the problem. A child's heart murmur may be very threatening to the parents and frightening to the child. Although this condition is abnormal and may be serious, it may not be serious for that particular child. Only medical help can determine the extent of the problem.

3. Help parents and pupils to understand the nature and significance of the problem by encouraging questions and by supplying information as requested. Be certain understanding and clarity occur.

4. Help parents and pupils to determine the various courses of action to be taken and discuss the consequences. The solution may be relatively simple if parents have a family physician. However, if parents do not know where to go or do not have a physician or funds, the problem may be more complex in resolving.

5. Encourage parents and students to choose a particular course of action, but indicate the decision will rest with them.

When contacting parents about student health problems that are not unusual, such as vision or hearing difficulties, the school nurse may send home a form notice because it is the quickest and easiest way to communicate with a large number of parents. The use of this reporting method has these limitations: the note may not reach home; parents may not read it; parents may not be able to understand or interpret it; and it may be cold, formal, and impersonal. Therefore, the procedures used to get in touch with parents must receive careful consideration.

From recent studies on effective ways of communicating with parents to get action, it has been found that children of parents in the high social ranks are more likely to receive attention than those in low social ranks; children whose parents give defects a high urgency rating are more likely to receive attention; notifications about a child's defect by more than one contact technique (written notice, telephone call, home or school visit, and others) are more likely to secure attention than if parents are notified by one contact only. Those contacts involving personal interaction by telephone or visitation are significantly more productive than those using a written medium. Also, parents who receive two notifications of children's defects are more likely to get attention than parents who receive only one notification. Three notifications do not appear to be worth the effort.

Research findings conclude the most effective techniques of communication for parent action are notices written by a physician and telephone calls by school nurses. However, a study in San Diego* of sixth grade pupils re-

*Brophy, H. E.: Project pursuit: a health defect follow-up activity, Journal of School Health **40**: April, 1970.

vealed that the face-to-face contact by a home call or a nurse-parent conference at school or at the parent's place of work resulted in over 70% of defects identified through health appraisals receiving attention.

WHICH COMMUNITY HEALTH RESOURCES ARE ESSENTIAL?

School personnel should be familiar with and use all local community health resources to help meet the health guidance needs of pupils. Schools must take the initiative to learn about the services available and establish communications with the various physicians, dentists, psychiatrists, and other health specialists in private practice, health clinics and hospitals, voluntary health agencies, health departments, child guidance clinics, social service agencies, family service agencies, civic and service organizations, welfare agencies, and religious services located in the community.

Health problems that schools experience when dealing with poor people are of greater magnitude and more complex in solution than for other students. Many children in ghetto areas do not receive basic health services needed to attain high levels of wellness. It will be necessary for schools to take the initiative to stimulate community action to provide such assistance or to enter into a cooperative arrangement for such services. In California the state Department of Education* developed a plan to provide health services for 29,000 children in 176 school districts in 27 counties. Medical services were provided by private physicians and part-time school physicians, and clinics were established for schoolchildren in migrant camps. Dental treatment was also made available through the use of a mobile unit. Nurses and nurses aides were based in the camps. Through the assistance of the Office of Economic Opportunity numerous neighborhood health centers have been established in deprived areas in an attempt to provide better systems for delivery of health care. These

centers have worked closely with school personnel. The drug and venereal disease problems demand additional community resources.

It will be necessary for at least one person in the school to be familiar with the kinds and variety of resources available so the best guidance can be provided to students and parents. Frequently the school nurse assumes this responsibility and is the best informed person.

HOW DO SCHOOLS ADJUST PROGRAMS?

After appropriate care or treatment has been received by a student, it may not always mean that the child has been cured or that the child's health problem has been corrected. A child with a severe vision problem may have to wear corrective lenses but still may not be able to read the type in a textbook. A pupil with a heart problem may be under treatment and need to control activities or have all classes on one floor. A student with epilepsy may be receiving medication to control seizures but may have to take the drug while at school. It therefore becomes necessary for schools to adjust programs to fit the needs of students with health problems.

Among the numerous ways schools have modified and adjusted educational programs are the following:

1. Special consideration for students in the regular classroom. The visually handicapped or hard-of-hearing child may need to be placed in the front of the room. Special rest periods during the day may have to be provided for some pupils. For others, midmorning snacks may be necessary.

2. Special teachers for certain handicapped children provided in the regular classroom. The partially sighted child may need to have special large-print textbooks and other materials prepared. The pupil with speech difficulties may need special attention. Children with learning disabilities may need special guidance.

3. Special classes in the regular school. Those who are mentally handicapped, blind, or deaf may be grouped into special classes

---

*Eisner, V.: Health services under the Elementary and Secondary Education Act, Journal of School Health **40:** Nov., 1970.

with specially prepared teachers. Greater attention to a curriculum to satisfy the needs of these children may therefore take place.

4. Special day schools. Cerebral palsied children, those who are emotionally disturbed, and those who are severely mentally retarded may be housed in a facility entirely separate from the regular school.

5. Special residential schools. Blind and deaf students may need to remain overnight for extended periods of time in these schools to receive the best education.

6. Home teachers. Those children who are ill or injured and who must remain at home for long periods of time may need to have teachers go directly to their homes.

7. Hospital teachers. Those students who must remain in hospitals for extensive periods of time may need service of hospital teachers.

Schools differ in the nature and extent of the educational services provided for handicapped pupils. The larger school districts and those with more funds are usually able to provide the greater services. Federal and state funds are frequently available to subsidize local programs.

It is essential to understand that health guidance is an important and essential part of the school health services program. It should receive adequate consideration in schools. Without follow-up procedures to obtain corrections, treatment, and care including the adjustment of school programs, health appraisals by themselves are not important to the educational process. Assistance in guidance should be forthcoming from a variety of school personnel. School nurses spend a considerable portion of their time in health guidance and are important resources not only for teachers, but also for parents, students, and others. Teachers should clearly understand their responsibilities in health guidance.

QUESTIONS FOR DISCUSSION

1. What procedures are necessary when children with health problems have been discovered in schools?
2. What is meant by the term "health guidance," and what is its relationship to informal health education?
3. What is informal health education, why is it necessary, and how can it occur in schools?
4. How would you differentiate between health guidance and health counseling?
5. What are some of the pupil health problems needing health guidance?
6. What are the major purposes of health guidance in schools?
7. How can the health problems of children needing health guidance be generally categorized?
8. What organizational and administrative factors must receive consideration when a school health guidance program is being introduced?
9. What are the guiding principles necessary for an effective school health guidance program?
10. What should be the role of the counselor in the health guidance program?
11. What are the responsibilities of a school drug counselor, and how can such a position be justified?
12. What are some of the duties of the school nurse as the nurse's responsibilities expand?
13. What are the responsibilities of the various school personnel in health guidance?
14. What are some of the effective techniques for health counseling?
15. What guidelines should be used when students or parents are being counseled?
16. What health resources may be available in the community to help with student health problems?
17. What ways have schools tried to adjust programs to help pupils with health problems?
18. What guidance can a school provide for children and youth in the ghettos with health problems?

SUGGESTED CLASS ACTIVITIES

1. Form a panel discussion group to consider the need for a health guidance program in a hypothetical school situation.
2. Prepare a list of problems in which children and youths need health guidance.
3. Take the part of a health counselor and counsel a member of the class concerning a hypothetical health problem (The rest of the class members should act as an audience and give the counselor constructive suggestions when the interview is completed.)
4. Invite various members of the school personnel including nurses, physicians, and guidance specialists to participate in a discussion concerning problems of health guidance and counseling in the elementary school.
5. Form a committee to survey a number of elementary schools to learn what they are doing concerning health guidance.
6. Identify a given student health problem (for example, vision defect) and trace the health guidance procedures that might be necessary in a given school to assist this pupil.

7. Plan a model health guidance program for a school or school district.
8. Prepare a group of seventh and eighth grade students in a school to develop a program of guidance about drugs for their peers.
9. Visit a school in the ghetto to discover the activities provided for the health guidance of its students.
10. Identify health areas in which informal health education can be introduced into the curriculum.
11. Have students plan informal health education for specific health problems, such as drugs, VD, and contraception.
12. Have students survey the community to determine the extent of the available personnel to guide parents and students with health problems.

REFERENCES

Anderson, C. L., and Creswell, W. H., Jr.: School health practice, ed. 6, St. Louis, 1976, The C. V. Mosby Co.

Angers, W. P., and Paulson, P. C.: Cooperation between counseling and health services, Journal of School Health 34: Feb. 1964.

Ayers, G. E. Communicating with inner-city children, School Health Review 3: Jan.-Feb., 1972.

Bernhagen, L.: Progress report of the health guidance in sex education committee, Journal of School Health 34: April, 1964.

Bryan, D. S.: School nursing in transition, St. Louis, 1973, The C. V. Mosby Co.

Brophy, H. E.: Project pursuit; a health defect follow-up activity, Journal of School Health 40: April, 1970.

Burney, L. E.: New missions in health service; to act or react, Journal of School Health 40: Jan., 1970.

Carroll, P.: School health and guidance services; a co-operative venture, Journal of School Health 30: Jan., 1960.

Caufman, J.: Factors affecting outcome of school health referrals, Journal of School Health 38: June, 1968.

Cornacchia, H. J., Smith, D. E., and Bentel, H. J.: Drugs in the classroom; a conceptual model for school programs, ed. 2, St. Louis, 1978, The C. V. Mosby Co.

Cowen, D. L.: Denver's preventive health program for school-age children, American Journal of Public Health 60: March, 1970.

Dinkmeyer, D. C.: Guidance and counseling in the elementary school, New York, 1968, Holt, Rinehart & Winston.

Eiseman, S.: The need for effective health counselors in schools, Health Education 6: Sept./Oct., 1975.

Eisner, V.: Health services under the Elementary and Secondary Education Act, Journal of School Health 40: Nov., 1970.

Griffin, J.: Follow through; parents, school, and community work together to provide health care for good classroom performance, School Health Review 5: July/Aug., 1974.

Harris, W. H.: Guidance in health education, Journal of School Health 35: May, 1965.

Hummel, D. L., and Bonham, S. J.: Pupil personnel services in schools–organization and coordination, Chicago, 1968, Rand McNally & Co.

Hutson, P. W.: The guidance function in education, ed. 2, New York, 1968, Appleton-Century-Crofts.

Knotts, G. R., editor: Guidelines for the school nurse in the school health program, Kent, Ohio, 1974, American School Health Association.

Langton, C. V., Allen, R., and Wexler, P.: School health organization and services, New York, 1961, The Ronald Press Co.

Meeks, A. R.: Guidance in elementary education, New York, 1968, The Ronald Press Co.

Meyer, H.: Guiding children to better health through health counseling, Journal of School Health 37: May, 1967.

Miller, C.: Foundations of guidance, New York, 1961, Harper & Row, Publishers, Inc.

Neil, H.: Better communications for better health, New York, 1962, Columbia University Press.

Nemir, A.: The school health program, ed. 3, Philadelphia, 1970, W. B. Saunders Co.

Oda, D. S.: Increasing role effectiveness of school nurses, American Journal of Public Health 64: June, 1974.

Paige, J. C.: Health programs for the disadvantaged; implications for school health, Journal of School Health 40: March, 1970.

Ratchick, I., and Koenig, F. G.: Guidance and the physically handicapped child, Chicago, 1963, Science Research Associates, Inc.

Robey, D. L., and Dickey, B. A.: Health counseling, Journal of School Health 36: April, 1966.

Rosencrance, F., and Hayden, V.: School guidance and personnel services, Boston, 1960, Allyn & Bacon, Inc.

Statts, A.: Complex human behavior, New York, 1963, Holt, Rinehart & Winston.

Stafford, R. L., and Meyer, R. J.: Diagnosis and counseling of the mentally retarded; implications for school health, Journal of School Health 38: March, 1968.

Stefflre, B.: Theories of counseling, New York, 1965, McGraw-Hill Book Co.

White House Conference, 1960: Goals for the next decade, Journal of Health, Physical Education, and Recreation 31: Sept., 1960.

Wilson, C. C., editor: School health services, revised, Washington, D.C., 1964, National Education Association and American Medical Association.

Woody, R. H.: Counseling in Health Education, Journal of School Health 41: Jan., 1971.

6 School safety

When we think of the health and well-being of elementary school children we must think of accident prevention and emergency care. It is simply a matter of probabilities. Year after year more children are killed and disabled by accidents than by all diseases combined. The rate for elementary school boys is four times that for girl students.

For all ages—and practically all people of any age group were once elementary pupils —accidents have consistently ranked among the top five leading causes of death. Accidents are the leading cause of death and disability for all persons age 1 to 38.

By and large elementary teachers have apparently been doing a good job in safety education. Over the past half century the accident death rate for children in the 5- to 14-year age range has dropped more than that of any other age group. Yet there is still room for improvement when we lose some 8,000 elementary school children each year through accidents. More tragic is the fact that approximately half of these accidents could have been prevented.

While it is true that major advances have been made in medical, surgical, and hospital care and rehabilitation of injured children, wouldn't it be better if these accidents had never occurred?

WHAT CAN TEACHERS DO?

Because health and safety are so closely related from the viewpoint of the optimum welfare of the school child, it is very important that teachers have a clear understanding of the relationship of health and safety education in the school program. Even though health and safety are related, nevertheless they also can be considered separate entities in that many parts of safety and accident prevention must be dealt with differently than is health education.

Teachers, parents, and others interested in and responsible for the optimum growth and development of children should be cognizant not only of the problems in health education, but also of those in safety education as well. For many years the schools have accepted responsibility in health education in attempting to help each child develop to his or her greatest possible capacity not only academically, but also emotionally and physically; naturally, teachers and others have attempted to do everything possible to educate the children concerning health as well as to try to help them maintain good health and to protect them from ill health and disabling diseases and disorders. Now it is recognized that safety ranks in the same category in the attempt to assure the optimum growth and development of children. If teachers think in terms of protecting and providing for the optimum health and growth of children, then they cannot fail to assume responsibility in safety education.

WHAT IS THE NATURE OF THE ACCIDENT PROBLEM?*

Although the problem of accidental deaths and injuries has assumed major proportions in the United States, many of us are not thoroughly conscious of the extent of the present problem of safety and accident prevention.

During the past 20 years approximately 2 million people were killed in accidents in the United States. In addition to those killed, more than 200 million received some type of disabling† injury.

---

*Data from National Safety Council.: Accident facts, Chicago, 1977, The Council.
†"Disabling beyond the day of the accident" (National Safety Council definition).

Although the total accidental death *rate* seems to have decreased slightly during the past few years, more than 115,000 people are killed in accidents each year, and approximately 400,000 received some type of *permanent disabling injury*. In addition to the many people killed and permanently disabled each year, according to the National Safety Council, approximately 11 million people sustain injuries that cause suffering, medical expense, and loss of time from school or work.

Many of the hazards that formerly existed are gone, but in their place have come others far more numerous and serious. Modern machines have become an element of major importance in the life of everyone. Motor vehicles (including mopeds), powered pleasure boats, airplanes, power mowers, electric appliances and tools, unsafe toys, chemicals, poisons, and explosives as well as nuclear energy are examples of modern developments that have introduced, created, and multipled hazards in the modern world. The hazards have become so numerous, the methods of meeting them so varied and complicated, and the intellectual and emotional preparation needed to live safely among the hazards so extensive, that safety has emerged as a major problem of our society.

WHAT ARE THE PURPOSES OF THE ELEMENTARY SCHOOL SAFETY PROGRAM?

The original aims of elementary school safety were largely protection of the child. It is now clearly understood that the schools must assume considerable responsibility for safety beyond merely protecting and sheltering pupils.

The infant must have almost complete care and protection. However, as the infant grows and develops, protection should be gradually reduced. At the same time, safety education should be provided as well as the inculcation of proper safety practices and habits. Since there are so many hazards in life and so many different degrees of risk, parents and teachers must seek a practical changing balance between protection and education.

If children are overprotected, their personal responsibility and adjustment may be retarded, thus leaving them more likely to be involved in accidents in situations where they are not personally protected. On the other hand, if children are underprotected, in the absence of proper safety education, they may be seriously injured or even killed.

The main aims of the elementary school safety program are to:

1. Prevent accidents
2. Eliminate hazards
3. Develop individual and group safety consciousness
4. Develop wholesome attitudes, habits, and practices pertaining to safety
5. Develop attitudes of personal responsibility for safety
6. Impart an understanding of environmental hazards in the modern world
7. Impart an understanding of safe conduct in the ordinary activities of life
8. Teach the relationship of safety to individual and group health at school, in the home, and in the community

HOW ARE ACCIDENTS CLASSIFIED?

The use of statistics in attempting to reduce the accidental death and injury rate have been questioned at times as somewhat inadequate. Nevertheless, statistics showing *how* and *where* people are killed and injured continue to be the basis upon which organized efforts are founded in educational and prevention programs.

To gain a proper perspective of the total accident situation, it is necessary to know as accurately as possible the number of people involved in accidents resulting in death, permanent disability, and disabling injuries. To deal intelligently with the accident problem, it is important to show also the many accidents occurring within the activities in which people participate from day to day. For example, if teachers in the schools are to help reduce the number of deaths and injuries to school children, it is very important that they know just where and how accidents occur not only in and about the school building and ground, but also on the way to and from school, in the community, and in the home.

The National Safety Council classifies accidents into four main divisions, which have been found to be useful in studying and clarifying accident statistics for use by those interested in and working with safety education. The four general classifications are *motor vehicle* accidents, *home* accidents, *work* accidents, and *public* accidents (exclusive of motor vehicle accidents). Of course, it is necessary to make many classifications within the four divisions if we are to know exactly where and how accidents happen. It is one of the duties of teachers and others in safety education to reclassify accidents in such a way that they will be meaningful to pupils for safe living.

By using the detailed breakdown data on specific types, locales, and time of day and season of accidents, teachers can make statistics in the four principal classes of accidents more meaningful to pupils. This practical information is available in the latest annual edition of *Accident Facts*, published by the National Safety Council.*

Motor vehicle accidents

Accidents involving both motor vehicles and pedestrians are responsible for a large number of deaths and injuries each year. During the 1950s and for the first 2 years of the 1960s traffic fatalities remained somewhat constant, ranging from a low of 35,568 in 1954 to a high of 39,628 in 1956. In 1962 the fatality toll went beyond 40,000. What has happened since then has been extremely serious. Traffic deaths soared to 49,163 in 1965 and an all-time high of 56,000 in 1972. However, with the energy crisis of the early and mid 1970s—and its attendant 55 miles per hour speed limit—the number of motor vehicle deaths dropped back to 46,000 in 1975. Yet, with increasing numbers of drivers violating the 55-mile limit, the motor vehicle death rate is rising again. Because of the nature of motor vehicle accidents, in

---

*National Safety Council, 425 N. Michigan Ave., Chicago, Ill. 60611.

Table 6-1. Deaths and disabling injuries by principal classes of accidents for a typical year (1975)*

	Deaths	**Disabling injuries**
Work	12,600	2,200,000
Motor vehicle	46,000	1,800,000
Home	25,500	4,000,000
Public	22,500	2,800,000

*Data from National Safety Council: Accident facts, Chicago, 1977, The Council.

which such heavy equipment and speed is involved, the injuries are usually severe, causing a large number of those injured each year to be permanently disabled in some way.

The first step for the elementary school is to have a strong, well-organized *to* and *from* school safety program. But traffic safety education should not end with this program because only about 5% of the children injured in traffic accidents are proceeding to and from school.

Pedestrian safety. Elementary school-age children seem to be particularly vulnerable to pedestrian accidents. Boys and girls in the 5- to 9-year age group in particular are involved in more pedestrian accidents than any other age group under 65. Pedestrian studies indicate that:
1. Crossing streets from between parked cars and crossing between street intersections are the principal actions of children involved in pedestrian accidents
2. September, October, March, and April are the most dangerous months for boys and girls as pedestrians
3. From 3 to 6 P.M. is the most dangerous pedestrian period for children

The elementary school pedestrian program should be based on local accident facts. To be significant, traffic data should include all pedestrian accidents, not just fatal accidents. These generally can be obtained from the local police or health department.

One major mistake we have made in pedestrian safety education is unknowingly leading pupils to believe that as long as they cross with the light or in the crosswalk, there is no need to watch for motor vehicles.

Passenger safety. More children are injured inside motor vehicles than in pedestrian accidents. Although this is basically a problem of parents and drivers, the elementary school teacher can help through the proper education of children.

In teaching passenger safety the teacher can develop with the class the many things with which a driver has to contend and the actions by passengers that lead to accidents. Children wrestling in a car or school bus make it difficult for drivers to concentrate on the complex driving situations that they face; they may even take their eyes from the road, creating extra hazards in the case of sudden stops, pedestrians stepping from the curb, or cars entering his path of travel. All drivers use their ears as well as their eyes in driving. Excessive noise masks the sound of cars overtaking and passing. Arms out the window and objects thrown from the car or bus provide distractions for both the driver and drivers of other cars.

Classroom teaching emphasis also should be placed on the fact that children should ride in the rear seat of passenger automobiles. The frequency and severity of injuries are lower for rear seat occupants. In addition, *the use of lap and shoulder belts will greatly reduce the injury to children.* The belts maintain the child in place, preventing the child from being thrown against the interior of the car or from being thrown outside of the car. Seat belts have also proved effective in preventing injury in nonaccident situations such as sudden stops. The belts are simple to operate, and even a kindergarten child can manage them.

Bicycle accidents

Every elementary school should have an effective bicycle safety program. Furthermore, elementary school teachers should take an active part in the program as approximately 85% of the bicycle injuries occur in the 5- to 14-year age group.

A National Safety Council study of fatal bicycle accidents showed that:

1. Riding on the left side of the street is more hazardous than riding on the right side
2. In one accident in three, the bicyclist struck the motor vehicle
3. In four out of five accidents the rider was violating the rules of safe riding

Also, the study showed that the most frequent violations of the bicycle riders were that the rider did not have the right of way, turned improperly, disregarded stop signs and signals, rode in the center of the street, and rode *against* traffic.

The first step in bicycle safety is to have the correct sized bicycle, properly equipped and maintained. For optimal safety a properly equipped bicycle should comply with specifications established by the Bicycle Institute of America (p. 323).

Although a bicycle of proper size, properly equipped and maintained is important to safety, the development of skill plus safe riding habits and attitudes is even more important.

Some of the most important rules for safe bicycle riding, which also apply to motorized bikes (mopeds), are the following:

1. Observe all traffic regulations (traffic signals, signs, one-way streets, never pass on a curve, pass another vehicle on the left, and so forth).
2. Look before executing a maneuver, before entering the street, before swinging out to pass a parked car.
3. Ride on the right with the flow of traffic (single file on busy streets, never more than two abreast, a safe distance behind the vehicle ahead).
4. Always use the proper hand signals for turning and stopping. All signals should be given with the left hand well in advance of a turn or stop.
5. In the city or town particularly
   a. Watch for car doors opening.
   b. Watch for pedestrians stepping from between parked cars.
   c. Walk your bicycle across busy intersections.
6. Give the pedestrian the right of way

(take special care coming out of driveways).

7. Park your bicycle in places provided (if no rack is available, place your bicycle out of pedestrian traffic, leave the bicycle upright so no one will trip over it).
8. If absolutely necessary to ride at night, wear white or clothing of reflective material.
9. Don't ride two on a bicycle.
10. Don't hitch rides on another vehicle.
11. Slow down at street intersections, and look both right and left before crossing.
12. Refrain from weaving in or out of traffic or swerving from side to side—ride in a straight line as much as possible.

Home accidents

Most people think of home as being a place of safety and security. Yet thousands of men, women, and children are killed, and hundreds of thousands are injured in home accidents each year. Home accidents account for the largest number of injuries each year.

The deaths and injuries that happen in the home are largely caused by three main factors (1) there are many objects and appliances in the home that are dangerous if they are not handled properly; (2) many people are careless; and (3) many people, and especially children, lack an understanding of the dangers involved.

Mechanical factors frequently are contributing causes of home accidents. Many people seem prone to use equipment improperly or to try to use something unsuited for the task or to use equipment that is rickety or broken.

Although mechanical factors often contribute to home accidents, the human element is involved more often. Poor judgment, haste, ignorance regarding safety practices, fatigue, and physical defects are personal elements responsible for a large number of home accidents. Appliances in and around the modern home, such as power mowers, irons, toasters, gas stoves, washing machines, refrigerators, sewing machines, knives, and cooking and eating utensils are a few of the items that, if not used properly, may lead to death or injury.

The *kitchen* is a place where injuries frequently occur. Many wounds are caused by the careless use of such items as knives, forks, and can openers. Water and grease on the kitchen floor are the cause of many falls resulting in injury. Hot grease and cooking utensils on the stove cause many burns. Many children are burned when pans of hot water or hot food are knocked off the stove. If gas is used for cooking, there is always danger of gas poisoning. Sometimes the flame goes out and lets the gas escape into the room, or the handle of the gas jet may be accidentally opened without the person knowing it. With the energy shortage causing many people to go back to the old-fashioned wood stove, it is important that special safety precautions be taken when such stoves are used.

Many injuries from burns and falls happen in the *living room*. Since falls from slipping on waxed floors happen frequently, waxed floors should be rubbed down well after the wax is applied to keep them from being too slick. Sometimes small rugs on a floor slip when stepped on and cause someone to fall. Also, running on slick floors is a frequent cause of injury by falls among children. Sparks from the fireplace often causes fires; consequently, a fire screen should be placed snugly before a fireplace to prevent sparks from starting fires.

Electric lamps and cords in a living room should be handled with care and should be placed so that children will not trip over them. "Amateur" attempts at fixing TV sets are an increasing cause of injury and death. Children often leave toys on the floor, causing serious injuries when people trip and fall over toys. Parents should teach children to form the habit of putting toys in their proper places when they are through playing with them.

Although the *bedroom* in the home is looked upon by most people as a safe place, nevertheless many serious injuries from falls happen in bedrooms each year. Many falls happen when people get out of bed in the dark and stumble over furniture. Lights should be placed so that they can be turned on before a person gets out of bed. Also, many babies and small children are seriously hurt when they roll out of bed. Accidents of this kind are caused by carelessness on the part of those caring for children. There should always be a railing on a small child's bed to keep the child from rolling out.

The *bathroom* in the home is a place where some serious accidents can happen. Many of these occur in the bathroom as a result of falls, electric shock, and poisoning. Touching electric switches or electric equipment when the body is wet can cause death. This is especially true if there happens to be a short circuit or broken insulation. Electric switches and equipment should be placed so that they cannot be reached when one is in the bathtub. Many deaths occur when radios fall from a chair or shelf into the water when someone is taking a bath. Serious falls frequently happen in the bathroom. Falls may happen when getting into or out of the bathtub or getting into or out of a shower. Rubber mats or safety mats placed in the bathtub and shower help to prevent falls. There should also be a sturdy handgrip fastened to the walls to grasp for support while getting into or out of a bathtub. Water on the floor in the bathroom causes many falls. Also, soap dropped on the floor may cause falls when it is stepped on. The family medicine cabinet is usually kept in the bathroom. Since many poisons, drugs, and medicines may be kept in the medicine cabinet, care must be taken by both children and adults to prevent accidental poisoning.

Injuries occur in the *halls* and on *stairways* in the home. Going up or down stairs in the dark or in a dim light may lead to falls. Carpets that are not fastened securely on steps may cause falls, as can toys and pieces of furniture left on a stairway or in a hallway. Therefore, both children and adults should keep one hand on the rail when going up or down stairways.

More and more families are installing smoke detector devices in halls and on stairways, as well as in other home locations, to assure the earliest possible warning of fire. This relatively new fire protection measure should be part of the teaching unit on fire safety.

There are many ways to be injured in the *basement* of the home. Many falls happen on the stairway leading to the basement. The steps of the stairway should be strong, kept in good repair, and kept free from objects that may trip or cause a person to fall. The stairway should have a good light, and the switches should be placed so that the light can be turned on either at the top or at the bottom of the stairway. The last step of the stairway leading to the basement should be painted white so that person known when he reaches the bottom. The basement should be kept free from waste or rubbish—fires start easily in piles of dry rubbish and waste.

Many serious injuries from electric equipment happen in the basement; therefore, one should always use great care in handling electric wires and switches. Usually the floors are wet or damp. Even a light electric shock may prove very serious if the person is standing on a damp floor.

Electric cords used on washing machines in the basement should be covered with heavy rubber insulation. An asbestos cord that is ordinarily used on a heating appliance, like an electric iron, is not satisfactory where there is water. When the asbestos covering of cords becomes soaked with water on a wet floor, the wire is no longer properly insulated since water makes electric shock stronger. Heavy rubber insulation on electric wire does not become water soaked. Many people have been killed by electric shocks when using an electric cord covered only with cloth or asbestos in a damp basement.

Outdoors, the ever-growing use of power lawn mowers has created additional hazards. The rotary type of power mower can be especially hazardous. Fingers, hands, feet, toes, and eyes are the parts of the body most frequently injured. Small stones, pieces of metal, and other objects thrown by a power lawn mower can be dangerous missiles.

The growing trend in American suburbia

to get out of the house and cook and eat in the back yard or patio has brought sharp increases in burn injuries to both adults and children. Often young children are allowed or even encouraged to build the fire, sometimes using dangerous flammable fluids. The recognized fact that many parents drink as part of the suburban "barbeque ritual" makes such home occasions even more dangerous to elementary school children unless they are apprised of the dangers and preventive measures. This is an important function of safety education in our schools.

Public accidents

Boating and water mishaps involving children have become increasingly tragic statistics with the marked growth in pleasure boat enthusiasts throughout the United States in recent years.

There are now some 8 million water pleasure crafts in the nation, almost all of which are under 26 feet in length. Most casualties occur in boats less than 20 feet long, and most operators are blithely ignorant of boat-safety standards, navigation, and handling. As in motor vehicle and private aircraft accidents, boating deaths are often the result of excessive drinking by parents or other adults. Though the new U.S. Coast Guard regulations are tougher and tighter, it still remains for the schools to teach boys and girls the basic rules of boating safety.

Camping safety is another area of growing concern since, with increased affluence, more and more elementary school children are going to camps during the summer months. Recent evidence indicates that a shocking lack of knowledge and concern for standards of health and safety prevails in America's camps for children. This is especially true of commercial camps, but it occurs to a lesser extent in camps run by nonprofit organizations. The reasons for the spreading incidence of summer camp accidents are greed on the part of some commercial camp owners, immature and inexperienced counselors, and unsafe facilities and equipment. Add to this the all too frequent outbreaks of food poisoning and food infection—caused by improper storage, preparation, or handling—and the old appeal "send this child to camp" becomes less and less convincing.

SCHOOL SAFETY

Every year thousands of accidents happen to school-age children, resulting in injury and death.

Among children from 5 to 14 years of age, accidental deaths decreased from a high of nearly 10,000 per year in the mid 1920s to about 8,000 in recent years. The substantial decrease has been accomplished despite the increase in number of children from 5 to 14 years of age.

One of the contributing reasons the death rate among children 5 to 14 years of age decreased is that in elementary schools throughout the country, teachers and others who come in contact with the child have placed greater emphasis on safety education and protection for the elementary school children.

Safe school environment

The school plant should be a safe place for children to live and work. Schools having well-organized and planned safety programs have a minimum of serious accidents.

Since the 1971 earthquake in southern California, parents, educators, and safety specialists have been concerned about protective school construction and survival plans. As is true in most dramatic occurrences where people are killed and injured, the public becomes alarmed. As time goes by, alarm become mild concern, followed by apathy. Apparently it is "human nature" to feel that a similar tragedy will not happen again, or if it does, it will happen somewhere else.

Regardless of public and political apathy, teachers and administrators can do much to improve chances for survival in the event of an earthquake, tornado, hurricane, and other natural disasters.

School safety patrols. School safety patrols provide a valuable adjunct to the school pedestrian program. Today there are many thousands of safety patrol boys and girls in the United States. However, in recent years there has been a trend toward increased use of adult guards at intersections close to the school. Law enforcement agencies can help in determining the need for and the location of guards or patrols. In addition, they can provide assistance in the selection and training of patrol members. The National Safety Council is also a resource for information on policies and procedures.

School bus patrols. Major responsibility for the safe transportation by school bus of children to and from school rests with the school bus driver. However, patrol members may be appointed for each bus. School personnel are responsible for helping children develop desirable attitudes and practices to be followed as bus passengers.

Procedures recommended for bus patrol members are as follows:
1. To assist the bus driver in seeing that all pupils board and leave the bus in an orderly manner.
2. To assist the bus driver in checking attendance and seeing that all passengers remain in a safe riding position while on the bus.
3. To assist the bus driver in seeing that passengers keep all parts of their bodies within the bus and that items carried by the passengers are correctly stored.
4. To assist the driver in safeguarding pupils required to cross streets or highways after alighting from or to board a school bus. The patrol member alights in advance of passengers about to cross the highway.
5. To assist the driver in the event of an emergency and in the use of the emergency door on the bus.

These procedures and precautions, along with the regulations and construction requirements considered in Chapter 3, should assure safe bus transportation for pupils.

How is the school safety program organized?

The program of safety within the schools should be directed and controlled primarily by the school authorities. Organizations and agencies outside of the school should be utilized to render services in the school safety program.

The organization and supervision of a safety education program will vary with the size of the school system and the nature of the program. No single organizational pattern can be prepared to fit all school situations. In the matter of supervision of safety, many cities have appointed a supervisor of safety who has direct responsibility for coordinating the total safety program. In smaller communities the supervisor may be a teacher on the staff particularly interested in and having a knowledge of safety and accident prevention. In some schools the director of health, physical education, and recreation also acts as supervisor of safety. The supervisor should work with school principals and teachers in planning, reviewing, and carrying out the program.

Nonteaching staff members, including the school custodian and bus drivers, have supporting supervisory functions in the safety and accident prevention program. Boards of education should prepare and issue regulations through the school administrators having to do with the responsibilities for the protection of school children and school property.

School safety councils. Some elementary schools have established school safety councils—with representation of teachers, pupils, school nurses, administrators, custodians, bus drivers, public safety personnel—to solve accident problems in and around the school. Other schools have included safety problems as part of the function of the school health council. The health council's makeup, purposes, and procedures have been discussed in Chapter 2. An excellent source of continuing information for teachers and others concerned with school safety is the National Safety Council's quarterly magazine, *School Safety.*

Who is liable and responsible for school accidents?

Although teachers have always been concerned about accidents involving school children, a study of the accident situation in the schools shows that in the past there has been a lack of the proper understanding on the part of some teachers as to their full responsibility in accidents involving school children.

The changing attitude of the public regarding the accident situation in the United States has caused greater emphasis than ever before to be placed on the responsibility of the schools for the safety of the school child. Also, the accident situation in schools is a greater problem than in earlier years because of the extended school program and wider variety of activities offered. Programs of physical education, athletics and recreation, science laboratories, bus transportation of pupils, and safety patrols are some of the additions within the modern school program that increase hazards for school children.

The question is frequently asked, "Why is there a greater tendency today to attempt to hold the teacher financially liable for injuries to pupils?" The answer to this question in part is that today most people have come to expect accidents to be paid for. When an accident occurs resulting in injury to an individual usually the first question asked is, "Who is to pay for the accident?" The growth of liability insurance for teachers as well as accident and health insurance for students and parents, together with the trend for people to recover costs due to accidents, have helped to develop the attitude that accidents should be paid for. It is only natural then that some parents may expect reimbursement for school accidents resulting in injuries to pupils.

Until a few years ago, the common law in the United States, in the absence of specific state legislation, held that boards of education or school committees could not be held financially liable for accidents to school children. In other words, the school funds, raised by taxation in most cases, could not be used for any purpose other than education. This left the teacher practically the only source through which remuneration could be gained. Increasingly, states have passed new legislation that permits individuals to file suit against a school district or board of education in cases of alleged negligence.

It is now commonly understood that a teacher or a school board, or both, in case of *negligence*, can be held responsible and financially liable for accidental injury to a pupil. Increasing numbers of court procedures and damage suits for injuries through accidents to school children are being recorded. Each year there are some 8,000 schools involved in lawsuits resulting in payments of over $15 million.

Teachers should familiarize themselves with the school law in their own state regarding negligence and liability to civil suit.

The law of negligence is partly based on the theory that everyone has the right to live safely and must be protected from the negligence of others in this right. In the school situation the teacher owes a duty to the school child. In many cases the failure to act to prevent an accident to a school child would be considered negligence on the part of the teacher.

The law of negligence implies, so far as the duty of the teacher to the pupil is concerned, that there must be *foreseeability*. The teacher acting as a reasonably careful and prudent person should anticipate danger or an accident.

Teacher or other school personnel negligence is generally predicated on (1) failure to foresee risks, (2) failure to take reasonable action to avert risks, (3) failure to give adequate warning or instruction in "difficult feats," and (4) failure to provide proper emergency care to the injured child, or increasing the severity of the injury through improper methods of first aid.

Some conditions that may make teachers liable to legal action include:

1. Permitting pupils to play unsafe, unorganized games
2. Maintaining attractive nuisances (conditions of school environment, apparatus, equipment, machinery, and the like)
3. Permitting pupils to use dangerous devices
4. Inadequate planning and organizing for field trips
5. Permitting use of defective equipment
6. Failing to provide adequate supervision for pupil activities

In addition to the possibility of the teacher's being held financially liable for the injury of a child, especially in a case of negligence, there is another factor that should be taken into consideration. In many cases, the teacher may not be vulnerable from the viewpoint of financial liability. However, the teacher may be quite vulnerable from the viewpoint of failing to take proper responsibility in case of an accident to a child. That is, although the teacher could not be held financially liable for the accident, nevertheless, the superintendent of schools or the board of education could hold the teacher negligent, perhaps resulting in censure or even discharge for failing to use reasonable care in providing safe conditions for the child.

What is the nature of safety education in the elementary school?

In elementary schools the classroom teachers form the nucleus for the teaching of safety. In a majority of the elementary schools throughout the country, the classroom teachers are the only teachers available for teaching safety. Even in the large city school systems where specialized safety educators are employed, the classroom teachers are the ultimate source of safety teaching for the children. However, in the schools where a safety educator or health coordinator is employed, the problems of a classroom teacher are materially simplified in that assistance is readily available in planning safety projects, determining teaching content, and selecting pamphlets, books, films, and other materials.

Safety education should have a place at each grade level throughout the elementary school. Details of content, objectives, methods, and techniques of teaching are found in Chapters 9 to 11.

Why do we need community cooperation for child safety?

Community understanding and cooperation are extremely important to the success of a school safety program. Taxes paid by members of the community play an important role in the creation of a safe school environment. They support safety measures in school construction, proper school equipment, maintenance and repairs to schools and equipment, school transportation, and school crossing protection. A good school safety program along with measures to see that the community appreciates the necessity for the many protective features involved in the program will help to make the people more receptive to financing the elimination or control of hazards.

The community has many resources upon which the schools can draw for assistance and support. The police and fire departments can provide accident facts for program planning, technical assistance and guidance in removing or limiting hazards, program stimulation through class visitation, and support with activities such as the school safety patrol program.

The PTA is generally an excellent medium for communicating to the parents and the community the objectives and activities of the school safety program. Members can be called on to conduct bicycle skill test programs, to survey home accidents, to give recognition to the work of safety patrols, to provide safety patrols with belts, badges, and rain coats, and to sponsor swimming programs. The PTA can also be a powerful force in supporting specific measures such as the control of traffic and parking in the vicinity of the school, improving recreational facilities, and the adoption of uniform laws and standards.

Some communities have safety councils or citizen committees that can provide accident data, resource material for teachers working on particular projects, program aids such as safety films and patrol handbooks, technical assistance on curriculum revision or program planning, organization of conferences and seminars for the exchange of information, and communitywide or areawide support for programs.

WHAT PROVISIONS SHOULD BE MADE FOR EMERGENCY CARE OF INJURED AND ILL PUPILS?

Every school regardless of size should have carefully organized plans and procedures for the proper care of injured and ill pupils. These plans should be made for emergency care of both mass and individual injuries and illnesses. When illnesses or injuries occur, school personnel frequently are not prepared to handle them properly.

Organization and administration of the school emergency care program is the responsibility of the board of education. This responsibility, however, is usually delegated to the superintendent, principal, and other school administrators.

Members of the school personnel should establish a uniform policy for the emergency care of the injured and ill. The policy established by a particular school will depend on a number of facts, including the size of the community and school; availability of nurses, physicians, hospitals, and ambulances; effective communications; and trained first-aid personnel. In formulating the emergency care policy, school administrators should seek the aid, advice, and cooperation of school and community safety councils, parents, local medical and public health groups, and any of the community organizations or agencies, such as the police department, fire department, and ambulance and auxiliary services that may be able to lend aid and assistance when necessary.

The main responsibilities of the school in emergency care are to give *immediate and proper first aid, to notify the parents, and to be certain that the injured or ill are placed under the care of parents or a physician designated by the parents.* The school policy including plans, procedures, and responsibility assignments should be made available in writing to all teachers and other members of the school personnel who may be involved in any way in emergency care. Also, it is advisable to make the *parents* acquainted with the policy for emergency care.

Since new teachers usually join the school faculty beginning with the fall term, it is advisable for school administrators to make them familiar with the emergency care program at the beginning of the term or before the school term begins. Also, the beginning of the fall semester is a good time to review the emergency care program for all teachers

and to acquaint them with any changes in policy, plans, or procedures. It is the duty of the school administrators to make teachers who join the faculty at times other than at the beginning of the fall season familiar with the policy concerning school emergency care.

In the final analysis a community's emergency care program depends on (1) availability of *trained first-aiders* at the scene; (2) quick and effective *communication;* (3) prompt, safe, well-equipped and attended *transportation;* and (4) access to *hospitals with specialized emergency care equipment and medical and nursing personnel.*

Plans for emergency care

Detailed plans and procedures should be decided upon to take care of any or all emergency situations. Although it is practically impossible to list all of the detailed plans that may be necessary for each and every community, nevertheless there are a number of common procedures to which all schools should be prepared to adhere.

Emergency transportation. Every school should have plans for transporting injured or ill children to their homes, to a hospital, or to physicians' or dentists' offices. Previous arrangements should be made to have available school buses, ambulances, or other suitable transportation such as private cars. Frequently it may be advisable for the school nurse or other members of the school personnel to transport children in private cars. When children are transported in private cars, proper insurance coverage should be carried on the cars. Regardless of the means, some acceptable type of transportation should be available to the school at all times when children are in attendance.

Facilities and equipment. Proper first aid and emergency care implies that there will be sufficient facilities and equipment in every school. There should be emergency rest rooms containing cots, blankets, lavatories, towels, chairs, and a table. The emergency room should be equipped with adequate first-aid supplies for any type of injury or sudden illness. The first-aid supplies should be maintained in accordance with the best standards for first-aid care. The kinds and amount of first-aid material will depend upon the size of the school and the availability of community resources for assisting with emergency care. In addition to the first-aid supplies found in the emergency room, classroom teachers should have on hand such things as soap and small dressings for minor wounds. A suggested list of first-aid supplies is found on p. 120.

Reports and records. An adequate report

STANDARD STUDENT ACCIDENT REPORT FORM
Part A. Information on ALL Accidents

1. Name: _____ Home Address: _____
2. School: _____ Sex: M ☐; F ☐. Age: _____ Grade or classification: _____
3. Time accident occurred: Hour _____ A.M.; _____ P.M. Date: _____
4. Place of Accident: School Building ☐   School Grounds ☐   To or from School ☐   Home ☐   Elsewhere ☐

NATURE OF INJURY

Abrasion _____	Fracture _____
Amputation _____	Laceration _____
Asphyxiation _____	Poisoning _____
Bite _____	Puncture _____
Bruise _____	Scalds _____
Burn _____	Scratches _____
Concussion _____	Shock (el.) _____
Cut _____	Sprain _____
Dislocation _____	
Other (specify) _____	

DESCRIPTION OF THE ACCIDENT

How did accident happen? What was student doing? Where was student? List specifically unsafe acts and unsafe conditions existing. Specify any tool, machine or equipment involved. _____

5.

PART OF BODY INJURED

Abdomen _____	Foot _____
Ankle _____	Hand _____
Arm _____	Head _____
Back _____	Knee _____
Chest _____	Leg _____
Ear _____	Mouth _____
Elbow _____	Nose _____
Eye _____	Scalp _____
Face _____	Tooth _____
Finger _____	Wrist _____
Other (specify) _____	

6. Degree of Injury: Death ☐ Permanent Impairment ☐ Temporary Disability ☐ Nondisabling ☐
7. Total number of days lost from school: _____ (To be filled in when student returns to school)

Part B. Additional Information on School Jurisdiction Accidents

8. Teacher in charge when accident occurred (Enter name): _____
   Present at scene of accident: No: _____ Yes: _____

IMMEDIATE ACTION TAKEN

9. First-aid treatment _____ By (Name): _____
   Sent to school nurse _____ By (Name): _____
   Sent home _____ By (Name): _____
   Sent to physician _____ By (Name): _____
   Physician's Name: _____
   Sent to hospital _____ By (Name): _____
   Name of hospital: _____

10. Was a parent or other individual notified? No:___ Yes:___ When:_____ How: _____
    Name of individual notified: _____
    By whom? (Enter name): _____
11. Witnesses: 1. Name: _____ Address: _____
    2. Name: _____ Address: _____

LOCATION

12.

Specify Activity		Specify Activity		Remarks
Athletic field _____		Locker _____		What recommendations do you have for preventing other accidents of this type? _____
Auditorium _____		Pool _____		
Cafeteria _____		Sch. grounds _____		
Classroom _____		_____ shop _____		
Corridor _____		Showers _____		
Dressing room _____		Stairs _____		
Gymnasium _____		Toilets and		
Home Econ. _____		washrooms _____		
Laboratories _____		Other (specify) _____		

Signed: Principal: _____ Teacher: _____

(National Safety Council—Form School 1)   Printed in U.S.A.   Stock No. 429.21
Rep. 100M106002

Fig. 6-1. National Safety Council accident report form. (Courtesy National Safety Council, Inc., Chicago, Ill.)

of each and every emergency injury or illness arising in the school should be made. The National Safety Council standard accident report form is shown in Fig. 6-1. Ordinarily, the principal, or sometimes the policy, may delegate the responsibility to the school nurse, the teacher, or some other member of the school personnel. In any case, teachers are likely to have a part in making reports, particularly when children are injured or become ill under their supervision. The report should contain such information as the name of the pupil; time, location, and nature of the accident or illness; witnesses, teachers, or other persons present; possible causes of the illness or injury; description of the illness or injury including the part of the body seemingly injured; first aid given; notification of parents; and disposition of the case.

School policy on emergency care. Minor injuries and illnesses happen frequently among school children. At such times, the classroom teacher should follow the policy of the school in caring for the pupil. If an illness is mild, the child should be kept on a cot and kept warm under constant or regular supervision. If the illness seems to be progressive, the parent should be called, and the usual procedure invoked for caring for more serious illness. The teacher should remember that no medication of any kind should be given. In minor injuries, the policy of the school often is that the classroom teacher care for them. First aid for such injuries as minor cuts and scratches usually can be safely cared for by the teacher. The teacher should stress the importance of cleanliness by washing the wound with soap and water and applying a sterile dressing.

For certain seemingly major illnesses, the school policy concerning the notifying of parents and taking whatever steps necessary should be put into operation immediately. The child should rest on a cot, and body temperature should be maintained. Someone should be in constant attendance with the child until the school has fulfilled its responsibility of carrying out the parents' instruction or, in case the parents cannot be contacted, in getting the services of the family

physician or taking the child to a hospital. In cases of major injuries the school policy for rendering first aid under such circumstances should be put into effect.

Information for emergencies

It is imperative that certain kinds of information be readily available to facilitate the rapid and proper handlng of emergency cases. The following kinds of information should be carefully listed, organized, and placed near a telephone in the principal's office where it is accessible to all teachers or other school personnel who may be expected to assist in any way with emergency care of injured and ill children:

1. A list of all pupils with full and correct names
2. The names of both parents
3. Home address
4. Home telephone number
5. Business address of both parents
6. Business telephone number of both parents
7. Name of family physician
8. Business telephone number of family physician
9. Home telephone number of family physician
10. Physician of choice, in case family physician cannot be reached
11. Telephone number of physician of choice if family physician cannot be reached
12. Relatives to be called in case the parents cannot be reached
13. Telephone number of relatives to be called in case parents cannot be reached
14. Hospital of choice
15. Hospital telephone number
16. Any special directions from parents concerning the handling of emergency injury or illness
17. List of homeroom teachers
18. List of pupil's daily class schedule
19. Telephone number of local ambulance services
20. Telephone number of fire department
21. Telephone number of police department

Recently an increasing number of communities have centralized their emergency communication systems. Through the efforts and cooperation of the telephone companies a growing number of towns and cities have begun an emergency communication plan, with **911** as the all-purpose number to dial. School administrators and teachers as well as other school personnel should be aware of the local emergency communication system.

Notification of parents

Some schools ask parents to sign a permit authorizing the proper emergency care of their children in case of injury and certain illnesses. This is particularly helpful in situations where parents or guardians cannot be immediately contacted. Then the school feels free to call the designated family physician or hospital or take any other action it thinks necessary for the best welfare of the child.

Parents or guardians should be notified immediately in case of serious injury or illness. When notifying parents by telephone, the person making the call should speak in a calm, reassuring voice to allay any fear or anxiety the parent may suddenly develop. A full description of the child's injury or illness should be given so far as it is evident and possible. Parents should be told whether immediate medical attention seems needed. Sometimes emergency room hospital care may be advised and stressed to the parent. The person making the call should learn from the parents whether they will come to school for the child or whether they wish him to be brought home. Parents should be encouraged to call for children whenever possible. Occasionally, it may be the desire of the parents that the family physician call at school if it seems necessary. If an ambulance is needed, parents should give permission to summon one before the school takes this action.

Sometimes it may be necessary for the child to go directly to the hospital emergency room or the family physician's office. In some cases the parent may wish someone from the school to accompany the child. Usually the nurse or principal will provide transportation

and render any other assistance necessary.

Since most physicians are not well prepared to provide emergency care in their office in critical life-death situations, it is usually most advisable to call 911 or another emergency phone number and have the child quickly transported to the emergency unit of the nearest hospital. It is important to call the hospital and to inform them of the nature of the injury or illness while the child is en route to the emergency room. This gives hospital personnel time to set up whatever equipment and medicines may be required for a specific case. It also alerts them to possible need for a surgeon or other specialists whom they may need to call to the emergency room.

Sick or injured children should never be sent home unless accompanied by a responsible adult and unless the parents or some responsible person designated by the parents is there to care for them. In cases in which parents or guardians cannot be immediately contacted, the school authorities must proceed according to their best judgment. It may seem necessary to call a physician or dentist directly, or in some cases it may be necessary to call an ambulance and take the child to a hospital. In every case members of the school personnel should give the parents every possible aid in caring for a sick or injured child. Often if specialized medical attention is indicated, the parents may be at a loss concerning the selection of a physician. In this case the school authorities should be prepared with a roster of names of various medical specialists available such as pediatricians, otorhinolaryngologists, orthopedists, ophthalmologists, surgeons, and dentists so that they can consult with the parent in making a selection.

It is advisable that the school, particularly from the viewpoint of public relations, follow up emergency cases. Parents or guardian should be called within from 24 to 36 hours to learn the condition of the injured or ill child. If the condition is serious, periodic telephone calls from the school might be made until the child is well on the way to full recovery. The follow-up of emergency cases costs little and usually brings a great deal of goodwill to the school.

TEACHER'S ROLE
IN EMERGENCY CARE

Every teacher should be prepared to assume some responsibility for the school emergency and first-aid care program. Even though physicians, nurses, and others highly skilled in emergency and first-aid care are available at practically all times, the teacher must be prepared to accept certain responsibilities, such as the following:

1. Assist with any emergency in which large numbers of pupils are injured or become suddenly ill
2. Render first aid or contact those who are officially designated to give first aid when a pupil under the teacher's direction is injured or becomes ill
3. Assist those who are officially designated to give first aid when necessary by doing such things as calling parents or physician
4. Give first aid for minor injuries such as small and insignificant wounds that do not require the attention of a physician, nurse, or others officially designated to give first aid
5. Render proper first aid for any and all injuries and illnesses when there is no other trained person available to help

Although the situations are likely to be relatively few in which the teacher does not have assistance with first aid, nevertheless, the teacher should be prepared to assume full responsibility for those few times when there is no immediate help. The teacher should keep in mind that giving first aid does not involve medication of any kind. The teacher should never use antiseptics on a wound unless it is an established policy of the school to use them. Then *only* those that are indicated in the written policy of the school should be used. The teacher should not give the child any type of medication, even including such seemingly harmless things as aspirin tablets, unless directed to do so by a physician. All first-aid supplies in the school should have the approval of those re-

sponsible for formulating the policy for emergency and first-aid care.

WHAT FIRST-AID PROCEDURES
SHOULD TEACHERS USE?*

The emergency care given at the time a person is injured or becomes suddenly ill is known as first aid. It is the care given before medical aid is available. Under most circumstances, medical aid is readily available. The duties of the person giving first aid end immediately when medical assistance is obtained.

It should be kept in mind by teachers that *first aid is the emergency care given at the time an injury or sudden illness first occurs.* It does not mean attempting to care for injuries or illnesses after medical aid has been obtained. Therefore, such actions as repeated bandaging of wounds or attempting to care for extended illnesses is not a responsibility of the teacher and should not, under any circumstances, be attempted. Every elementary school classroom teacher should have a knowledge of first aid. Some states now require that elementary teachers have completed a university credit course in first aid or have had comparable Red Cross instruction. Every man and woman employed in an office, ship, or factory, every parent in the home, every boy and girl in junior and senior high school should have some understanding of first aid.

The following basic points should be kept in mind in giving first aid:
1. First aid is given to an injured person for the purpose of preventing further harm.
2. First aid is given for the purpose of reducing suffering and discomfort.

---

*Adapted in part from American National Red Cross: Advanced first aid and emergency care, Garden City, N.Y., 1973, Doubleday & Co., Inc.; Standard first aid and personal safety, Washington, D.C., 1973, American National Red Cross; Fishbein, M., and Irwin, L. W.: First-aid training, Chicago, 1961, Lyons & Carnahan; Kennedy, R. H., editor: Emergency care, Philadelphia, 1966, W. B. Saunders Co.; U.S. Department of Health, Education, and Welfare, and the U.S. Department of Defense: Family guide emergency health care, Washington, D.C., 1966, U.S. Government Printing Office.

3. Many children injured in accidents receive further injury through improper emergency care.

4. Sometimes the failure to receive proper first aid may result in permanent injury or even death.

5. The first-aider should know what *not* to do, as well as what to do.

6. Hurry is seldom necessary, especially if it is likely to cause further damage to the injured person, except in cases of severe bleeding, stoppage of breathing, and poisoning.

7. If the injury is serious, a check should be made for suspended breathing, hemorrhage, shock, obstructions to breathing caused by a foreign body in the mouth or throat, back and neck injuries, and broken bones.

8. If the child is vomiting, the head should be turned to one side to facilitate breathing.

9. Clothing should be loosened about the neck and chest, particularly if breathing is difficult.

10. The child's body temperature should be maintained by covering with blankets or coats to reduce or prevent shock.

11. An injured person should not be moved, unless it is absolutely necessary, until the exact nature of this injury is known and provisions have been made to prevent further damage.

12. An unconscious person must not be given liquid, food, or medication of any type, since the child may strangle on it.

The teacher or person responsible for giving first aid should remember that there are three emergency situations that require immediate and instant action to save life (hurry cases): serious bleeding, suspended breathing, and poisoning. Although shock may be extremely serious, the first-aider usually has more time to act.

Serious bleeding

Severe bleeding must be stopped immediately. In addition to danger due to loss of blood it is likely to bring about serious shock. Furthermore, children are usually frightened by the sight of their own blood if it is serious. Fright may add to the seriousness of shock. If a large blood vessel is severed, a quart of blood can be lost from the body within 1 minute. Consequently, in an emergency of this kind the teacher must act instantly.

Pressure is the method recommended to stop bleeding. In most cases hand pressure with a sterile dressing or clean napkin, towel, or cloth is the accepted procedure. A compress directly on the wound with a tight bandage will control the blood flow in a majority of wounds. Blood flow from the head and face can usually be controlled in this way.

If a large artery of the arm or leg is cut, it may be necessary under some circumstances to apply a tourniquet. A tourniquet is used only on an arm or leg when a large artery is cut. Because a tourniquet is an extremely dangerous piece of equipment in the hands of the average first-aider, its use is highly restricted. Some results of improper use of a tourniquet are the following:

1. The artery may be permanently damaged through crushing by too much pressure.

2. Keeping the supply of blood from a part of the body too long may cause gangrene.

3. Additional bleeding resulting from removing the tourniquet too soon may prove serious.

4. Removing the tourniquet after an extended period of application may increase shock.

A tourniquet can be applied to the arm about midway or slightly above the midpoint between the elbow and the shoulder. For the leg, it can be applied about 3 inches below the groin. It should not be too close to the edge of the wound. Any material fairly thick and soft that can be tied around the arm or leg and twisted tight enough to stop the bleeding can be used as a tourniquet. *It must not cut or bruise the flesh.* Such materials as wire or rope should never be used as a tourniquet.

It is important to remember that a tourniquet should be used *only in case of very serious bleeding that threatens life* and cannot be stopped by other recommended means; also, that a tourniquet is seldom necessary and that if a tourniquet is applied, it should not be released other than by a physician.

Artificial respiration

A person cannot live more than a few minutes without breathing. Most people would die within 5 or 6 minutes if breathing completely ceased. It is extremely important to begin artificial respiration immediately after the cessation of breathing because the heart continues to beat only a short time after breathing has stopped.

Some of the causes of complete or partial cessation of breathing or serious interference with the oxygen supply of the body are electric shock, drowning, certain gases, choking, strangling, certain chemical fumes, and some drugs such as morphine, barbiturates, and alcohol. From the viewpoint of the school situation, however, mechanical obstruction is likely to be the most common cause of suspended breathing or serious interference with breathing. The mechanical causes include foreign bodies in the throat and windpipe, submersion in water involving drowning, and strangulation.

There are many ways of administering artificial respiration. However, the mouth-to-mouth or mouth-to-nose method is recommended as the most efficient and usually the most practical. The following directions briefly explain how to give mouth-to-mouth and mouth-to-nose artificial respiration.

Place the person on his back with his arms at his side. Check the mouth to be sure that it is free from any kind of foreign matter. Remove anything from the mouth that may obstruct breathing by wiping it out with your finger or with a cloth. Place one hand under the person's head and your other hand on the forehead. Move the head so that the chin is pointed upward with the lower jaw in a jutting position as shown in Fig. 6-2 A. In this position the base of the tongue tends to move away from the back of the throat to give clear passage to the air.

In the mouth-to-mouth technique close the person's nostrils with your fingers or cheek. Place your mouth tightly over the person's mouth as shown in Fig. 6-2, B. If you do not wish to come in contact with the person, place a handkerchief over his nose and mouth. If you use the mouth-to-nose technique, close the person's mouth and place your mouth over his nose as shown in Fig. 6-2, C. Exhale into the person's mouth or nose. Remove your mouth and turn your head to one side while you inhale. Repeat the exhaling of air into the person's nose or mouth and remove your mouth to inhale. The rate of breathing in this way should be about *12 times per minute*. Exhale vigorously in giving artificial respiration to an adult or older child.

If at any time obstruction to breathing develops that makes it difficult to get air into and out of the person's lungs, quickly turn the victim on the side and slap several times between the shoulders with the palm of your hand. Then quickly resume artificial respiration.

There are a few differences in using the mouth-to-mouth method of artificial respiration on small children and on grown people.

Place a small child on his back with his chin pointed upward and his lower jaw in a jutting position. Place your mouth over *both* the child's nose and mouth tightly enough so that air cannot escape as shown in Fig. 6-2, *D*. Hold the child's lower jaw in position with one hand and then place your other hand on his stomach just below his ribs. Exhale gently and smoothly into his nose and mouth until his chest rises. While breathing into his nose and mouth, with your hand apply a little pressure to his stomach to keep it from filling with air. When you have breathed enough air into the child's lungs, as indicated by his rising chest, raise your head and allow the air to pass from his lungs. Keep one hand under his jaw and the other on his stomach and *repeat this cycle about 20 times a minute*.

If there is any obstruction to getting air into the child's lungs, quickly bend the child over with the head down and administer three or four quick pats between the shoulders. Then continue artificial respiration immediately.

If no pulse can be felt in the carotid ar-

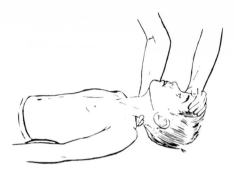

A, Move the head so that the chin is pointing upward.

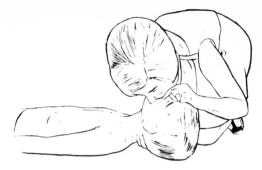

B, Close the child's nostrils and place your mouth tightly over his mouth.

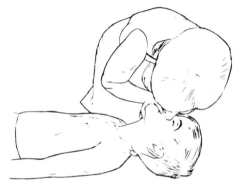

C, If the mouth-to-nose method is used, close the child's mouth and place your mouth over his nose.

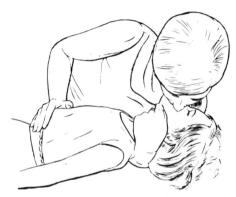

D, In the case of a young child hold the child's jaw in place with one hand and place your other hand on her stomach. Place your mouth over both the nose and mouth of the child.

Fig. 6-2. Administering artificial respiration.

tery on the neck under the angle of the lower jaw, the *CPR technique* should be used as described below.

ABC of life support*

This emergency first-aid procedure consists of recognizing stoppage of breathing and heartbeat—then applying cardiopulmonary resuscitation (CPR), which involves: (A) opening and maintaining victim's *Airway;* (B) giving rescue *Breathing;* (C) providing artificial *Circulation* by external cardiac compression (heart massage). CPR should be performed by people with special training. For information, get in touch with your local

---

*From the Metropolitan Life Insurance Co., New York, 1974.

Heart Association or Red Cross. To refresh your memory, these are essential ABCs:

A *Airway open.* Turn victim on back and quickly remove any foreign matter from the mouth. Place your hand under person's neck and lift, tilting head back as far as possible with other hand. This provides an airway.

B *Breathing restored.* If person is not breathing, place your mouth tightly over his mouth, pinch nostrils, and blow into airway until you see chest rise. Remove your mouth. Give four breaths and check for neck pulse (Fig. 6-3). If pulse is present, continue rescue breathing at 12 times a minute. For small child or infant, cover nose and mouth tightly with your mouth. Blow gently 20 times a minute.

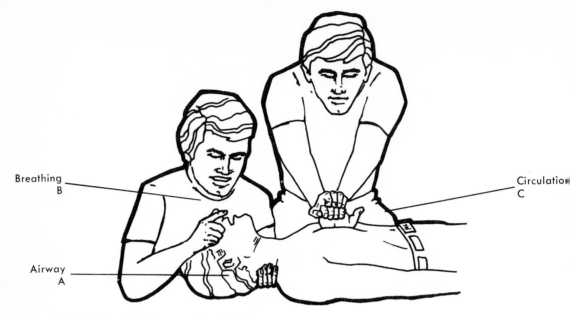

Breathing
B

Circulation
C

Airway
A

Fig. 6-3. The ABC life support (Cardio-Pulmonary Resuscitation, CPR). (From the Metropolitan Life Insurance Co., New York, 1974).

C *Circulation maintained.* Quickly feel for neck pulse; keeping victim's head tilted with one hand, use middle and index fingers of other hand to feel for carotid pulse, in neck artery, under side angle of lower jaw. If no pulse, start rescue breathing and external cardiac compression.

Victim's back should be on firm surface. Place heel of your hand on center of lower breastbone with fingers off chest and other hand on top. Gently rock forward, exerting pressure down, to force blood out of the heart. Release pressure. Alternate (B) Breathing with (C) Circulation.

Two rescuers: Give 60 chest compressions a minute—one breath after each five compressions. *One rescuer:* Perform both artificial circulation and rescue breathing giving 80 chest compressions a minute—two full breaths after each 15 compressions.

FOR SMALL CHILDREN AND INFANTS: Use only the heel of one hand and, for infants, only the tips of index and middle fingers. Give 80 to 100 compressions per minute with two breaths after each five compressions.

REMEMBER: These basic ABCs only briefly outline what to do for a person unconscious from drowning, electrocution, suffocation, accident, heart disease or stroke. Time is crucial. Rescue efforts must begin at once and continue until professional help arrives. To be fully effective, special training and periodic refreshers are vital.

There are a few other measures that should be followed in suspended breathing:

1. The body temperature of the person should be maintained.

2. Artificial respiration should be continued without interruption.

3. The person should not be moved until normal voluntary breathing returns.

4. If it is necessary to move the person, resuscitation should be carried on during the time the child is being moved.

5. When the person is revived, body temperature should be maintained. The victim should remain quiet for a while and should be treated for shock by a physician.

6. Since in some cases of suspended breathing recovery is unusually slow and discouraging to those giving first aid, artificial

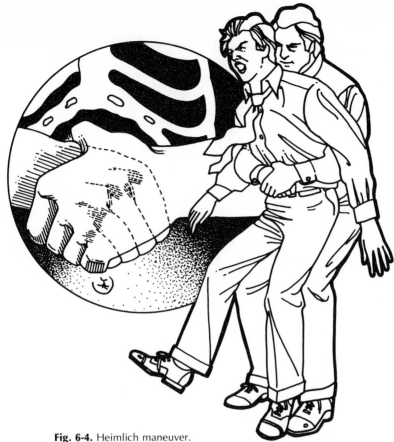

Fig. 6-4. Heimlich maneuver.

respiration should be continued for at least 3 hours, or longer, or until rescue squad or hospital emergency personnel and equipment are available.

Choking

The following article, authored by Henry J. Heimlich, is adapted from *Emergency* and is reprinted with their written authorization.

Heimlich maneuver: the thrust of life*

The effectiveness of the Heimlich maneuver in saving the lives of those choking on food and other objects is based on its simplicity. The technique was not easily discovered but resulted from extensive scientific investigation.

*Adapted from Heimlich, H. J.: Heimlich maneuver; the thrust of life, Emergency, Carlsbad, Calif., 1977, pp. 64-67.

The principle of the Heimlich maneuver is easily understood from the following definition:

Heimlich maneuver Technique for saving the life of a person choking on food or another object; consists of external compression of the air in the lungs in order to provide a flow of air from the larynx sufficient to expel the obstructing object.

Diagnosing a choking victim. There should be no difficulty in differentiating a choking victim from one having a heart attack because there are clearly distinguishing factors. In more than 90% of instances the victim is seen to choke on food or another object. The choking victim cannot breathe or speak, becomes cyanotic, and collapses. The heart attack victim, on the other hand, is able to breathe and usually can talk. Furthermore, it has been shown that over 98% of persons dying suddenly in an eating establishment have choked on food and only slightly more than 1% have had a heart attack. There is obviously a life-threatening danger to the choking victim if the Heimlich maneuver is not applied because an observer thinks only of heart attack. There should be little possibility that the Heimlich maneuver will be performed unnecessarily in a heart attack victim.

In an article in the *Journal of the American Medical Association*, Dr. Heimlich introduced a signal that has come to be known as the "Heimlich sign," which indicates, "I am choking on food." Victims grasp their neck between their thumb and index finger to indicate the choking situation (Fig. 6-5). Should this sign become universal, the diagnosis of food choking will be 100% accurate.

Heimlich maneuver. To be safe and effective, the Heimlich maneuver should be performed in one of the following prescribed manners:

1. When the rescuer is standing and the victim is standing or sitting (Fig. 6-4), the rescuer takes these steps.
   a. Stand behind the victim and wrap your arms around the victim's waist.
   b. Place your fist, thumb side, against the victim's abdomen slightly above the navel and below the rib cage (Fig. 6-6).
   c. Grasp your fist with your other hand and press into the victim's abdomen with a quick upward thrust.
   d. Repeat several times if necessary.
2. When the victim is sitting, the rescuer stands

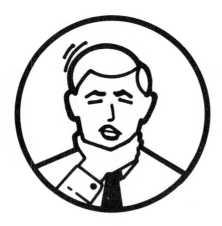

Fig. 6-5. Heimlich sign.

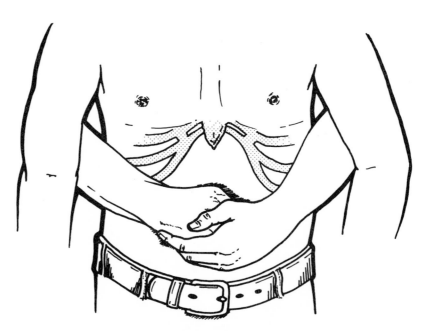

Fig. 6-6. Rescuer standing when using the Heimlich maneuver.

behind the victim's chair and performs the maneuver in the same manner as on opposite page.

3. When the rescuer is kneeling and the victim is lying face up (Fig. 6-7), the rescuer takes the following steps:
   a. With the victim lying on his back, face the victim, and kneel astride his hips.
   b. With one of your hands on the top of the other, place them on the victim's abdomen slightly above the navel and below the rib cage (Fig. 6-7).
   c. Press into the victim's abdomen with a quick upward thrust.
   d. Repeat several times if necessary.

The standing and sitting positions are used most often; however, it is extremely important that rescuers learn the supine position (victim lying down, face upward). Only in that position, with the rescuer astride the victim's thighs, can a small person—slight woman or child who cannot reach around the victim's waist or who is not strong enough to press a fist upward around the diaphragm with sufficient force—save a heavy victim. In the supine position, the rescuer uses his weight, not strength, to press upward on the diaphragm.

The choking victim has 4 minutes to live from the onset of choking; however, when a victim is on the floor unconscious, he does not have the full 4 minutes but only a matter of seconds. It is necessary to straddle the victim's thighs immediately and apply the Heimlich maneuver without delay. Back-slaps, fingers in the mouth, or mouth-to-mouth resuscitation will cause delay and diminish the possibility of rescue.

Community involvement. The Heimlich maneuver is similar to a vaccine—unless the entire population receives it in adequate repeated doses, some people will die. Communitywide Heimlich maneuver teaching programs have led to the saving of many lives. Individuals and organizations have started such ongoing programs by involving an entire city through advance TV and newspaper publicity and participation of officials, devoting a full day to the programs. Dr. Heimlich has had the privilege of speaking at many such "opening day" meetings. Since

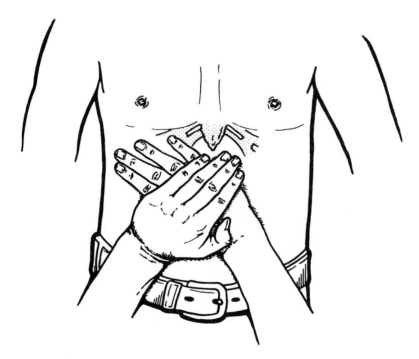

Fig. 6-7. Rescuer kneeling when using the Heimlich maneuver.

children not only are 25% of choking victims but have saved lives (an 8-year-old saved his 6-year-old brother, a 13-year-old saved his mother's life), schools should be involved.

Shock

In a state of shock the body processes are usually greatly reduced. Broken bones, poisoning, severe burns, hemorrhage, perforation or inflammation of internal organs, reactions to drugs or proteins, or strong emotions may cause shock. Intense pain, loss of blood, tissue destruction, and sometimes strong emotions may interfere with the nervous system's control of the circulatory system. There may be a fall in blood pressure to a level so low that circulation is inadequate. The brain fails to get enough blood to supply sufficient oxygen and nutrition, and, as a result, consciousness may be lost.

Shock may not be clearly noticeable following most minor injuries. However, some degree of shock may follow any injury, particularly if it is accompanied by strong emotional reactions.

Some people are much more subject to shock than others. An injury that causes only slight or moderate shock in one person may cause serious shock in another. Severe shock usually follows serious injury. Consequently, the teacher should always be alert and expect shock in giving first aid to pupils who are accident victims. Shock may appear soon after an injury, or it may appear many hours later.

The question is often asked as to how it is possible to prevent shock. The answer is that it may not be possible to prevent shock, but the proper first-aid care may greatly reduce its seriousness. There are a number of ways by which shock can be detected. Some of the signs are the following:

1. The lips and fingernails are blue or grayish.
2. The skin is cool to the touch, yet it is covered with moisture, making it feel clammy.
3. The injured child may be nauseated.
4. The injured child may vomit.
5. The victim may be partially conscious and complain of feeling cold.

6. The face becomes pale, almost a gray color.

First aid for shock consists of keeping the person lying in a supine position with the head lower than the feet. Precaution should be taken, however, in placing the head lower than the feet. *In head or chest injuries, or if breathing becomes more difficult* with the head low, the *child's head and shoulders should be raised a few inches* higher than his feet. This can be done by placing a pillow or coat under the victim's head and shoulders. If the child develops difficulty in breathing with the head and shoulders elevated, lower them. The pupil should be kept comfortably warm with blankets or coats *but not overheated.* Pain contributes to shock. Unnecessary movement of an injured person makes unnecessary pain. Fear may increase shock. The child should be reassured and should not be bothered with unnecessary questions. The first-aider should never give a person in shock any kind of liquids or stimulants.

Poisoning

Once poison is swallowed and reaches the stomach, it is only a matter of time until it is absorbed. In most cases of poisoning it is important that the poison be diluted and as much of it as possible emptied from the stomach by vomiting. Poisoning from foods occurs frequently. Food poisoning may be caused by spoiled or partially spoiled foods. Certain types of mushrooms are poisonous; also, some kinds of wild berries, roots, and some types of leaves. The poisonous types of mushrooms are frequently called toadstools. Small children are frequently poisoned by aspirin and petroleum products, such as kerosene and gasoline.

The symptoms of poisoning may vary greatly, depending on the substance swallowed and the time elapsed after taking. Some of the general symptoms are nausea, stomach cramps, pain, and sometimes vomiting. Sometimes poisons are absorbed before symptoms become evident. The corrosive poisons, such as acids and alkalis, may burn the lips and mouth and cause very marked shock. Poisoning caused by foods may cause vomiting, diarrhea, and collapse. There is usually some degree of prostration present.

When first aid for poisoning is given, the first step is to call the hospital emergency room or the nearest poison control center. When first aid for poisoning other than strong acids, petroleum products, and alkalis is administered, an attempt should be made to dilute the poison and to induce vomiting. Fluids suitable for use in diluting the poison and filling the stomach are plain water and milk. If baking soda is available, a few teaspoons should be added to each glass of water, because it tends to induce vomiting. Although water is always the most readily available fluid, milk is good to use, because it gives some protection to the lining of the digestive tract. Four or five glasses of fluid should be given. Vomiting should not be induced if acids or alkalis were swallowed, because the poison coming up may do further damage to the lining of the food passages.

With the rapid increase in the number of over-the-counter and prescription drugs available to children in the home, opportunities for poisoning or dangerous overdose are much greater today than in past years. Sometimes children will ingest medicines or drugs in the home, yet effects may not be noticed until later in the day while at school. An up-to-date, useful guide for teachers, school nurses, and administrators is provided on p. 116.

Diabetic reactions

Diabetic reactions occur as the result of too much (insulin reaction) or too little (diabetic coma) insulin. In an insulin reaction, the first sign noted in the child is general irritability in which the pupil may be despondent, cry readily, or be exuberant or belligerent. In addition, the student may be hungry, perspire excessively, tremble or be unable to concentrate, and complain of dizziness. The symptoms vary in duration and will often disappear in 10 to 15 minutes by providing the child with any of the following: sugar cube, pop, candy, raisins, fruit juice with sugar, or any other carbohydrate. If the symptoms do not subside after this action, then the pupil's parents should be notified. A diabetic coma, a rather rare condition, is

caused by the failure to take insulin, an illness, or neglect of a proper diet. It is slow in onset and may be observed by these symptoms: thirst, frequent urination, flushed face, labored breathing, nausea, and vomiting. The teacher should keep the child in a resting state and maintain body temperature. In addition, the school nurse, the principal, or the parents should be immediately notified.

Epileptic convulsions

Most elementary school classroom teachers at one time or another are confronted with the problem of dealing with epileptic convulsions in children. The minor form of epilepsy is not a particular problem for the teacher. The seizures in major or grand mal epilepsy require emergency care on the part of the teacher. The seizures are usually marked by loss of consciousness, convulsions, and thrashing about. The convulsive state is then followed by prolonged stupor.

In giving a child first aid for a seizure, the teacher should not resist his thrashing about. Keep calm and let the convulsion run its course, which it will do in 2 to 5 minutes. The child should be kept in the open where he will not injure himself by striking any hard or sharp objects. *Do not force anything between the patient's teeth.* His collar should be loosened to prevent breathing from being obstructed. Turn the victim's face to one side so that liquid emitted does not fall back into his throat. Place something soft, such as a rolled-up coat, beneath the person's head. After the convulsion the child should be taken to the emergency room to lie down and sleep. However, the parents should be notified because they may wish to call for the student at once. Ordinarily, if it is known that the child is epileptic, prearrangements should have been made with the parents and physician concerning the routine to follow.

Fainting

Just before fainting, a child is likely to feel weak and dizzy. Vision becomes blurred, the face becomes pale, and the victim may be covered with a cold sweat. When a child faints, he or she should be placed on his back with head lowered. The color of the face in-

To find the correct counterdose, first locate the substance causing the trouble in one of the lists printed immediately below. Next to that substance is a number, which refers to the corresponding counterdose (bearing the same number) in the section below the dotted line.*

POISONS | OVERDOSES

Acids—18
Bichloride of mercury—6
Camphor—1
Carbon monoxide—16
Chlorine bleach—8
Detergents—8
Disinfectant
  with chlorine—8
  with carbolic acid—12
Food poisoning—11
Furniture polish—17
Gasoline, kerosene—17
Household ammonia—10

Insect and rat poisons
  with arsenic—2
  with sodium fluoride—14
  with phosphorus—5
  with DDT—11
  with strychnine—15
Iodine tincture—4
Lye—10
Mushrooms—11
Oil of wintergreen—9
Pine oil—17
Rubbing alcohol—9
Turpentine—17

Alcohol—9
Aspirin—9
Barbiturates—3
Belladonna—15
Bromides—11
Codeine—13
Headache and cold compounds—9
Iron compounds—7
Morphine, opium—13
Paregoric—13
"Pep" medicines—2
Sleeping medicines—3
Tranquilizers—3

- -

1

Induce vomiting with:
- Finger in throat, *or*
- Syrup of ipecac, *or*
- Teaspoon of mustard in half glass of water, *or*
- 3 teaspoons of salt in warm water.

2
- Give glass of milk, or
- Give 1 tablespoonful of activated charcoal, or
- Give "universal antidote" (obtain from drug store and keep on hand at home).
- Induce vomiting. (See No. 1)

3
- Induce vomiting (See No. 1)
- Give 2 tablespoons epsom salt in 2 glasses of water.
- Then give large quantities hot coffee or strong tea.
- Do not give coffee or tea for tranquilizer overdose.

4
- Give 2 ounces thick starch paste. Mix cornstarch (or flour) with water.
- Then give 2 ounces salt in quart of warm water. Drink until vomit fluid is clear.
- Finally, give glass of milk.

5
- Induce vomiting. (See No. 1.)
- Then give 4 ounces mineral oil. Positively do *not* give vegetable or animal oil.
- 4 ounces hydrogen peroxide.
- 1 tablespoon sodium bicarb in quart of warm water.

6
- Give glass of milk, *or*
- Give 1 teaspoon of activated charcoal, *or*
- Universal antidote. (See No. 2.)
- Induce vomiting. (See No. 1.)
- 1 ounce of epsom salts in a pint of water.

7
- Induce vomiting. (See No. 1.)
- 2 teaspoons of bicarb in a glass of warm water.
- Give glass of milk.

8
- Give patient 1 or 2 glasses of milk.

9
- Give a glass of milk.
- Induce vomiting. (See No. 1.)
- Tablespoon sodium bicarb in quart of warm water.

10
- Give 2 tablespoons vinegar in 2 glasses of water.
- Give whites of 2 raw eggs or 2 ounces of olive oil.
- Do *not* induce vomiting!

11
- Induce vomiting. (See No. 1.)
- Give 2 tablespoons epsom salt in 2 glasses of water.

12
- Induce vomiting. (See No. 1.)
- Then give 2 ounces of castor oil.
- Next give glass of milk or whites of 2 raw eggs.

13
- Give glass of milk, *or*
- Universal antidote. (See No. 2.)
- 2 tablespoons epsom salt in 2 glasses of water.
- Keep patient awake.

14
- Give 2 tablespoons of milk of magnesia.
- Give glass of milk.
- Induce vomiting. (See No. 1.)

15
- Give glass of milk, *or*
- Universal antidote. (See No. 2.)
- Induce vomiting. (See No. 1.)
- Give artificial respiration.
- Keep patient quiet.

16
- Carry victim into fresh air.
- Make patient lie down.

17
- Give water or milk.
- Give 2 ounces vegetable oil.
- Do *not* induce vomiting!

18
- Give 1-ounce milk of magnesia in large quantity of water.
- Do *not* induce vomiting!

*From American druggist magazine, 1966.

dicates to some exent the amount of blood being supplied to the brain. If the face is very pale, the head should be kept lowered until the color of the face improves. If, on the other hand, the face is extremely red, it may be desirable to keep the head level or slightly raised. After the fainting victim has recovered consciousness, the victim should lie quietly for a few minutes. The child should then sit up for a few minutes before taking a standing position. The fainting person should have plenty of fresh, cool air. After regaining consciousness, a cool, wet cloth may be applied to the face or chest as a stimulant to recuperative action.

Nosebleed

Nosebleed is frequent following a blow on the nose, although there may be other causes. Some of the small blood vessels in the mucous lining of the nose can be ruptured very easily. It is often unnecessary to give first aid for nosebleed as many, if not most of them in children, will stop without emergency care. For minor cases pressure can be applied by closing the nostrils with the fingers. In giving first aid for more persistent nosebleed, it is preferable to place the child flat in a prone position. It keeps the blood from flowing back into the throat. Cold packs may be applied to the nose, or it may be temporarily packed with sterile gauze. If a nosebleed cannot be readily stopped, a physician is required.

Wounds

Any injury to the skin or tissue is classed as a wound. The person giving first aid is largely concerned with wounds in which the skin or mucous membrane is broken. Any tiny break in the skin is considered a wound if germs are allowed to enter.

Wounds may be classified according to the way the injury occurs, the type of wound made, and the kind of first aid required. The general types of wounds with which the first-aider is likely to be concerned are incisions or clean-cut wounds, torn or lacerated wounds, abrasions or scraping, or rubbing types of wounds made by the body sliding on the floor or on a rough surface. Puncture or stab wounds are made by such objects as pins, needles, and nails.

Clean-cut wounds usually bleed freely, and they are not so likely to become infected. Wounds made by machines or other rough objects, however, are more likely to become infected. They may not bleed freely, and frequently there are dirt and grease in the wound. Puncture wounds are ordinarily more serious than other types of minor wounds. They usually do not bleed freely, and they are hard to cleanse properly. Furthermore, there is danger of tetanus, or lockjaw, from puncture wounds.

Infection is a chief danger from a majority of wounds. Although thousands of germs may enter even a tiny wound, not all wounds in which germs enter become infected. The body may resist and overcome the germs, depending on a number of factors, or the germs may not have the strength to grow and multiply.

In giving first aid for wounds in which serious bleeding is not a factor, a main purpose is to prevent infection if possible and to keep germs from entering a wound once it is made. If a physician will be available soon, all the first-aider will need to do as far as the wound itself is concerned is to cover it with a sterile dressing. The first-aider should never try to clean a wound or to apply an antiseptic if the services of a physician are needed and readily available. If it is necessary to cleanse a wound, use plain soap and running tap water adjusted to room temperature. The first-aid care of ordinary small wounds requires only that the first-aider apply a sterile compress and bandage to keep dirt from entering the wound.

Punctures and stabs are particularly dangerous types of wounds for the following reasons:

1. Tetanus, or lockjaw germs, may grow readily when there is a lack of air, such as in a puncture wound.
2. Punctures do not bleed freely; consequently, dirt and germs are not washed out as in an open wound.
3. It is extremely difficult to clean the

wound, and germs may have been deposited in the bottom of it by the instrument making the wound.

A physician is needed to treat a puncture wound as he may wish to take protective measures against tetanus. If a physician cannot be secured for some time, the first-aider should encourage bleeding without bruising the tissue.

Eye injuries

Since the eyes are very delicate organs, they should be treated with the greatest of care. Children should not be allowed to use most sharp-pointed instruments because of the danger of injuring the eye or falling on the instrument. The following points should be remembered in caring for eye injuries:
1. If any type of chemical gets into the eyes, it should be washed out immediately with plenty of water.
2. The use of any kind of sharp object should be avoided in removing foreign particles from the eye.
3. The first-aider should *never* attempt to remove an embedded object from the eye.
4. If a foreign object gets into the eye, the eye should not be rubbed. Rubbing the eye with a foreign object in it, especially if it is a sharp particle, such as a cinder, may drive it into the eyeball tissue.
5. If a child gets an object in the eye, the teacher should attempt to remove it with a sterile cloth. If the object cannot be removed readily, a physician is needed.

Burns

There are three general types of burns—*chemical*, *thermal*, and *solar*. Burns and scalds are from heat of such a degree as to cause injury to the skin and tissue of the body. Burns from hot liquids or steam are classified as scalds. Burns are sometimes classified as follows: first-degree burns are those in which the skin is reddened; second-degree burns are those in which the skin is blistered; third-degree burns are those in which there is a destruction of deeper tissue and are very serious since growth cells that form new skin are destroyed.

Giving first aid for a burn depends somewhat upon the extent of the burn. If it is extensive or if tissue has been destroyed, a physician is needed as soon as possible. The main duty of the first-aider in this case is to try to prevent and care for shock until a physician is in charge of the individual. Nothing should be put on the burned area. Relief of pain and control of tissue damage can often be achieved in first- and second-degree burns by application of ice, "instant cold" chemical bags, or immersion in ice water. Chemical cold sprays should not be used because of the danger of frostbite and possible tissue damage.

Fractures

Although there are many classifications of fractures, for the purpose of first aid they can be classed as (1) simple fractures, in which a bone is broken but the skin is not broken and (2) compound fractures, in which a bone is broken and a wound extends from the break through the tissue and skin.

Physicians have classified fractures into many different varieties, depending on the extent of the injury in most cases. For example, in a simple fracture the bone is broken, and there has been some injury to tissue around the bone, but the skin is not broken. In a compound fracture the bone is broken, and the skin is also wounded so that the wound communicates directly with the area of the broken bone. Sometimes a portion of the bone itself will penetrate the skin. A complicated fracture is one in which the bone is broken, the skin is broken, and there may be serious damage to blood vessels or organs around the broken bone.

Fractures are also described in relation to the nature of the injury to the bone. In a greenstick fracture the bone is split. In a comminuted fracture the bone may be broken into several pieces; for example, there may be a combination of several kinds of fractures, so that one may have a compound comminuted fracture.

The symptoms of fracture include swelling, pain, and bruising. If a portion of a limb

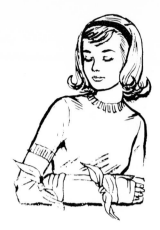

Fig. 6-8. Board splint for fractured arm.

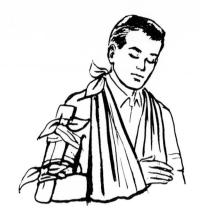

Fig. 6-9. Splint and sling for fracture of upper arm.

swings in any direction that it could not do unless the bone were broken, that is sure proof that there has been a fracture. If a bone that ordinarily appears straight suddenly assumes an angular position, the irregularity of the line indicates a fracture. Not all symptoms will necessarily be present in every fracture.

If fracture is suspected, a physician is needed. The usual policy of the school should be followed in this case. Shock may follow a broken bone. The first-aider should give first aid for shock. If medical aid is readily available the child should not be moved. If it is necessary to move the patient, a splint should be applied if the arms (Figs. 6-8 and 6-9) or legs are involved; if the neck or back is involved, extreme care should be used in handling the person. If it is necessary to move the injured person with a neck or back injury before medical aid is available, it should be remembered that the body should never be allowed to sag, especially the head or neck. The child should be prevented from moving in any way if at all avoidable. Some rigid material should be used on which to move the person. A wide flat board or door will keep the body straight and prevent it from sagging. Plenty of help should be available for carrying the injured person.

Skull fracture may result from any type of hard blow on the head or by the head striking a hard surface. Some of the symptoms of skull fracture are bleeding from the nose, mouth, or ears, unconsciousness, pupils of the eyes unequal in size, and face flushed or pale, depending on the seriousness of the injury, and there may be evidence of a blow on the head, such as a cut or a bump. All of the symptoms may not be present in every case.

First aid for skull fractures involves keeping the person in a lying position with the head and shoulders *slightly elevated if the face is flushed.* If the face is pale or ashen, the head and shoulders should not be elevated. The child's body temperature should be maintained, but no heated object should be applied. A physician should be secured as soon as possible. If a person must be moved before medical aid is available, the victim should be kept in a lying position.

Dislocations

A dislocation is a bone out of place at a joint. The ligaments may be injured by being torn, the blood vessels and nerves may be injured, and the ends of the bones may be chipped. A physician is needed to reduce a dislocation safely. The parts of the body that may be dislocated are the fingers, shoulders, jaw, elbows, knees, and hips. The first-aid care for a dislocation consists of placing an ice bag or cold compresses over the joint and securing a physician. There should be no movement of the joint, since there is danger of chipping the bone.

Frostbite

In some areas of the country, schoolchildren may occasionally suffer from frostbite. It results from loss of circulation because of constriction of arteries at low temperatures. Consequently, the tissues are deprived of oxygen. Injury from frostbite varies with circumstances, and the kind of emergency care given.

The fingers, toes, nose, ears, and cheeks are the parts of the body most likely to be frostbitten. The signs of frostbite are a sensation of intense coldness, then numbness, then finally almost complete loss of sensation in the frozen part. The frostbitten part may be flushed at first and then become very white or grayish white. Because of numbness and loss of sensation, people may not realize that their nose, cheeks, or ears are frostbitten until someone calls attention to it.

In giving first aid for frostbite, the teacher should be careful not to damage the tissue. Rubbing or careless handling of a frozen part may bruise the tissue and cause further damage. If a person is outdoors, the frozen part should be covered with the hand or with cloth, preferably woolen. The child should be brought indoors and placed in a warm room, and the frostbitten part should be covered with a warm cloth such as a blanket. However, hot objects of any kind should be kept away from the frostbitten part.

Sprains

In sprains, ligaments and other tissues may be damaged. Wrists and ankles are most frequently sprained. In giving first aid for a sprain, the teacher should apply cold compresses or an ice bag for 20 or 30 minutes after the injury. The injured part should be kept elevated, and the child not allowed to put any weight on the sprained part. A sprained ankle may be helped by a crisscrossing bandage, elastic bandage, or adhesive around it to keep it immovable. The usual school procedure should be followed in contacting the parents concerning a physician.

First-aid supplies

Every elementary school should have adequate first-aid supplies, depending on the enrollment as well as the location of the school and the availability of medical assistance. In most elementary schools the first-aid supplies are likely to be under the care of the principal. They should be kept in a central place, such as the health service room, emergency room, or the principal's office. Periodic stock taking should be done to assure that first-aid kits are complete and up to date. The following list shows the usual first-aid supplies needed by the school:

Absorbent cotton
Adhesive tape
Compresses of various sizes
Sterile gauze of various sizes
Roller bandage of various sizes
Triangular bandages
Cotton swabs sterilized in packages
Scissors
Eye dropper
Aromatic spirits of ammonia
Tourniquet
Tincture of green soap
Meat tenderizer (for bee stings)
Wooden applicators
Hand brushes
Elastic bandages, 2 and 3 inches wide
Blankets
Splints
Pillows
Paper cups
Safety pins
Tweezers
Hot-water bottle
Ice bag
"Instant cold" chemical bags

It is important to remember that *no medicines of any kind* are part of a first-aid supply cabinet!

QUESTIONS FOR DISCUSSION

1. How do the yearly numbers of deaths caused by accidents to children compare with those caused by diseases each year in the United States?
2. What is meant by the statement that proper safety habits and desirable safety attitudes are based upon safety education?

3. What are some major causes of children's accidents?
4. Who should be responsible for the school safety education program?
5. What are the major functions of the school safety program?
6. To what extent is the home a factor in the total accident problem?
7. What are some important steps that may be taken to reduce the frequency of accidents in schools?
8. Under what conditions is the teacher liable in the event of a serious accident involving a schoolchild?
9. Why is it important that planning for safety teaching take into account all grades of the school?
10. What groups are ordinarily involved in city safety councils or committees?
11. What are the advantages of considering school safety as a phase of total community safety?
12. How can accident statistics be used to advantage in teaching safety?
13. Why are elementary school-age children particularly vulnerable to pedestrian accidents?
14. Why are the months of March, April, September, and October the most dangerous for child pedestrians?
15. How can teachers help in preparing children to avoid accidents as passengers in cars and buses?
16. Why should every teacher assume responsibility for a safe bicycle program?
17. What is the teacher's part in providing a safe school environment?
18. Why should safety education have a place in every grade of the elementary school?

SUGGESTED CLASS ACTIVITIES

1. Obtain figures showing the numbers of accidents caused by various factors (a) in the home and (b) in the community.
2. Form a committee to prepare a sample checklist of possible home hazards, room by room, which may be used by children in evaluating the safety status of their own homes.
3. Form a committee to prepare a sample checklist for a safety survey of the school plant and grounds.
5. Prepare a list of safety measures employed in a school that is well known to you. Evaluate this list and indicate how it might be made more adequate.
5. Form committees to outline topics on home, traffic, and other community safety subjects that may be used at the various school levels with which class members are most concerned.
6. Prepare a list of major sources of safety materials suitable for use in the elementary grades.
7. Form a panel to discuss and evaluate the various plans for teaching safety, that is, as a separate subject, by integration, by utilizing opportunities (teachable moments) as they arise.
8. Prepare a plan for teaching safety in a school that is well known to you. Take into account the special circumstances of that school that are likely to influence the type of safety education program that would be most feasible at least in the first stages of its development.
9. Outline a detailed plan for teaching safety for one grade level in which you are most interested.
10. Develop a plan for the formation and conduct of an elementary school safety council.
11. Visit a law enforcement agency and prepare a report regarding school safety patrols.

REFERENCES

American Alliance for Health, Physical Education, and Recreation: Safety education review, Washington, D.C., published annually, The Alliance.

American Alliance for Health, Physical Education, and Recreation: School safety policies, (Report of the Joint Committee on Health Problems in Education of the National Education Association and the American Medical Association) Washington, D.C., 1968, The Alliance.

American National Red Cross: Standard first aid and personal safety, Washington, D.C., 1973, American National Red Cross.

Baker, S.: Injury control; accident prevention and other approaches to reduction of injury. In Sartwell, P., editor: Preventive medicine and public health, New York, 1973, Appleton-Century-Crofts.

Consumer Product Safety Commission: Banned products, vol. II, Part 1, Washington, D.C., Oct. 1, 1973, The Commission.

Craig, A. B.: Some hazards of aquatics, American Journal of Diseases of Childhood, June, 1973.

Green, M. I.: A sigh of relief; the first-aid handbook for childhood emergencies, New York, 1977, Bantam Books, Inc.

Hartley, J.: First aid without panic, New York, 1977, Popular Library.

King, B. G.: Man and the control of accidental injuries, Public Health Review, Dec., 1973.

Market Facts, INC.: Household safety study, Chicago, 1971, Market Facts Inc.

McFarland, R. A., and Moore, R. C.: Childhood accidents and injuries, Boston, 1970, Harvard School of Public Health.

Meyer, R.: Childhood injury and pediatric education; a critique, Pediatrics (Suppl.), 1969.

National Safety Council: Accident facts, Chicago, 1978, The Council.

National Safety Council: School safety magazine, Chicago, published quarterly, The Council.

Smith, V.: A study of injuries, Journal of School Health, Feb., 1971.

Stack, H. J., and Elkow, J. D.: Education for safe living, Englewood Cliffs, N.J., 1972, Prentice-Hall, Inc.

Westaby, J. R.: A bookshelf on injury control and emergency health services, American Journal of Public Health, April, 1974.

7 Mental health and the teacher

If a child lives with criticism, he learns to condemn.
If a child lives with hostility, he learns to fight.
If a child lives with fear, he learns to be apprehensive.
If a child lives with pity, he learns to feel sorry for himself.
If a child lives with jealousy, he learns to feel guilty.
If a child lives with encouragement, he learns to be confident.
If a child lives with tolerance, he learns to be patient.
If a child lives with praise, he learns to be appreciative.
If a child lives with acceptance, he learns to love.
If a child lives with approval, he learns to like himself.
If a child lives with recognition, he learns to have a goal.
If a child lives with fairness, he learns what justice is.
If a child lives with honesty, he learns what truth is.
If a child lives with security, he learns to have faith in himself and those about him.
If a child lives with friendliness, he learns the world is a nice place in which to live.
ANONYMOUS

When John Locke used the phrase, "mens sana in corpore sano"—a sound mind in a sound body—he expressed the interrelationships that exist between physical and mental health. He envisioned mental health as a condition of the whole personality, not as an entity separate from physical health. He stressed the importance of the total health of children. Current concepts of health also include reference to social and spiritual aspects introduced in Chapter 1.

The mental phase of health today has never had greater meaning. The tremendous anxieties, pressures, and concerns in the world have their effect on children and youth. The young people living in poverty and among bias and prejudice are especially subjected to extensive biologic, psychologic, sociologic, and economic stress. The cultural, ethnic, racial, and economic inequalities, the tensions over world peace, the dichotomy of moral and social values, the stress on materialism, the need for good grades, the conformities to outmoded and antiquated practices and traditions in schools, and the inadequacies of educational opportunities

create a social climate conducive to mental illness. The Joint Commission on Mental Health of Children stated*:

The major crisis of our time is a crisis of human relations . . . we have lost our capacity for mutual trust, love and responsibility. . . . Social changes on a major scale are required if all our children and youth are to . . . enjoy optimal mental health.

It is imperative that schools recognize these conditions and that teachers become aware of their roles in the promotion and maintenance of good mental health.

In Chapter 4 reference was made to the significance of the teacher continuously observing pupils for signs and symptoms of health deviations. These observations of boys and girls often lead to the following questions:

"Why is Bill always boisterous and rude?"
"Why does Ann cry so easily?"

---

*Report of Task Force VI and excerpts from the Report of the Committee on Children of Minority Groups by the Joint Commission on Mental Health of Children, New York, 1973, Harper & Row, Publishers, Inc.

"Why is Susan so hard to reach?"
"Why is Jack so nervous?"
"Why does Sam use drugs?"
"What can I do to help Bob whose parents are alcoholics?"
"Why is Nancy frequently truant?"
"Why is Mary always so quiet and withdrawn?"
"Why does Bill become frightened so easily?"
"Why is Jane always sullen and unhappy?"
"Why is Ed constantly picking on other children?"
"Why is Marion having trouble getting along with her classmates?"
"How can I help, and what should I do to best understand and to help children with behavior problems?"

This chapter has been designed to enable the teacher to better understand the behavioral problems exhibited by pupils, to discover ways to assist children in need of help, and to aid pupils to grow into happy, productive, and useful individuals who will make worthwhile contributions to the society in which they live.

WHAT IS MENTAL HEALTH?

Although it is very difficult to define mental health to the satisfaction of everyone, for the purpose of this chapter it is defined as the adjustment of the individual to self and to society so that the realities of life can be faced and the individual can function most effectively with the greatest satisfaction, cheerfulness, and socially acceptable behavior. Mentally healthy persons are able to control their emotions and adequately meet situations that occur in their environment; they are possessed of a sense of self-esteem, insight, and self-acceptance. The observable features of this adjustment may be identified in what is called personality or the individual's personality—the sum total of traits and characteristics that make each person a unique individual. Children have numerous combinations of traits and characteristics. There are many types and varieties of personalities.

Mental health is affected by the environment in which a person lives and by that person's experiences. It is an outgrowth of one's total life. It is dependent on the satisfaction of a person's physiologic and psychologic needs. The physiologic needs include food, air, water, warmth, rest and sleep, clothing, and freedom from disease and other health hazards. The psychologic or emotional needs include the following:

1. Affection—love
2. Security—to belong, to have roots, to have protection
3. Acceptance as an individual—free of prejudice or bias, concern for individual differences
4. Achievement—success experiences, recognition
5. Independence—create and develop things, be on one's own, do things under one's own guidance and direction
6. Authority—guidance and direction by adults
7. Self-respect—courteous, fair, and just treatment

Mentally healthy individuals exhibit these characteristics:

1. Pursue reasonable goals using their talents and abilities.
2. Have a sense of self-respect, self-reliance, and achievement; feel worthwhile; have a high level of self-esteem.
3. Know they are liked, loved, and wanted.
4. Have a sense of security and are reasonably at peace with themselves and their environment; enjoy life.
5. Can think and act rationally and realistically when seeking solutions to problems; are able to withstand frustration and anxiety, to persevere despite difficulty, and to ask for help without loss of self-esteem.
6. Can distinguish between feelings and facts.
7. Can maintain integrity in work and play; exhibit confidence and orderliness.
8. Are able to work in groups; are interested in others.
9. Respect the rights of others.
10. Face the realities of life and are able to accept responsibilities; are self-disciplined.

The normal individual has a satisfactory self-concept and concept of the culture in which that person lives. The individual can accept bigness or smallness of size, good or poor looks, artistic talent or lack of it, intellectual capacities or limitations. The individual can get along with children and adults in school, at home, in the neighborhood, and elsewhere. Normal individuals can function in the world about them by being able to adjust to its rules and conformities, to express their feelings by behaving in personally gratifying ways that the social order will accept, and to contribute to a changing and challenging society.

Mental health is usually considered a positive aspect of health. If it were placed on a continuum, it would be located at the extreme end and would represent the highest level of health to be achieved. However, it may also be considered to be negative in nature and on the continuum would be found at the other extreme. It would be the lowest level of health, or mental illness. There are varying degrees of positive mental health just as there are varying degrees and kinds of mental illness. Often these variations are difficult to define or identify.

WHAT IS MENTAL ILLNESS?

Maladjusted individuals, persons unable to get along with themselves and with others, may be considered to be mentally ill. They cannot or will not adjust to socially acceptable norms for behavior. These pupils are said to be unsocial, emotionally disturbed, and disruptive, with behavior and personality problems. The extent of illness is a matter of degree as well as of kind. Some people have mild emotional disturbances, whereas others have severe mental health problems. Teachers should not interpret every maladjustment or expression of unacceptable behavior as an indication of illness. At times everyone experiences mild disturbances. Students and adults may be unhappy, frustrated, anxious, depressed, angry, rude, boisterous, quiet, withdrawn, worried, unable to resolve problems; they may act irrationally, find it difficult to work with some people, or resort to the use of defense mechanisms without being what is usually thought of as mentally ill or emotionally disturbed.

It is the frequent, repeated, and consistent manifestation of such behavior that may lead one to suspect mental or emotional disorder.

The types of mental illness may be categorized as follows:

psychoses Acute or chronic illnesses, the "insanities," that require intensive treatment in hospital settings; affect total personality, can be either organic or functional in origin; characterized by severe mood disturbances with serious changes in thought and feelings, by behavior withdrawal from reality, or by persistent delusions and hallucinations; include such conditions as schizophrenia, paranoia, general paresis, and senile psychosis.

neuroses Less severe disturbances that affect only portion of personality; include anxiety states, fears, phobias, hypochondriases, hysterias, obsessions, and compulsions.

personality disorders Psychosomatic problems of individuals (emotional problems expressed through physical ailments), drug addiction, chronic alcoholism, and delinquencies.

Mental illness is found in children as well as in adults. It is estimated that approximately 10% of pupils (5 million) have emotional problems and maladjustments requiring psychiatric help, with an additional 3% having seriously psychotic or prepsychotic conditions. In the average class of 32 boys and girls, a teacher may expect to recognize emotional difficulties in three or four pupils and to identify one child needing psychiatric assistance.

Mental illness is considered to be the leading health problem in the United States. The following estimates have been made:
1. That approximately 20 million people are suffering from some form of mental or emotional illness; approximately one in ten people is afflicted
2. That one person in fifteen of those mentally ill will need hospitalization
3. That 30% to 60% or more of the patients who consult doctors have complaints in part due to emotional disturbances
4. That 500,000 children suffer from psychoses and borderline psychotic conditions
5. That 1 million children are afflicted with personality disorders

6. That one in three of the 15 million youngsters reared in poverty have serious mental and emotional problems
7. That 6 million children and adults are mentally retarded—30 per 1,000; approximately 2 million are under 16 years of age; most are mildly retarded; estimated 40% have personality disorders
8. That approximately 250,000 to 600,000 children and youth are neglected and abused, with an estimated 6,000 deaths yearly. These pupils are subject to physical neglect, emotional neglect and abuse, physical abuse, and the battered child syndrome.

Mental illness is frequently a component of the following:

1. Alcoholism—alcohol is the most abused drug in the United States; there are 7 to 10 million alcohol abusers; approximately 200,000 develop each year; more than 20% of men admitted to mental institutions are alcoholics; problem drinking is a causal factor in almost half of the 58,000 traffic deaths yearly; in some Indian reservations the rate is 25% to 30% as against 6% to 7% in the total United States.

2. Drug addiction—there are approximately 500,000 narcotic addicts; use of amphetamines, barbiturates, hallucinogens (including LSD), and the sedative-hypnotics (marijuana) have greatly increased in recent years; some 30 million Americans have tried marijuana at least once; there are probably 300,000 to 400,000 daily users, with 2 to 4 million occasional users; in 1975 over $46 billion was spent on legal drugs ($225 for every man, woman, and child); large numbers of young people are using a variety of drugs.

3. Juvenile delinquency—over 750,000 young people are in juvenile courts yearly; 30% to 40% have been there before; the rate is rising particularly among those in the ghetto and the poor.

4. Broken homes—one marriage in two ended in divorce in 1975 to 1976; the ratio is higher in teenage marriages.

5. Suicide—25,000 suicides occur yearly, with 500,000 attempts being made; 6.6% are 15 to 19 years old; boys try three times more than girls; American Indians rate is five times the national average; it is one of the ten leading causes of death in the United States and is the fourth leading cause of death among 15- to 19-year-olds; rates have greatly increased.

6. Emotional maladjustment and personality disorders—these are related to job maladjustments in industry and accidents; mental stress, school failures, criminal behavior, divorce, and absenteeism play an important precipitating role.

WHAT ARE THE CAUSES OF MENTAL ILLNESS?

Mental illness is caused by a multiplicity of complex factors. It may be related to heredity, to environment, and to the reciprocal interaction of these factors. It may develop in a context of interpersonal relations, starting with mother and later with other persons. Disturbances are more likely to occur during children's critical growth periods.

Although mental illness is usually not inherited, it is believed that schizophrenia and some types of neuroses, or a predisposition to them, may be inherited. Also, the bodily strengths or weaknesses with which individuals are born may lead to problems that result in illness. The person who is very small or very large in stature, who is unusually obese or thin, who has poor vision or hearing, or who has a deformed limb or body part may not be able to satisfy physiologic or psychologic needs. Therefore, the individual may not be able to make suitable adjustments to these conditions.

Environmentally there are interrelated physical and psychologic conditions and situations that may cause illness:

1. Physical or biochemical components
   a. Infections—brain inflammation
   b. Nutritional deficiencies—diabetes, anemia, nervous disorders
   c. Accidents—nervous system damage, loss of limb, physical deformity
   d. Glandular deficiencies or imbalance—abnormal body size and shape, excess nervousness and anxieties
   e. Alcohol—brain softening

f. Anemia—lack of oxygen to brain, death, or damage to brain
g. Drugs—death or damage to brain
h. Physical defects—facial disfigurement, paralysis
i. Birth problems—premature births, early pregnancy trauma
j. Excess physical punishment for misbehavior

2. Psychologic components
   a. Social relations with group or other persons—cultural and social differences, overly competitive society, peer culture—outgroup, prejudice, insecurity, status, lack of self-esteem
   b. Love and marriage—unhappiness, maladjustments, sustained rejection
   c. Family conflicts—constant quarreling, divorce, housing, broken homes
   d. Occupational—work adjustments and pressures, economic status, job, money
   e. Sexual adjustments—ability to satisfy need
   f. Religious conflicts—within family or social group
   g. Parental attitudes—mother domination, rejection, overprotectiveness, discipline, expectations
   h. Parent personalities—chronic alcoholic, neurotic, parental fear and distrust of people, lack of care
   i. School experiences—grade placement, teacher competency and personality, discipline, competition for grades, inappropriate curriculum

After an accident a child may suffer a severe injury, resulting in the loss of a limb. The pupil may not be able to regain a feeling of security or status with peers; the student may not be able to accept or adjust to the physical deformity. Likewise, a student whose parents are chronic alcoholics may not receive adequate nutrition, which may lead to anemia, nervousness, and other conditions.

The heredity and environmental factors in mental illness have a social relationship. The pupils, teachers, and other school personnel; the ministers, priests, rabbis, and others at church; the friends, physicians, adults in the community; and the parents, grandparents, brothers, and sisters in the home play significant roles in the affection received, the stresses, tensions, and anxieties developed, the security provided—in fact, the total environment of a boy and girl. These people furnish the experiences that help or hinder children in satisfying their physiologic and psychologic needs. The lack of, or the improper, experiences result in the failure of these needs being fulfilled. The signs of maladjustment referred to previously may then begin to appear and be the behavior incipient to more serious mental health problems.

The incidence of mental illness among low-income native Americans, blacks, and other cultural and ethnic groups is greater. The poor are those deprived of the basic necessities of food, housing, medical care, education, and employment. They also experience bias, prejudice, and inequality of opportunity. Such omissions and attitudes are related to family conflicts, instability, frustration, failure, lack of personal dignity, and other stresses and problems.

Mental illness is a condition that grows over a period of time; it results from the exposure to many experiences and environments. A teacher viewing the behavior of a student in class must remember that the child has been exposed for from 6 to 8 years to parents and others before the child reaches school. Therefore, the roots for mental illness may have already been planted and may blossom forth in school when the pupil is faced with an additional unsatisfying or trying atmosphere.

Mental illness is a condition whose start is difficult, if not impossible, to determine. The body can withstand, within reason, fear, anxiety, worry, and other stressful conditions. However, when stress becomes extreme, the individual can no longer tolerate these conditions and consequently becomes disorganized, disoriented, and maladjusted. This disturbance is often difficult to determine without expert help.

WHY SHOULD SCHOOLS BE CONCERNED WITH THE MENTAL HEALTH OF PUPILS?

The school is usually thought to rank second to the family as the most important unit in society affecting the mental health of children and must be concerned for these reasons:

1. The effectiveness of the educative process will be seriously hampered, since approximately 10% of pupils (5 million) are afflicted with emotional disturbances.

2. Educational failure, or the "failure syndrome," is one of the underlying factors that triggers acting-out in schools, depression, drug abuse, truancy, and other maladjustments. Children who exhibit such behavior have a lower self-concept, or self-identity.

3. The experiences to which a child is exposed can help prevent serious difficulties or hasten such problems. Hence, schools play a role in both primary and secondary prevention of mental illness—before conditions occur and in the control of existing conditions. Early identification of children with emotional difficulties is important because remedial help can hopefully be provided at a time when intervention is maximally effective. The increase of problems and the great shortage of community mental health services and facilities add to the need for emphasis on prevention.

4. Behavior is more readily modified at the elementary level than later in life.

5. Children in ghetto and deprived areas must experience success in school with special attention given to their physical and psychologic needs. In one big city reported by Abrams and associates* 48% of the children were already educationally handicapped in terms of readiness, or probable readiness, to enter school as compared with a black school where 76% of the pupils were affected and a white school of middle income families where 10% were affected. Many will perform poorly in school.

6. The school is the only agency outside the home that reaches practically all children and youths.

The school program in mental health should attempt to achieve the objectives

*Abrams, R. S., Vanecko, M., and Abrams, I.: A suggested school mental health program, Journal of School Health **42:** March, 1972.

previously referred to by promoting positive mental health in all students, preventing mental illness and emotional disturbances, and assisting children with mental health problems.

WHAT SHOULD THE SCHOOL MENTAL HEALTH PROGRAM INCLUDE?

Mental health should permeate the entire school curriculum. Every activity in school has mental health implications—the atmosphere in the classroom and in the total school program, the relationships of pupils to teachers, nurses, and principals, the relationships of the school with parents, the methods used in teaching, the content of the curriculum, the procedures used to handle accidents and emergencies, and the use of health examinations and health screening tests. The nature and scope of this program could be patterned after the components of the total school health program and include the following:

1. Mental health services
   a. Locating problem children
   b. Helping problem children
      (1) Counseling and guidance
      (2) Use of community resources
      (3) Adjustment of school program
2. Mentally healthful environment
3. Mental health instruction
4. Coordination of mental health program

Mental health services

The kinds of mental health services available vary widely, with well-equipped schools having one or more of the following: a central child study bureau or guidance or pupil personnel department, guidance counselors, physicians, psychiatrists, psychologists, mental health specialists, nurses, social workers, remedial instruction teachers, and special classes. Large school systems usually have some consultant psychiatric help either on a part-time basis or on a case referral basis; suggestions have been made that psychiatrists be employed full-time. The basic mental health team that should be found in school systems includes consulting psychiatrists, psychologists, and psychiatric social workers. Several states require that children be given special services for emotional problems.

Locating problem children. Children who are emotionally disturbed or who exhibit behavior that causes one to suspect mental illness need to be identified and located early if they are to receive the greatest help. The teacher is the main contact person with pupils and is in a strategic position to render valuable service. The importance of teacher observations has been stressed in Chapter 4; however, the specific signs of maladjustment that the teacher must know and recognize are found on p. 54. It has been estimated that teachers can select 70% of the emotionally disturbed children, and with a clinic team, 90% of their problems can be discovered. The deviant behaviors observed are generally the result of pupil needs (p. 16) not being fulfilled. Teachers must be alert throughout the entire school day and be observant in their informal contacts, conferences, and interviews with pupils and parents for clues that will help to identify the problems of their pupils. Should the teacher desire to more objectively identify children in need of help, the Teacher Observation of Classroom Adaptation (see chart on p. 130) will provide a useful instrument.

Some other procedures teachers may use to help identify disturbed children include the following:

1. Sociometric technique—the teacher may ask pupils to list the three classmates they would like to have sit next to them in order of preference. This information can then be plotted on paper, and those pupils with few, if any friends, can be readily identified. The isolates are easily located through the use of this method.

2. Examination of school records including health records—these contain chronologic reports of children's performances and health status.

3. Written autobiographies—the teacher may have pupils write compositions on such topics as the following:

> "What I criticize about myself"
> "What others criticize about me"
> "What makes me mad"
> "The person I would like to be"
> "My life 10 years from now"

4. Student survey—the procedure shown in Fig. 7-1 should provide helpful clues when

	Always 3	Seldom 2	Never 1
1. I can get extra help from the teacher when I need it.	_____	_____	_____
2. The teacher praises me when I do well.	_____	_____	_____
3. The teacher smiles when I do something well.	_____	_____	_____
4. The teacher listens attentively.	_____	_____	_____
5. The teacher accepts me as an individual.	_____	_____	_____
6. The teacher encourages me to try something new.	_____	_____	_____
7. The teacher respects the feelings of others.	_____	_____	_____
8. My work is usually good enough.	_____	_____	_____
9. I am called on when I raise my hand.	_____	_____	_____
10. The same students always get praised by the teacher.	_____	_____	_____

Fig. 7-1. Student survey. (From Gearheart, B. R., and Weishahn, M. W.: The handicapped child in the regular classroom, St. Louis, 1976, The C. V. Mosby Co.)

completed by pupils and reviewed by the teacher.

5. Thinking about yourself—an activity useful in grades 3 to 7 to show the degree of discrepancy between a child's perception of self and as the pupil would like it to be.

Finding problem children is also the responsibility of other school personnel, including nurses and psychologists. Their specific responsibilities vary in schools, but they should be observant of pupil behavior, should assess pupil records, and should use a variety of formal procedures.

School psychologists may use personality adjustment tests, such as the California Test of Personality (elementary series), which covers five levels of personality, including self-relevance, feelings of belongings, and social skills; the California Test of Mental Maturity; the Goodenough Draw-A-Man test; a semiprojective story completion instrument called "Secret Stories," which is an adaptation of Roger's use of "Wishes"; the Brown Personality Inventory of Children; or Roger's Test of Personality Adjustment, in addition to evaluating the information from school personnel to find emotionally disturbed students.

A variety of other instruments identified by Reinert* as useful devices include: (1) Bower-Lambert Scales (grades K to 12), a semiprojective technique; (2) Deveraux Elementary School Behavior Rating Scale (grades K to 6); and (3) Walker Problem Behavior Identification Checklist (grades 4 to 6) for teacher use. Greenberger and associates† developed a Psychosocial Maturity (PSM) Inventory, a self-reporting attitude instrument for use with 8- to 11-year-olds.

Counselors, physicians, nurses, psychiatric social workers, psychologists, and psychiatrists may individually or collectively be involved in case studies of pupils. Teachers

---

*Reinert, H. R.: Children in conflict, St. Louis, 1976, The C. V. Mosby Co.

†Greenberger, E., Josselson, R., Knerr, C. and Knerr, B.: The measurement and structure of psychosocial maturity, Journal of Youth and Adolescence 4: June, 1975.

and other personnel may also be requested to report their observations. This is a technique whereby the conclusions of a variety of people are brought together to help identify and understand deviant children, to determine needed action to help children, and to suggest school adjustments.

The assessment of the mental health status of pupils is both difficult and complex. Accurate, objective observations of behavior together with the pooling of information obtained from many sources are necessary.

Helping problem children. When schools have located pupils who may have mental health problems, the question arises, "What shall we do with them?" The action taken by the school is referred to as the follow-up procedure and may include counseling and guidance, the use of community health resources, and adjustment of the school program to the needs of the pupil.

Counseling and guidance (see also Chapter 5) refers to that help rendered to pupils and parents for any or all the following reasons:
1. To understand the problem
2. To encourage parents to obtain further diagnosis or treatment
3. To assist parents with the location of, and the contact with, community health resources
4. To aid in adjustment of the school program

Counseling and guidance may take place at an unplanned or a planned meeting with the pupil or parent, or both, at school or in the home, by telephone, by note or letter sent home, or by other procedures. Any of the school personnel, including teachers and nurses involved in the identification of problem pupils may perform this function. In addition, there ought to be someone in school to whom a student with problems may go who will listen in a nonjudgmental fashion. There might be a place and time so that young people may talk with their peers, or anyone available, about their problems and where appropriate help can be provided if desired.

Teachers have a responsibility to under-

Teacher observation of classroom adaptation*

Please rate each pupil from 0 to 3 for each of the following kinds of maladaptive behavior observed in the classroom, using the rating scale below. The examples given for each category of maladaptive behavior are merely illustrative suggestions, and should not be thought of as an exhaustive list.

Rating scale (0-3)
0 = Within minimal limits of acceptable behavior
1 = Mildly excessive
2 = Moderately excessive
3 = Severely excessive

_____ 1. Excessively lacking in involvement with classmates: e.g. shy, timid, alone too much, day-dreamer, friendless, aloof
_____ 2. Excessively aggressive behavior: e.g. fights too much, steals, lies, resists authority, is destructive to others or property, obstinate, disobedient, uncooperative
_____ 3. Excessively immature behavior: e.g. acts too young physically and/or emotionally, cries too much, has tantrums, sucks thumb, is physically poorly coordinated, masturbates, urinates in class, seeks too much attention
_____ 4. Excessively not working up to his ability: e.g. does not learn as well as your assessment of his ability indicates he is able to
_____ 5. Excessively restless: e.g. fidgets, is unable to sit still in classroom
_____ 6. Global rating of classroom adaptation: This is not a summary of the other behavior ratings but a general overall rating of the child's state of classroom behavior adaptation. However, if a child has been rated as maladapted in one of the classroom behavior categories, he should have a maladapted rating in the global category. If he has received a '0' in each of the boxes above he should have a '0' in this box.

*From Kellam, S. G., and others: Mental health and going to school, Chicago, 1975, University of Chicago Press.

stand and to help fulfill the physical and psychologic needs of their pupils. Therefore, if they recognize symptoms of mental or emotional disturbance in a child, they should initially examine their own activities in class or their relations with the pupil to determine whether they may be the cause of, or a factor contributing to, the behavior exhibited. It is conceivable that student maladjustments may be prevented by teachers modifying their activities or pupil relationships. The teacher may find it advisable to provide additional help to a child who is having difficulty in reading or to motivate the gifted student with additional responsibility. They may have to help pupils who have trouble controlling their emotions. Teachers may have to provide success experiences for a boy or girl. They may need to be friendlier with a pupil. They may have to try to gain acceptance of a child rejected by his peers. These are some of the considerations that teachers must make before determining that the problem is one needing referral to others.

Each school or school district determines its own procedures for counseling and guidance with much difference in nature and extent. The teacher usually has the responsibility for the observation of symptoms and the referral of the suspected deviant children to the school nurse, social workers, guidance counselor, school psychologist, or other appropriate school person. The nurse or counselor may be the intermediate person between the psychologist and the psychiatrist. The social workers, nurses, or counselors may have the responsibility for contacting the home. The psychologists and psychiatrists may also be expected to get in touch with parents. At what point and to what extent mothers and fathers become involved in the discussion, appraisals, and action is a matter that must be determined in each individual case and only after very careful analysis of the data.

In the community outside the school, the resources that are usually available to help mentally ill or emotionally disturbed children may include privately practicing psychologists and psychiatrists, child guidance clinics, general and mental hospitals with inpatient and outpatient care, youth agencies, associations for the physically handicapped, special schools, family service agencies, welfare agencies, and a variety of professional and voluntary organizations.* They offer services including diagnosis, treatment, transition, rehabilitation, education, information, and consultation. In several states, public health departments make available some or many of these services. The extent of community mental health services differs in school districts, with many of them being in short supply. Services for the poor are frequently inadequate. The cost for help may be part or full pay, depending on the need of the patient. Some organizations provide free services.

Individuals counseling or guiding children in schools must be familiar with the community resources providing mental health services. They will be better prepared to help refer children to the appropriate individual or agency and will be better able to guide parents who need assistance.

It is important that schools and the health personnel outside of the schools providing mental health services communicate with one another. The school has a great deal of information about problem students that would be useful to psychologists, psychiatrists, or child guidance clinics. By the same token, if the pupil's environment in school needs to be changed, or if he or she must receive special attention in the classroom, the child's needs can be understood better and given greater attention if the community experts make these needs known to the school. The schools and the community must work cooperatively if the best interests of the children are to be served adequately.

After problem children have been identified and are under care, it may be necessary to adjust the school program to their needs. This may be done by providing special services for disturbed children in the regular classroom with the help of extra or special teachers, by establishing special classes, by having special schools, or by making home instruction available.

Schools are beginning to segregate children with the more severe handicaps into special classes with specially trained teachers. Gary, Indiana, schools have several classes for children with severe emotional problems, with the local child guidance clinic supplying psychiatric supervision. In Chicago, classes are held for boys less than 12 years of age with normal intelligence and severe problems of truancy and classroom disorder. New York City has the "600" schools, also referred to as social adjustment schools, with the curriculum devised to fit the needs of the pupils. Classes are also being formed for brain-injured or brain-damaged pupils, hyperactive children, and those with perceptual difficulties who need medical supervision and who are educable. Many schools have special classes for the mentally retarded and the severely mentally retarded children. Some residential institutions for mentally ill children, especially those with severe emotional problems, are sending their pupils frequently to the local public schools. Other educational approaches include having a school in a psychiatric hospital, an entire school for narcotics, and programs of play therapy for younger children. In addition, there are now appearing so-called opportunity classes and schools for unsuccessful and emotionally disturbed pupils.

Instruction for children who are confined to their homes for psychiatric diagnosis and treatment is difficult. Many schools with home instruction programs do not provide for these children because teachers are seldom qualified for this assignment.

---

*Professional organizations include: American Academy of Child Psychiatry, American Association for Mental Deficiency, American Association of Psychiatry Services for Children, American Orthopsychiatric Association, American Psychiatric Association, American Psychological Association. Voluntary organizations include: National Association for Mental Health, Child Study Association of America, Council for Exceptional Children, National Society for Autistic Children, Inc., Al-Anon Family Group Headquarters and Alateen.

Healthful environment

Some teachers are great. . . . They put bandages on my hurts—on my heart, on my mind, on my spirit. Those teachers cared about me, and let me know it. They gave me wings.*

The single most important contribution to student mental health is the development of a wholesome emotional climate in the classroom. This atmosphere affects students' personal goals, their gaiety and depression; in fact the moods of the pupils in the room have great influence on all the students. What teachers say, do, and think has great significance on the patterns of behavior that are exhibited by students. Teachers have profound and lasting influences on children. The extent to which teachers can develop good human relationships with their pupils largely determines the extent to which a wholesome classroom atmosphere will exist. The setting in which children work together and are secure in the knowledge and feeling that they are accepted by the group and the teacher is what teachers should strive to achieve. This environment is influenced by teachers' preconceptions of pupils, concern with self, fear of witnessing emotion, values, biases, prejudices, and feelings of social class barriers.

The learning that takes place in school is affected by how people feel and believe, and what they value as well as how people treat each other. Teachers must be concerned with individuals and not just subject matter. There is a need to focus on the learner in the classroom. It is important not only to be merely concerned with what takes place in school, but also more importantly, to be concerned with what happens to students. An emphasis on humanism or humaneness must take place. Teachers must be concerned with justice, equality, friendship, tolerance, respect for the individual, self-expression, and decision making. These few suggestions should help to provide ways to achieve such a climate:

*McLeod, A.: Growing up in America; a background to contemporary drug abuse, Rockville, Md., 1973, National Institute of Mental Health.

1. Maximize individual learning through the recognition of individual differences.
2. Encourage and increase student involvement in the education process.
3. Provide a meaningful curriculum that satisfies the needs of students.
4. Provide opportunities for success experiences.
5. Permit freedom of expression in the classroom.
6. Listen to students in a nonjudgmental fashion.
7. Help students to assess their own value systems.
8. Make grades and grading procedures noncompetitive.
9. Aid young people to improve their abilities to cope with the complex world.
10. Aid young people to assume responsibility for own behavior.

The teacher who is interested in developing the best atmosphere must do the following:

1. Want to help children; establish a classroom environment free from fear and tensions; include an atmosphere of warmth and friendliness; aid in improvement of self-concept.
2. Believe that children are trying to do the best work possible.
3. Get acquainted with children and attempt to develop friendly relations: know their health and guidance records, be cheerful, let children talk, call students by name, talk with pupils, do not be shocked easily, provide warmth to the room by color and displays, using children to help.
4. Avoid ridicule, sarcasm, belittling remarks and help pupils to do likewise.
5. Accept the emotional problems of children and not condemn or reproach hostility; everyone gets angry sometime.
6. Understand the many factors that affect the mental health of children, including the family and the home, peer group relations, socioeconomic class, communications media, and the tensions of the times.
7. Be alert for indications of latent skills and interests and encourage pupils in their development.

8. Arouse interest in cultures and religions of all groups and accept pupils regardless of race, creed, or color.

Additional factors affecting the emotional climate in the classroom include the following:

1. Clarity and meaning of school activity
2. Excessive competition
3. Curriculum not adjusted to the needs of pupils
4. Uneven and unfair distribution of rewards and punishments; is the teacher always negative to some students?
5. Biases regarding students in terms of race, creed, color, or ability
6. Authoritarianism or permissive environment
7. Grades and their uniformity
8. Liberal use of praise and encouragement
9. Attainable goals within pupils' abilities

Anxieties and tensions are acquired and can quickly and easily become evident in class. The teacher can help to ease these conditions by being cognizant of the factors previously mentioned and also by providing relaxation outlets through music, art, drama, play, dance, or creative reading or writing.

Well-adjusted teachers are needed if the most wholesome emotional climate is to be found in the classroom. The teacher who suffers from anxiety and lack of self-confidence will communicate this to children. The teacher's personality is extremely important, since a maladjusted teacher is in a strategic position to do great harm to young people. It is estimated that mentally ill or maladjusted teachers are found in about the same proportion as in the general population—about 10%. One study reveals that 4% of teachers sampled in one school system were severely mentally ill. It has been stated that in the course of 12 elementary and high school years, a student will encounter two badly adjusted teachers. Teachers, therefore, need to give attention to their personal needs and to make adequate provision for sleep, rest, exercise, appropriate diet, and time for relaxation and need to maintain the highest level of health possible. The precursors of mental illness include prolonged stress, irritability, loss of sleep, withdrawal from social contacts, and somatic symptoms. Teachers should seek help when these symptoms appear.

The Gallup poll* reveals the following qualities desired in teachers:

1. Ability to communicate, to understand, to relate
2. Ability to discipline, be firm and fair
3. Ability to inspire, to motivate the child
4. High moral character
5. Love of children, concern for them
6. Dedication to teaching profession, enthusiasm
7. Friendly, good personality
8. Good personal appearance, cleanliness

Health instruction

The need for an educational program as part of the curriculum has been frequently mentioned as a means of promoting positive mental health and of preventing mental illness. Education can help pupils to understand themselves, their drives, their prejudices, their emotions, their ambitions, their growth and personality development, and their values as well as to help them learn how to get along with others, how to live in society, and how to be socially acceptable members of the world in which they live. Satisfaction that comes with self-esteem and self-concept leads to feelings of confidence, worth, strength, capability, and adequacy. Children who attain such attitudes are able to learn with increased interest, enthusiasm, and efficiency. In recent years, *death education* (see Chapters 9 and 11) has been introduced into curriculums to help pupils to be able to cope with losses and to better comprehend the meaningfulness of life.

Instruction should include both formal and informal programs (see Chapters 1 and 5). The suggested outline of content for mental health, the concepts that should receive consideration, and the objectives to be achieved through grade level groups in the formal

---

*Gallup, G. H.: Eighth annual Gallup poll of the public's attitudes toward the public schools, Phi Delta Kappan, **58:** Oct., 1976.

phase may be found in Chapter 9. They can be integrated into all phases of the curriculum, or specific units can be prepared and taught as part of health education using a variety of techniques (see Chapter 11).

Informally, mental health concepts and understandings of self can be learned and modified indirectly through interpersonal relations between teachers and pupils. The wholesome classroom atmosphere provides numerous opportunities for incidental teaching through informal discussion, counseling and guidance, and working with children in many ways. In addition, awareness groups can be convened voluntarily to permit students to express opinions and feelings on a variety of topics through verbal and other forms of communication.

Parent educational programs need consideration for inclusion in schools. Family understandings of children and youth needs and the need for communication are extremely important for positive mental health.

Coordination

The variety of phases of the school program in mental health discussed in this chapter must be coordinated if there is to be an effective program. The many segments are interrelated and must function harmoniously if the best program is to be arranged. There is need for satisfactory interaction among staff members, between parents and school personnel, and between the school and its community. Schools or school districts will need to delegate this coordinating responsibility to a director of guidance or special services, a physician, a psychologist, or someone at the administrative level if it is to be achieved.

It is common practice in schools to find a variety of people who are responsible for parts of the program rather than one person in charge of all segments. The mental health services may be handled by the director of guidance, a psychologist, or some other individual. In those schools where an instructional program exists, the responsibility for its construction and implementation may be delegated to the director of health, the direc-

tor of curriculum, or some such person. The environmental phase of the program usually has many people involved, with no one person specifically identified to administer it because of its complexity and diversity.

Some schools are now establishing advisory school mental health committees as one method of achieving coordination. Membership on this committee may include physicians, psychiatrists, psychologists, nurses, social workers, counselors, mental health association and health department personnel, teachers, and principals. There is need to relate school mental health programs with community mental health programs, pupil personnel services with school health services. Some of the problems this group might attempt to solve include the following:

1. Preparation of justification for the need for an administrative person to be responsible for the total mental health program
2. Development of policies and procedures to improve communications among the school, the home, and the community
3. Evaluation of the existing mental health program
4. Development of an instructional program
5. Improved identification of students with emotional disturbances
6. Better coordination between the schools and the community

SUMMARY

In summary, it can be stated that teachers' role in mental health is to understand and provide for the physical and psychologic needs of children, to be alert in their observations for symptoms of emotional disturbance, to refer problem pupils to the appropriate school authorities, to aid in the followup program for deviant students through counseling and guidance and the adjustment of the school program, to provide adequate and appropriate educational experiences for all pupils, to help provide particular educational experiences for special students, to develop a wholesome mental health classroom atmosphere, and to serve on an advisory school mental health committee on request.

QUESTIONS FOR DISCUSSION

1. What is the meaning of the term "mental health"?
2. What are the characteristics of a mentally healthy student?
3. What is the meaning of the term "mental illness"?
4. Why is mental illness a leading health problem in the United States?
5. What are the causes of mental illness?
6. What are the reasons that justify the school's concern for the mental health of pupils?
7. What should be the objectives of the school mental health program?
8. What should constitute an adequate school mental health program?
9. What kinds of mental health services should be included in the school program?
10. What are some of the procedures teachers may use to help locate children with emotional disturbances?
11. What might the school do to help children with mental health problems?
12. What can the teacher do to provide an emotional climate in the classroom that promotes good mental health?
13. What are the signs and symptoms that may lead to mental illness that teachers should be able to recognize?
14. What should the goals of the mental health instruction program include?
15. What might teachers do to be more humane in their dealing with pupils?
16. What can the schools do to better coordinate the segments of the mental health program?

SUGGESTED CLASS ACTIVITIES

1. Have students form buzz groups to discuss action to be taken with children who exhibit behavior such as always boisterous and rude, always quiet and withdrawn, very hard to reach, unable to get along with classmates.
2. Have a panel discussion of the needs of children and the characteristics of mentally healthy and mentally ill children.
3. Have a school psychiatrist discuss the nature of children's emotional problems.
4. Discuss the causes of mental illness.
5. Debate the issue "Should schools be concerned with the mental health of students?"
6. Survey one school or more to determine the nature of their mental health programs.
7. Have a school psychologist discuss the role of the teacher in identifying children with emotional disturbances.
8. Have the school counselor, nurse, or psychologist discuss the role of the school in helping students with mental health problems.
9. Discuss the role of the teacher in the mental health program.
10. Survey the community resources for mental health services for children.

11. Prepare reports on classes and schools for emotionally disturbed children.
12. Show a film illustrating student behavioral problems. Have the class attempt to determine teacher and school responsibilities.
13. Have students attempt to establish the ideal emotional classroom climate that the teacher might establish.
14. Visit a school to investigate the nature of the mental health instruction program.
15. Have students discuss the special attention that may be necessary for ghetto children and have them identify the rationale for same.
16. Prepare reports of the services community mental health resources make available to school children.

REFERENCES

Allinsmith, W., and Goethals, G. W.: The role of schools in mental health, New York, 1962, Basic Books, Inc. Publishers.

American Medical Association: Mental health and school health services, Chicago, 1965, The Association.

Association of State and Territorial Health Officers, Association of State and Territorial Mental Health Authorities, and Council of Chief State School Officers: Mental health in schools, Washington, D.C., 1966, The Council.

Association for Supervision and Curriculum Development: Learning and mental health in schools, Washington, D.C., 1966, yearbook, The Association.

Bernard, H. W.: Mental health in the classroom, New York, 1970, McGraw-Hill Book Co.

Burnes, A. J.: Laboratory instruction in the behavioral sciences in the grammar school. In Getz, B., editor: Behavioral sciences in the elementary grades, Second Annual Graduate Symposium, Cambridge, Mass., 1966, Lesley College.

Canfield, J., and Wells, H. C.: One-hundred ways to enhance self-concept in the classroom, Englewood Cliffs, N.J., 1976, Prentice-Hall, Inc.

Caplan, G.: Types of mental health consultation, American Journal of Orthopsychiatry **33:** April, 1963.

Charles, C. M.: Individualizing instruction, St. Louis, 1976, The C. V. Mosby Co.

Cornacchia, H. J., Smith, D. E., and Bentel, D. J.: Drugs in the classroom; a conceptual model for school programs, ed. 2, St. Louis, 1978, The C. V. Mosby Co.

Cowen, E. L., and others: A preventive mental health program in the school setting; description and evaluation, Journal of Psychology **56:** Oct. 1963.

Cowen, E. L., and others: Emergent approaches to mental health problems, New York, 1967, Appleton-Century-Crofts.

Crow, L., and Crow, A.: Mental hygiene for teachers, New York, 1963, Macmillan Publishing Co.

Cummings, S.: An appraisal of some recent evidence dealing with the mental health of black children and adolescents and its implications for school psychologists and guidance counselors, Psychology in the Schools **12:** April, 1975.

Deutsch, A., editor: Encyclopedia of mental health, vol. 5, New York, 1961, Franklin Watts, Inc.

Fishtein, R.: Classroom psychology, Brookly, 1973, Book-Lab, Inc.

Gallup, G. H.: Eighth annual Gallup poll of the public's attitudes toward the public schools, Phi Delta Kappan **58:** Oct., 1976.

Glasser, W.: Mental health or mental illness? New York, 1960, Harper & Row, Publishers, Inc.

Greenberger, E., and others: The measurement and structure of psychosocial maturity, Journal of Youth and Adolescence **4:** June, 1975.

Guinn, R.: Promoting mental health in the bicultural classroom, Health Education **8:** May/June, 1977.

Harris, C. W., editor: Encyclopedia of educational research, ed. 4, New York, 1969, Macmillan, Inc.

Klagsburn, F.: Preventing teenage suicide, Family Health/Today's Health **9:** April, 1977.

Martin, L.: Mental health/mental illness, New York, 1970, McGraw-Hill Book Co.

National Health Education Committee: Facts on major killing and crippling diseases in the United States today, New York, 1971, The Committee.

National Institute of Mental Health: Mental health of children, PHS 1396, Washington, D.C., 1965, Superintendent of Documents.

National Society for the Study of Education: Mental health in modern education, Fifty-fourth yearbook, Part II, Chicago, 1955, University of Chicago Press.

Reinert, H. R.: Children in conflict, St. Louis, 1976, The C. V. Mosby Co.

Report of the Committee on Mental Health in the Class-

room, American School Health Association: Mental health in the classroom, revised, Journal of School Health **38:** May, 1968.

Report of Task Force VI and excerpts from the Report of the Committee on Children of Minority Groups by the Joint Commission on Mental Health of Children: Social change and the mental health of children, New York, 1973, Harper & Row, Publishers, Inc.

Report of Task Forces IV and V and the Report of the Committee on Clinical Issues by the Joint Commission on Mental Health of Children, The mental health of children; services, research, and manpower, New York, 1973, Harper & Row, Publishers, Inc.

Rogers, D.: Mental hygiene in elementary education, Boston, 1957, Houghton Mifflin Co.

Schulman, J. L., and others: Mental health in schools, Elementary School Journal **74:** Oct., 1973.

Smith, D. F.: Adolescent suicide; a problem for teachers, Phi Delta Kappan **57:** April, 1976.

Stickney, S. B.: Schools are our community mental health centers, American Journal of Psychiatry **124:** April, 1968.

ten Bensel, R. W., and Berkie, J.: The neglect and abuse of children and youth; the scope of the problem and the school's role, Journal of School Health **46:** Oct., 1976.

U.S. Department of Health, Education, and Welfare: The protection and promotion of mental health in schools, PHS mental health monograph 5, Washington, D.C., 1964, Superintendent of Documents.

Zolcynski, S. J., and McKee, J. M.: The development of a student mental health record, Journal of School Health **32:** June, 1962.

PART FOUR

Health education

8 Health education today

Health education today in America's schools is on the threshold of growth and emphasis not unlike that of science education in the 1960s. More and more states, such as New York, Florida, Texas, New Mexico, Tennessee, Virginia, Arkansas, Oregon, Illinois, Hawaii, New Jersey, Michigan, Maine, South Carolina, Nebraska, and Maryland, have mandated *comprehensive* health education in the state's public elementary schools. The trend continues and indicates that in the not too distant future all fifty states will follow with legislative or state board of education decisions requiring specified time in the curriculum for health instruction. It is important that these mandates are for a comprehensive curriculum in health education, not just the fragmented "crisis" areas of drug education, smoking and health, and alcohol education. Yet in some states failure to also allocate adequate funds has tended to slow down maximum implementation of statewide programs of quality health education.

Elementary school health education is not without support from allied professional groups. A most significant position paper, *Education for Health in the School Community Setting,* was adopted by the Governing Council of the American Public Health Association on October 23, 1974 at its annual meeting in New Orleans. In part this major exposition of the Association's viewpoint held that*:

The school is a community in which most individuals spend at least twelve years of their lives . . . the health of our school-age youth will determine to a great extent the quality of life each will have during the growing and developing years and on throughout the life cycle.

The American Public Health Association supports the concept of a national commitment to a comprehensive, sequential program of health education for all students in the nation's schools, kindergarten through the twelfth grade. The Association will exert leadership through its sections and affiliates to assure for health education:

1. Time in the curriculum commensurate with other subject areas.
2. Professionally qualified teachers and supervisors of health education.
3. Innovative instructional materials and appropriate teaching facilities.
4. Increased financial support at the local, state, and national levels to upgrade the quantity and quality of health education.
5. A teaching/learning environment in which opportunities for safe and optimal living exist, and one in which a well-organized and complete health service is functioning.

In an earlier classic report the National Commission on Community Health Services —comprised of many national authorities in the health field—had this to say about the importance of health education in our schools*:

This nation is currently concerned with the improvement of all kinds of education for all kinds of people. It is imperative that, while bringing the three "R's" to more people, education about the big "H"—health—be included in our new plans for learning.

Health education must become a fundamental part of the basic, balanced curriculum; it can be effectively taught in school, and *no other public agency today offers health instruction to children of school age*. State Departments of Education and local school boards should assume greater responsibility for the development of health curriculums.

---

*From American Public Health Association, School Health Section: Position paper; education for health in the community setting, Washington, D.C., 1975, American Public Health Association.

*From the National Commission on Community Health Services: Health is a community affair, Cambridge, Mass., 1966, Harvard University Press.

THE CURRICULUM

The heart and soul of education is the curriculum. When all is said and done about methods, techniques, materials, supervision, evaluation, and administration, we return to the road of values, the curriculum. The elementary school curriculum is the hub of the entire process of educating children.

The modern interpretation of the term "curriculum" includes all of the educational experiences that children have in school. This broad concept of curriculum goes beyond the boundaries of subject content or courses of study. It recognizes and provides for a variety of valuable learning activities that take place outside of the classroom routine. Yet, few would seriously question the view that subject matter—*what* we teach—is the basic ingredient of the curriculum. Most of the educational outcomes and values we seek depend on the development of understanding, attitudes, skills, and behavior patterns associated with the learning of subject matter.

In recent years health education has become more and more accepted as one of the essential subjects in the elementary school curriculum. The curriculum content areas that are to be found in the better elementary schools across the nation include *language arts, social studies, arithmetic, science, health and safety, music, art,* and *physical education,* each of which has a significant place in the general education of elementary pupils. Regardless of a child's present or future role in our society, the child will find that these areas of learning provide the basis for a happy, useful life.

WHY IS HEALTH EDUCATION NEEDED?

Time is of the essence in our modern elementary schools. We cannot possibly teach everything; hence, what we teach should prepare the child for the highest quality of living in a free democratic society. We must provide those learning experiences that will enable pupils to appreciate and benefit from the good found in our culture. At the same time we must help pupils to avoid or overcome problems and defects in our society that tend to limit the quality of living.

In today's space age we are constantly influenced by social, political, economic, and technologic developments that occur with the speed of figures moving through an old-time newsreel. With progress we conquer some old problems and create some new ones. Yet, in many instances the age-old beliefs and superstitions persist. People and their motives remain fairly constant.

Recognizing then that the health needs of children and adults represent a unique combination of the old and the new, let us look at some of the major factors and trends that point out the urgent need for health teaching in our elementary schools.

Acceleration of research in health sciences

It is rather common knowledge that scientific inquiry in the fields of medicine, dentistry, public health, nutrition, biochemistry, basic biology, genetics and heredity, physiology, anthropology, psychology, pharmacology, biophysics, and other health sciences has progressed with rapidity and vigor. As a result, the storehouse of human knowledge in these disciplines increases with each passing day. For the layman to be able to understand and appreciate new developments in the health sciences, some knowledge of the fundamental concepts of healthful living is necessary. Health teaching must prepare children not only to be informed of the advances in health science, but also to know enough about these advances to accurately evaluate and appraise them in terms of their application to daily living.

Increase in health information

Partly as a result of intensified health research and partly as a reflection of the aroused interest of the "man in the street" in health problems, there has been a sharp growth in amounts of space and time given to health and safety in newspapers, magazines, radio broadcasts, and television programs. Some of this information is scientifically accurate, some is premature and only partially established, some is misleading, and some is outright falsehood. A background of basic learning experiences in health and safety is essential to intelligent analysis and interpretation of information and opinion released through public media.

More aggressive advertising of health products and services

Health services and products, as well as those that have implications for health (for example, cigarettes, liquor, sports cars) today are big business. Modern advertising, getting its cues from research in motivational psychology, is highly effective in persuading people to buy these products and services. The trend is distinctly away from the hard sell of the past, the blatant cure-all appeal. Instead, copywriters often base their material on sound health principles. At some point in the written or verbal appeal there is a subtle departure from scientific truth. The application favoring a certain product or service is frequently unsound. Advertising copy is flavored with such impressive words as "research," "science," "laboratory," "doctors," and "clinical." Even the more literate of our population are influenced by the siren song of the huckster—a combination of dramatic pseudoscience, status symbolism, and emotion. The chances of impairment of health, budget, or both, are substantially lessened when people have the background of health education necessary to intelligent, objective analysis of such advertising. The need for a fundamental understanding of both the content and the method of health science is obvious. Clearly, this must begin in the elementary grades.

Citizenship and health

Citizenship has long been a primary concern of elementary schools. Today, people and their governments (local, state, and federal) are increasingly aware of and sensitive to problems in health and safety. The growing cost of local, state, national, and international legislation makes it necessary that the individual voter be able to comprehend all the implications of the issues to participate intelligently in the democratic process. In this respect the public is frequently called on to support pending legislation sponsored by medical groups, public health authorities, labor unions, and politicians concerned with the nation's health. Such questions as federal aid to medical education, compulsory health insurance to provide for the needs of older citizens, fluoridation of public water supplies, immunization requirements for school children, required tuberculin tests or chest x-ray examinations for government employees (including teachers and school staff), increased taxes for official health departments, and the role of the voluntary health agency in our society demand an informed citizenry on health matters. To appraise intelligently and to decide on candidates, platforms, referenda, and campaigns involving public health issues, the voting citizen of today and tomorrow must understand the basic principles of safe and healthful living.

Remaining health problems

Despite marked progress against most of the infectious diseases the status of health in America is not what it should or could be. We know, for example, that more than a quarter of a million people lose their lives each year as a result of cancer and leukemia. Medical science is able to save one patient in three; yet with early treatment the cure rate could be one out of two.

Almost a million Americans die every year of heart disease, circulatory disorders, and related kidney conditions. Many of these would be alive today if certain known principles of healthful living could be put into practice. One person in ten in the United States is presently in need of professional help for emotional disturbance; yet only one in nine of these people is under treatment.

Accidents continue to take their toll each year to the extent of wiping out enough men, women, and children to populate the combined cities of Mount Vernon, New York, and Beverly Hills, California. Major advances have been made in reducing infant mortality in this country; however, we still lose more than 50,000 infants annually before they see their first birthday.

The surveys tell us that some 20% to 25% of our population is not covered by any kind of health insurance. Most of these are people in the aged and low-income groups. Millions of Americans do not have access to adequate public health services, and the production of new physicians continues to fall behind the needs of a bulging population.

In the face of markedly improved treatment by antibiotics, the venereal disease rate continues to be high, although there was a leveling off in 1977. Although the death rate for tuberculosis has dropped sharply in the past 20 years, the incidence of new cases has not shown a comparable decline.

Some seven to ten million alcoholics continue to make up 10% of all cases of mental illness and, combined with social drinkers, contribute to some 50% to 60% of motor vehicle accident fatalities. In the midst of agricultural and economic plenty the nutritional status of American children and adults is unbelievably bad; dietary studies show with alarming consistency that only one child in three is getting an optimally nutritious diet, one in three a barely adequate diet, and one in three a frankly poor diet. Research also indicates that children's diets become poorer as they grow into adolescence. Reporting a major study of a large sample of American families, the U.S. Department of Agriculture recently announced that approximately one half of our population is not getting a proper diet.

While Americans often fail to eat a well-balanced diet, they apparently do not stint on calories. This living on fat and starch has produced some 55 million overweight people in this country. Physicians agree that many cases of adult obesity begin in childhood.

The incidence of infectious hepatitis, a virus infection of the liver, continues to rise alarmingly. This hand-to-mouth disease now ranks high among all reportable communicable diseases and affects some 60,000 persons each year. Although death seldom results from infectious hepatitis, recovery takes at least 6 weeks and often much longer.

The status of the nation's dental health is deplorably low, with greater than 98% of the population suffering from dental defects, and the problem of tooth decay in the elementary grades is particularly serious.

The problem of use and abuse of drugs continues to be a critical one. Marijuana, LSD, amphetamines, tranquilizers, barbiturates, tobacco, alcohol, PCP (or "angel dust"), and cocaine are the more common substances used. Elementary pupils have shown a growing interest in and desire for information about a variety of drugs, and children at this level have been experimenting with drugs that just a few years ago were only a problem at the secondary school level.

To make any real progress against these and other health problems, we must bridge the gap between what is known about prevention and treatment and what is done by people to preserve health. To accomplish this we must have a citizenry that understands, appreciates, and practices the best principles of healthful living. The task for our elementary schools is obvious.

Selection of health services

Closely related to the fundamental problem of reducing the distance between available knowledge and how people behave in health matters is the problem of preparing people to utilize health services intelligently. Millions of people in communities throughout the United States are not aware of the kind or extent of health services available. Furthermore, a great many people who are somewhat aware of available health services are reluctant to take advantage of them because of a lack of knowledge and understanding concerning the role of such services in protecting and improving personal and family health. One of the basic units in health education, even at the primary grade level, is concerned with health specialists and facilities in the community.

Tendency toward health neuroses

It is now generally recognized that there is a tendency for both children and adults to become overconcerned about their health. The ever-growing number of people in this category points to another need for health education, a need for considerable emphasis on the proper kind of health education. Experience shows that the number of children who become overconcerned and neurotic about their health increases almost in direct proportion to the amount and extent of unorganized and haphazard health teaching to which they are exposed. The need here for a planned, progressive curriculum in elementary school health education is abundantly clear.

Gullibility of the public. Each year the American people spend billions of dollars on thousands of questionable health products and services. About a billion dollars is spent annually by people who are hopefully trying to lose excess fat; the results are at best disappointing, at worst harmful. The money goes for reducing salon memberships, drugs, appetite depressants, diet formulas, and similar gimmicks. The common cold, which defies the efforts of our best medical researchers to develop a vaccine or an effective treatment, results in Americans spending more than $750 million each year for remedies that are generally worthless. Both dollars and lives are lost every year by people who patronize quack "doctors" for treatments for cancer and other serious diseases. Medical authorities agree that a health-educated public is the best defense against the sale of useless, dangerous products and services.

The relationship between emotions and physical health

Although it has been vaguely known for centuries that there is a close relationship between emotional and physical health, limited use has been made of this knowledge in the maintenance of optimum health.

As a result of study and research in recent years, there is now a better understanding of the relationship of the emotions to the maintenance of good health. Rapid developments in psychosomatic medicine bring to light one of the main reasons it is so difficult for the individual to maintain optimum health under the stresses, strains, and tensions of present-

day life. The social, economic, and geographic mobility of our contemporary society has its effect on the emotional health and development of many elementary school children. The fact that 70% of our population is concentrated in 1% of the nation's land mass means that most elementary school children cannot escape the emotional stresses of urban and suburban living. The economic, social, marital, and occupational stresses of suburbia are sure to rub off on some of the children.*

It is known that a host of physical disorders are psychogenic in origin; that is, they are basically caused and brought on by the emotions. Further, most illnesses that are physical in origin become highly complicated by the emotions to the point where recovery is greatly impeded.

Specialists skilled in the science of psychosomatic medicine state that the more knowledge and understanding the individual has about the close relationship between emotional and physical health, the easier it is to maintain good health, and the easier it is to help the child or the adult to recover following a physical disorder brought on by the emotions.†

Health and safety misconceptions

Nowhere does the observer find more urgent reasons for health education in the elementary schools than in the research on misconceptions in health and safety. Studies in the areas of health misconceptions clearly show that both pupils and teachers hold many serious misconceptions about health and safety.

THE SCHOOL HEALTH EDUCATION STUDY

The School Health Education Study‡— a classic effort directed by Dr. Elena Sliep-

---

*Gordon, R. E., Gordon, K. K., and Gunther, M.: The split-level trap, New York, 1962, Dell Publishing Co.
†Dunbar, F.: Psychosomatic medicine, New York, 1955, Random House, Inc.
‡Sliepcevich, E. M.: School health education study; a summary report, Washington, D.C., 1964, School Health Education Study.

cevich—showed, with shocking clarity, the inadequacy of health instruction in elementary schools across the land. This investigation, begun in 1961 under a grant from the Samuel Bronfman Foundation of New York City, included more than 1,100 elementary schools spread over 38 states, with a total enrollment of more than half a million pupils. On the basis of tests given to sixth-grade children, it was found that only one pupil in five brushed his teeth or rinsed his mouth after eating, nine pupils in ten tended to repress unhappy feelings, and many scored poorly in safety. Pupils did best in the areas of exercise, sleep, and relaxation; cleanliness and body care; and nutrition. They demonstrated marked lack of understanding in the areas of dental health, mental health, and safety education.

The report urged that emphasis be given to the following topics that currently appear to be neglected:

1. Alcohol education
2. Community health programs
3. Consumer health education
4. Environmental hazards
5. Health careers
6. International health activities
7. Nutrition and weight control
8. Sex education, family life, parenthood, and child care
9. Smoking
10. Veneral disease education

Obviously, this is not a complete list of topics for elementary school health teaching. However, these areas were singled out for increased emphasis and, in some instances, earlier grade placement.

WHAT ARE THE ADMINISTRATIVE PROBLEMS?

Much impetus for the inclusion of health education in elementary schools has taken place in recent years. Numerous schools and school districts have added to and improved their health education programs. However, much remains to be done because many uninformed school administrators and school board members are giving little or no attention to the subject field, while others are conducting inadequate and ineffective programs. Elementary schools today face a variety of administrative problems that interfere with the inclusion and development of health instruction programs. Some of these problems include grade placement, time in the curriculum, how and where to include health education in the curriculum, use of current methods of teaching, provision for adequate teaching and learning aids, responsibility for the program including administrative role, finances, in-service preparation of teachers and other personnel, and parent education.

Essential to a quality school health program is the establishment and specific statement of policies by the central school administration. School health policies must not only keep abreast of new developments and nationally recognized authoritative recommendations, but they must be clearly stated in writing for school administrators, teachers, parents, school boards, school nurses, nonprofessional school employees, and health professionals in the community.

A recent survey by Henry A. Lasch of New Mexico State University disclosed wide disparity in the content and mode of publicizing school health policies. From this study of 144 public school districts in 46 states it seems clear that many school systems have not given proper priority to establishing, putting in writing, and disseminating sound policies for effective school health programs. The study makes it obvious that there is a pressing need for improved public relations within the school system, as well as throughout the community, regarding the philosophy, aims, and activities of school health instruction, health services and guidance, and healthful school environment. Lasch concludes that the following points should be adopted as standard practice*:

1. School health policies should be in writing so that fair and consistent decisions will be assured.
2. Policies should be publicized or at least made available upon request.

---

*Lasch, H. A.: A study of health policies in public school administration, Journal of School Health, April, 1976.

3. The schools should make it known to students, school personnel, parents, and community groups that administrative decisions are governed by a definite set of policies, procedures, and regulations.
4. Existing policies should provide the basis for decisions until such time as it is deemed necessary to change or discontinue a policy.
5. Democratic procedures must be followed whenever policies are added, deleted, or revised.

What about grade placement?

The problem of planning an orderly sequence of topics or units in health and safety throughout the elementary grades is not an easy one. Much has been said and written by health educators about the danger of overlapping and repetitious subject matter from one grade to another. Certainly, without proper planning and intergrade coordination, needless repetition of the same health and safety concepts will surely stifle pupil interest and motivation. When this happens, pupils quickly become bored, irritated, and often develop negative attitudes toward safe and healthful behavior. Yet again, as with curriculum organization, the issue boils down to this: do we stress subject matter or the developmental needs of children?

If the greater emphasis is placed on logical organization of subject matter, then a specific sequence of health units is decided on and followed. One successful method of organizing subject matter is the cycle plan. Under this plan learning experiences concentrate on selected health and safety units at 3-year intervals from grades 4 through 12. Originally, the four-cycle plan covered the total 12 school years. However, experience showed that a wide diversity of health units should be provided for in grades 1, 2, and 3 rather than stressing selected units. Thus, most schools now following the cycle plan begin with the fourth grade. For example, community health and sanitation receive special emphasis in grades 6 and 8 of the elementary school, nutrition is stressed in grades 5 and 7, and so with the other basic areas of instruction. All units are covered to some extent in each of the primary grades. The cycle plan is generally based on areas such as the following:

> Your body and how it works
> Nutrition and you
> Mental health and your personality
> You and your family
> Your skin, hair, and teeth
> Balancing exercise, play, and rest
> Alcohol, tobacco, and other drugs
> Choosing health services and products
> Control of diseases
> Your vision and hearing
> Living in a safe and healthy community

Perhaps the chief advantages of the cycle plan are these: (1) it minimizes undesirable duplication of subject matter and (2) it helps ensure continuity of learning experiences and comprehensive coverage of health and safety concepts. There are, however, two possible drawbacks: (1) it is both difficult and undesirable to formularize the health and safety needs of children grade by grade (for example, who is to say that nutrition is more crucially important to fifth graders than to fourth or sixth graders?) and (2) pupil sharing in setting goals and planning activities is somewhat limited.

Some elementary schools follow the year-to-year plan from kindergarten through the sixth or eighth grade (depending on local school organization), with attention given each year to learning experiences in most of the major areas. Thus, such topics as nutrition, rest, exercise, and physical fitness, safety, mental health, dental hygiene, alcohol and other drugs, tobacco, and control of diseases may be part of the content at every grade level.

Under this year-to-year plan, learning experiences are organized so that children will develop understandings and appreciations in a wide range of health and safety topics. The problem of overlapping, although always a possibility, can usually be avoided by adapting content to the developmental needs, interests, concerns, purposes, and learning capacity of boys and girls in each grade. For instance, in the primary grades (K, 1, 2, 3) emphasis is placed on developing desirable habits and attitudes in many aspects of safe and healthful living. Learning activities are, of necessity, brief and quite specific in terms of the child's world, and the approach is geared largely to the personal problems of the child.

At the intermediate grade level more thorough study of basic concepts is possible, and broader generalizations can be developed. Scientific explanations in depth are increasingly brought into the scheme of learning experiences to undergird the desired attitudes and practices. In the upper grades still further gains are made in pupil understanding of scientific data and method in health and safety. Pupil inquiry and problem solving are increasingly emphasized as the child advances through the grades.

Throughout all of this planned progression from grade to grade two essentials must be recognized: (1) teachers must be familiar with learning experiences in grades other than their own to assure continuity and to avoid unnecessary duplication or serious omission of content and (2) subject matter within a basic area must be appropriate to the major needs, concerns, and goals of boys and girls at their current developmental level. For example, the fifth-grade teacher who knows that children have studied about the four basic food groups in grade 4 is able to make the most of this previous learning by providing new experiences in wise choice of diet based on what is already known about the essential food groups. Some transitional overlapping here is not only necessary but also highly desirable in following the thread of continuity.

To illustrate the importance of aligning unit content at a given grade with the chief problems of pupils at that level, the area of safety provides a good example. Traffic safety, one of the most important aspects of safety education, should be included in the teaching at every grade level. Yet traffic safety has different meanings and implications at different grade levels. For the kindergarten or first-grade child traffic safety

means walking and crossing safely, understanding the value of seat belts in the family car, and behaving safely on the school bus. For the second or third grader safe cycling assumes new significance in light of the child's increasingly wider range of bike riding in the community. For the fifth or sixth grader traffic safety takes on a broader application with relation to licensing, social responsibility of auto manufacturers, state and federal highway construction, law enforcement, alcohol and traffic accidents, and motor vehicle legislation.

What about time allotment?

We really have very little research to justify our decisions on the length of class, or subject, periods in the elementary school. However, adequate time must be allotted for health education in the total school program. Authoritative recommendations, state and local proposed schedules, and the observations and experiences of individual teachers generally indicate that about 15 minutes daily is best in the primary grades, 25 to 30 minutes in the intermediate grades, and 30 to 35 minutes in grades 7 and 8. Of course, teachers will adjust time allotment to suit their pupils, the degree of difficulty of a unit of study, the interest of the class in a particular topic, and the materials and facilities including community resources available. What, then, can we say about time allotment that will serve the teacher as a sound guide? Briefly and concisely, this: *the time provided for health teaching at any grade level should be roughly equivalent to that given to any other basic subject or area of learning in the elementary school curriculum.*

How can health and safety be included in the elementary school curriculum?

Here we are concerned with the formal aspects of health education. This refers to the typical learning activities that take place in the classroom. Earlier we considered the informal approach to health education through health counseling and guidance (see Chapter 5).

To best fit health into the curriculum, we

must first know the prevailing plan in a given school. However, at the elementary level, health education should include both *integrative* and *direct* patterns of instruction. Education for health must receive specific time in the curriculum, just as social studies, science, language arts, arithmetic, and other areas, and must be identified as a distinct and specialized subject.

Integrative teaching. Numerous opportunities exist for correlating health with other subject fields. It may be related to *social studies* (for example, community health agencies, organizations, and personnel—doctors, nurses, dentists); *arithmetic* (for example, add, subtract, and multiply apples and oranges, determine the cost of a week's supply of cigarettes); *science* (for example, structure and function of the eye, ear, muscles, and other body organs); *language arts* (for example, show and tell about dental visit, prepare experience chart on use of milk, write story entitled "Who am I?"); *physical education* (for example, safety on apparatus and playground, exercise and health); *art* (for example, graphs, charts, murals, dioramas); and *music* (for example, compose lyrics about safety, nutrition, and other health areas).

Two important problems arise in using the integrative pattern of instruction. First, there may be a tendency for the teacher to fail to place proper emphasis on the health behavioral objectives desired. This leads to the second problem, which is the misplaced stress on the mere acquisition of factual data and information by pupils. For example, when teachers provide a reading lesson on nutrition in a health textbook, they may falsely assume that they are getting children to eat the proper foods. Yet this may be simply exposing children to understandings about foods needed for a healthful diet without motivating pupils to actually improve their eating habits.

Direct teaching. Direct teaching of health and safety in the elementary school calls for (1) specific time allotment comparable to that provided for other subjects, (2) teachers who know what and how to teach about health and safety, (3) up-to-date textbooks and other materials, (4) a syllabus or course outline, and (5) appropriate credit for pupil progress in health and safety within the framework of the school's grading system.

Direct teaching follows the age-old practice of compartmentalizing human knowledge and behavior into well-defined subject areas. Although from time to time some criticism has been leveled at direct teaching in health and safety, experience has shown that when properly conducted, this approach can be an effective one. It is true that health education is especially concerned with attitudinal and behavioral outcomes, but these learning products cannot be effectively achieved without a firm basis of knowledge. Direct teaching, with its provision for logical and coordinated arrangement of subject matter, tends to assure that understandings, attitudes, and practices will be best developed by pupils. Of course, favorable results depend upon sound teaching methods and the use of learning materials that are scientifically accurate, up to date, and motivating.

What teaching methods and materials should be used?

For teachers to emphasize attitudinal and behavioral changes, it will be necessary to utilize a variety of teaching techniques that actively involve students in a variety of ways. Chapters 10 and 11 provide details regarding principles of learning, methods, and specific teaching techniques. The traditional procedures in use that focus on cognitive learning generally do little more than place emphasis on knowledge and regurgitation of subject matter in health education.

Schools should provide an adequate supply of films, filmstrips, books, models, and pamphlets for teachers. The nature of such materials and their sources can be found in Chapter 12.

Who is responsible for the health education program?

A variety of persons must be involved in the health instruction program, including teachers, nurses, and administrators.

The *role of teachers* has previously been

discussed in Chapter 2. However, preservice preparation through course work and experiences where possible should be provided. In addition, while on the job, teachers will continually need to be reading journal articles and books, attending college courses, and participating in a variety of activities to keep up to date with current information in health education and the health sciences.

Often overlooked by teachers and administrators is the important contribution to be made by the *school nurse* to the elementary school health instructional program. Although we tend to think primarily of the nurse's functions in the health service activities as those of inspecting pupils referred with symptoms of illness, administering first aid, advising teachers about pupil health defects, maintaining pupil records of accidents and illnesses, advising parents of pupil health problems and encouraging appropriate treatment, giving screening tests, and referring parents and pupils to appropriate health specialists or agencies in the community, the school nurse is usually capable of playing a major role in health education.

Here are some of the ways school nurses contribute to elementary school health education:

1. Helping teachers with materials and aids for health units
2. Helping teachers plan the health curriculum
3. Serving as a member of the school health council
4. Assisting in the selection of health textbooks and other materials for health instruction
5. Serving as a consultant and advisor to the teacher
6. Helping teachers relate health instruction to the pupil health problems
7. Helping to prepare pupils for medical examinations and screening tests
8. Assisting in the teaching of units on first aid and home nursing
9. Helping teachers arrange for health specialists in the community to come to the school and speak to classes on health problems

Of course, nurses differ somewhat in their professional education and experience, but most school nurses have much to offer classroom teachers in helping them to do a better job of health education in the classroom. Classroom teachers should not overlook this valuable source of information and assistance.

A serious omission in many schools and especially in school districts is a lack of individuals with *administrative responsibility* to stimulate, develop, and improve health instruction programs. Without such persons the chances of programs emerging or continuing in schools are remote. One solution to this problem is for more colleges to require students majoring in school administration to complete at least one course in school health education.

What about financing?

As in all educational programs there must be adequate financial support for health education. Funds must be budgeted and made available for supervisory personnel (health coordinator), teacher salaries, up-to-date textbooks, and other teaching and learning materials.

What provisions are made for in-service preparation of school personnel?

To encourage teachers, school nurses, and health coordinators to keep abreast of new developments in health education, planned in-service preparation must be provided. New teachers to the system must also receive orientation regarding their responsibilities in health instruction. Without such motivation and updated information, teachers and other personnel cannot provide effective and stimulating health education programs.

What about parent education?

The question often is raised as to why it is so extremely difficult to get a large majority of elementary pupils to form the proper and correct health habits. On first consideration it would seem that with proper emphasis and motivation during teaching, a majority of the children may form the correct practices al-

most at once. One main reason it is so difficult for the teacher to get immediate results
is that a large part of her teaching is dissi-
pated when the children mingle in adult society. The children come in contact with
adults who fail to observe even the most fundamental health practices. The example set
by adults tends to minimize the importance
and the need for proper health habits in the
minds of children. Too, the home conditions
of some children are such that it is next to
impossible to follow the teachings of healthful living.

While parent education is far from easy
to make operational, it can be done through
planning and concerted effort. Formal education of parents can be accomplished
through lectures, films, group discussions,
and other programs arranged specifically for
parents. Such programs should deal with the
more critical and realistic problems of pupils
and the community.

Perhaps the most effective way of reaching parents is through informal education,
through counseling and guidance. This method must be given considerably much more
attention than schools have been willing to
do previously. Such programs may take the
form of teacher-parent and nurse-parent conferences, communication between parents
and school administrators, newspaper articles, radio and television presentations, and
other public relations techniques.

SUMMARY

All in all, then, health and safety education must be considered an essential and
vital part of the total curriculum of our
modern elementary schools. As we recognize
the challenge to sound elementary curriculums in this age of the astronaut, we can
look forward with measured confidence to
the continued increase in teacher time and
effort devoted to the pupil needs for safe and
healthful living in an increasingly complex
society.

QUESTIONS FOR DISCUSSION

1. What evidence is there to substantiate the increasing need for health teaching in elementary schools?
2. What are the essential administrative problems con-
   fronting health education in elementary schools
   today?
3. What are the ways in which health education can be
   included in the elementary curriculum?
4. What can the schools do to educate parents regarding the health of their children?
5. What considerations must be given in making decisions about the grade placement for health instruction?
6. What factors influence time allotment for health
   education in the elementary grades?
7. What are the major advantages and disadvantages of
   the cycle plan of health teaching?
8. What are the major advantages and disadvantages of
   the progressively graded year-to-year plan of health
   instruction?
9. What are some arguments for and against the *direct*
   approach to health teaching?
10. What are some arguments for and against teaching
    health through *integration?*
11. How can the school nurse help the classroom
    teacher in health instruction?

SUGGESTED CLASS ACTIVITIES

1. Analyze your own elementary school situation or one
   that is well known to you, and prepare a list of problems that indicate a need for health teaching.
2. Select a school that is well known to you. List the factors in that school that are conducive to sound health
   curriculum and teaching and those that are not.
3. Conduct a panel discussion and debate the relative
   merits of health teaching by the direct approach and
   by integration.
4. Conduct a panel discussion and debate the relative
   merits of the cycle plan and the year-to-year plan for
   grade placement of units in health and safety.

REFERENCES

American Academy of Pediatrics: School health; a guide
for health professionals, Evanston, Ill., 1977, The
Academy.
American Alliance for Health, Physical Education, and
Recreation Committee: Needed improvements in ele-
mentary school health programs, Journal of Health,
Physical Education, and Recreation, Feb., 1967.
American Association of School Administrators: Curriculum handbook for school executives, Washing-
ton, D.C., 1973, The Association.
American Public Health Association, School Health Sec-
tion: Education for health in the school community
setting, Washington, D.C., 1975, The Association.
Anderson, C. L., and Creswell, W. H.: School health
practice, St. Louis, 1976, The C. V. Mosby Co.
Byrd, O. E.: School health administration, Philadelphia, 1964, W. B. Saunders Co.
Cornacchia, H. J.: Elementary health education curriculum, Journal of Health, Physical Education, and
Recreation, April, 1958.

Culliton, B. J.: Preventive medicine; legislation calls for health education, Science, Sept. 26, 1975.

Don't teach us what you want to teach, teach us what we want to know, Journal of School Health, May, 1969.

Eisner, V., and Callan, L. B.: Dimensions of school health, Springfield, Ill., 1974, Charles C Thomas, Publisher.

Fodor, J. T., and Dalis, G. T.: Health instruction; theory and application, ed. 2, Philadelphia, 1974, Lea & Febiger.

Hill, P.: Health education needs of preschool and school age children, School Health Review, Sept.-Oct., 1972.

Joint Committee on Health Problems in Education: Why health education in your school? Washington, D.C. and Chicago, 1974, National Education Association and the American Medical Association.

Levin, H. M., editor: Community control of schools, New York, 1976, Simon and Schuster.

McGavran, E. G.: The role of primary prevention in public health, Health Education, July/Aug., 1977.

Metropolitan Life Insurance Company: Physical fitness tset; seven years experience, Statistical Bulletin, April, 1977.

Metropolitan Life Insurance Company: Longevity in the United States at a new high, Statistical Bulletin, May, 1977.

Miller, A. C.: Health care of children and youth in America, American Journal of Public Health, April, 1975.

National Commission on Community Health Services: Health is a community affair, Cambridge, Mass., 1966, Harvard University Press.

National Committee on School Health Policies: Suggested school health policies, ed. 4, Washington, D.C., 1966, National Education Association and the American Medical Association.

Nemir, A., and Schaller, W.: The school health program, Philadelphia, 1975, W. B. Saunders Co.

Pollock, M. B., and Oberteuffer, D.: Health science and the young child, New York, 1974, Harper & Row, Publishers, Inc.

Read, D. A., and Greene, W. H.: Creative teaching in health, New York, 1975, Macmillan, Inc.

Read, D. A., Simon, S. B., and Goodman, J. B.: Health education; the search for values, Englewood Cliffs, N.J., 1977, Prentice-Hall, Inc.

Russell, R. D.: Health education, Washington, D.C., 1975, Joint Committee on Health Problems in Education of the National Education Association and the American Medical Association (available from the American Alliance for Health, Physical Education, and Recreation, Washington, D.C.).

Sliepcevich, E. M.: School health education study; a summary report, Washington, D.C., 1964, School Health Education Study.

Sliepcevich, E. M.: Curriculum development; a macroscopic or microscopic view? The National Elementary Principal, Nov., 1968.

Why teachers are under fire, U.S. News & World Report, Dec. 12, 1977.

Willgoose, C. E.: Health education in the elementary school, Philadelphia, 1974, W. B. Saunders Co.

9 Organizing for health teaching

There is general agreement among the authorities on the importance of planning and organizing for health education. This is critical if objectives are to be attained in the cognitive (knowledge), affective (attitudes), and action (behavior) areas of child development. It is necessary in curriculums that clear definitions be provided in terms of what pupil goals teachers should be seeking, what content should be included, what methods and materials are to be used, and whether the purposes established have been achieved. Ideally, experiences for pupils should be provided that are both scientifically fact oriented and pupil inquiry oriented in a humanistic setting. This chapter attempts to give information and direction to this end.

Health education must be organized in both formal and informal ways if the differing needs and interests of students are to receive proper consideration. Pupils with drug problems, including alcohol and tobacco, with sex concerns, and with emotional and psychologic difficulties frequently cannot be helped except on one-to-one or small group arrangements. To date, insufficient attention has been given to the informal approach in schools. Chapter 5 provided a variety of ways to guide and counsel young people. This chapter and succeeding chapters focus on organizing for formal health teaching.

Curriculum development and implementation is basic to organizing for formal health and safety teaching. A variety of tasks need attention, including determination of what shall be taught and the preparation of units for teacher reference and use. In addition, teachers need help in developing their own plans for teaching and guidance through illustrative units.

Before presenting material in regard to curriculum development and teacher planning, it is important to understand some basic principles involved, to be familiar with the conceptual approach, to be aware of the usefulness of values clarification as a strategy in health education, and to have knowledge about personnel responsibility for the preparation of the curriculum.

WHAT ARE THE BASIC PRINCIPLES FOR CURRICULUM DEVELOPMENT IN HEALTH EDUCATION?

For any educational function to proceed on a sound basis, it must be predicated on certain valid principles or assumptions. If we begin with a firm foundation of fact and philosophy, we cannot stray far from the path of excellence. To choose learning experiences on the basis of established principles is to assure worthwhile education for pupils; to select on the basis of popularity, newspaper headlines, tradition, personal bias, and yesterday's problems is to run the risk of failure in preparing children to live most and serve best in a complex, changing society.

Fundamentally, a sound curriculum must be based on the needs, problems, and opportunities of society and the individual. Beyond this broad approach are certain principles and assumptions that may be used as guidelines for curriculum planning and development in health education:

1. Provision for a sequential, comprehensive program of instruction that includes the ascending spiral effect allowing for an increasing depth of information from kindergarten through grade 12
2. Provision for repetition of content areas without excessive duplication through the cycling of such areas, or in other appropriate ways
3. Adaptability and flexibility to allow for changes and modifications, introducing

151

new content, new information, and new materials as they develop and emerge in society

4. Utilization of the concept approach in curriculum development with particular emphasis on health, key concepts, concepts, and objectives

5. Emphasis on the preventive aspects of health in the instructional program

6. Health emphasis that includes physical or physiologic, sociologic, psychologic, and spiritual aspects

7. Emphasis on the needs and interests of students in forming the basis for the curriculum so it will be appropriate to the local community or communities and the social climates in which pupils reside; special consideration must be given to the children and youth problems of minorities and those with ethnic and cultural differences

8. Provision for writing goals in behavioral terms, including cognitive, affective, and action domains*

9. Where it is appropriate and possible, provision for goals observable in the classroom, nonobservable, and delayed in their attainment in the action domain

10. Provision for goals, with the following differential emphasis at the grade level groups indicated whenever possible:
    a. Primary grades—focus on physiologic aspects of health with limited psychologic and social aspects
    b. Intermediate grades—focus on physiologic aspects of health with greater inclusion of psychologic and social aspects and limited spiritual emphasis
    c. Upper grades—focus primarily on psychologic and social aspects with decreasing emphasis on the physiologic aspects but with concern for the spiritual phases

11. Provision for inclusion of all the alternatives to action so that students can make intelligent decisions regarding behavior

12. Allowance for students to make their own decisions regarding behavior

13. Current content, accurate and nonbiased, derived from scientific sources; both positive and negative aspects to be included whenever possible

14. The methods or techniques of teaching for behavioral changes that stress student involvement, decision making, critical thinking, discussions, problem solving, self-direction, development of values, and responsibility, which should provide for principles of learning (see Chapter 10)

15. Use of a variety of resource materials that are interesting, current, accurate, carefully screened, and appropriate for the grade level intended

16. Provision for periodic assessment of various aspects of the curriculum

These principles and assumptions may seem to be self-evident, yet so often elementary school programs of health education bluntly ignore one or more of these guidelines. The material that follows is based on these principles and their application.

THE CONCEPTUAL APPROACH

For many years researchers in psychology and education have attempted to better understand how children learn. To help pupils organize and learn effectively we need to know something about both the processes and the products of thinking. We do not think in a vacuum. We must have something to think about. So when we talk about the teaching-learning process we must recognize the importance of *what* children learn in relation to *how* they learn.

Thinking is a process that may be of one or more of these six types: *perceptive, associative, inductive-deductive, creative, critical,* and *problem solving.*

---

*The drug problem resulted in new educational terminology, such as humanistic, affective, and confluent education, and emphasis being introduced in schools. The need for students to develop positive self-concepts, to express feelings and aspirations, to reach social maturity, and to participate in values clarification has led authorities to support affective-humanistic education. It is believed such emphasis will enable persons to more effectively cope with life's problems. Confluent education refers to the integration of affective and cognitive elements in learning. These are worthwhile directions for inclusion in health education. The clearly written objectives found in the units in this chapter include these new ideas.

Concept formation

Percepts are simplified conclusions that students obtain from seeing, hearing, touching, tasting, and smelling. They are the raw materials of thinking that result from environmental stimuli. In the classroom these stimuli are generally provided and controlled by the teacher and may include the teacher's oral presentation, other pupils' comments, content of health textbooks, films, bulletin board information, and a host of others. Perception is essential to concept formation.

Inhelder and Piaget* indicate that children's ability to understand broad concepts, or generalizations, and abstractions depend on their ability to have direct sensory experiences. These experiences help them to construct and reconstruct percepts. Modern research shows that sensory-motor experiences (for example, manipulation and construction) are most effective in developing percepts. Then, through use and application of these raw materials of health science, children can understand and deal with more abstract concepts. For example, "use of substances that modify mood and behavior arises from a variety of motivations," is a rather obtuse statement that necessitates specific sensory experiences for understanding and comprehension. Pupils may need to discuss, hear comments by drug abusers, and review literature about why people use drugs to grasp the meaning of the concepts.

Thus, children are exposed to, screen, and select stimuli. The stimuli produce percepts that lead to the formation of concepts, which are conclusions of generalizations.

Conceptual framework of health curriculum

There is no best way to organize the health education curriculum. However, the concept approach introduced by Sliepcevich† was developed utilizing current educational philosophy, was innovative, and continues to be useful. It is fundamental to the eclectic plan identified in this text that gives consideration to a variety of other significant prevalent ideas, including: wholistic health (physiologic, psychologic, social, and spiritual), needs and interests, prevention, and ecology.

In the School Health Education Study three categories of concepts were organized into a hierarchy for the health education curriculum known as The Conceptual Framework: *key concepts, concepts,* and *subconcepts.*

The key concepts are (1) growing and developing, a dynamic life process by which the individual is in some ways like all other individuals, in some ways like some other individuals, and in some ways like no other individual; (2) interacting, an ongoing process in which the individual is affected by and in turn affects certain biologic, social, psychologic economic, cultural, and physical forces in the environment; and (3) decision making, a process unique to man of consciously deciding to take or not to take an action, or of choosing one alternative rather than another.* Stated more simply, students must decide whether to use or expose themselves to environmental influences that affect their bodies.

The concepts are as follows:

1. Growth and development and structure and function of the body are interrelated.
2. Growth and development can be predicted but are uniquely individual.
3. Protection and improvement of health is a responsibility of the individual, the local community, the state and nation, and the world community of nations.
4. Each environment holds the possibility of accidents.
5. Mutually reciprocal relationships exist among man, disease, and environment.
6. The family is essential to the continu-

---

*Inhelder, B., and Piaget, J.: The growth of logical thinking from childhood to adolescence, New York, 1958, Basic Books, Inc., Publishers.
†Lieberman, E. J., editor: Mental health; the public health challenge, Washington, D.C., 1975, American Public Health Association.

*Means, R. K.: The conceptual approach in structuring the health education curriculum, National Conference for School Health Education Curriculum Development, Washington, D.C., Feb. 10, 1967.

Table 9-1. Conceptual approach

Concepts are the bases for the goals and serve to identify the content of the drug education curriculum. Objectives give direction to teaching and learning. They should stress prevention, emphasize behavioral changes, and be written in behavioral terms.

CONCEPT: Use of substances that modify mood and behavior arises from a variety of motivations

Subconcepts	Content dimensions			Behavioral changes	Objectives
	Physical	Mental	Social		
Drugs range from mild to strong, have multiple uses, and produce many and varied effects on individuals who use them.	Effect on the body	Elevate mood; aid relaxation; reduce inhibitions; produce unpredictable and dangerous behavior	Used in society Development of laws	Practices or action domain—overt behavior	Refrains from regular use of drugs that lead to dependency. Avoids use of drugs that reduce ability to think clearly and act normally. Refuses to use illegal drugs.
Use of drugs may result in health and safety problems.	Effect on the circulatory and nervous systems; physical dependence possible	Modify perceptions of reality; lower emotional control	Use encouraged in some social situations	Attitudes or affective domain—feelings, interests, values	Is aware of a variety of drugs and their differing effects. Realizes the unpredictability of emotions and behavior when using drugs. Realizes the habit-forming and dependency possibilities of drug use and abuse.
Many factors and forces influence the use of drugs.	Alleviate fatigue; produce pleasure; reduce boredom, pain, craving for	Permit relaxation and loss of inhibitions	Promoted by social customs, family customs, desire for group approval	Understanding or cognitive domain—knowing, applying, analyzing	Knows differing effects of various drugs on the body. Understands diminished ability to control behavior when affected by drugs. Analyzes the mental and social factors involved in the use and misuse of drugs. Understands drugs can be habit forming and the potential of dependency is greater with some drugs and some individuals.

ance of life and the meeting of certain physical, mental, and social health needs.

7. Individual health behavior is affected by a variety of influences.
8. Personal use of health services, products, and information is influenced by perceptions and values.
9. People have diverse reasons for using chemical substances that modify mood and behavior.
10. Dietary patterns are affected by physical, mental, social, economic, and cultural factors.

The subconcepts are more detailed and are related to the concepts. An illustration of the development of subconcepts from one of the few major concepts previously mentioned may be found in Table 9-1.

Application of the approach

In carrying through this conceptual idea underlying the School Health Education Study, a health instruction curriculum is developed from the major concepts with subconcepts and content or subject matter emerging into teaching-learning units. These units include objectives, content, activities or experiences, resource materials, and evaluation. The units are arranged in four levels of progression (primary grades, intermediate grades, upper–junior high school grades, and high school grades) to provide a comprehensive health evaluation program that has graded subject matter proceeding from elementary to advanced levels.

Examples of realistic and effective application of the conceptual approach are the health education curriculum sample illustrative partial units, which are represented on pp. 167-222.

VALUES IN THE CURRICULUM

Family life-style changes, the influence of the mass communication media, technologic innovations, world events, materialism, conflict of conformity and self-reliance, ethics, and affluence among others are creating difficulties in the establishment of values by young people. As a result, youth are search-

ing for meaning in life. They are asking: "Who am I? Why am I here? What really matters?" They desire to cope with daily problems, to develop life coping skills, understand selves, and to be able to make wise decisions. Because of the failure to answer these questions a variety of patterns of behavioral problems have been appearing in schools. Such problems include apathy, inconsistent behaviors, drifting, dropping out, overconforming, and overdissenting. Schools have a major role in helping children and youths at early ages to begin to clarify their values.

Raths and his associates,* among other leaders in the field of psychology, have indicated the need for individuals to have a sense of purpose in their lives. People actively search for meaningfulness and identity in life, although some may never be able to clearly define or to achieve such a goal. The achievement or failure of achievement of a sense of purpose may affect an individual's mental health either positively or negatively.

There is no single, clear definition of values. They have been said to be deep, long-lasting commitments to a concept or doctrine that is highly prized and about which action will be taken in satisfying ways. They are characteristics or attitudes about human experiences that are strongly desirable to an individual or group of individuals. Values give direction to life and may be considered to be determinants of behavior. They aid in the making of decisions and judgments. They have been identified in the concept of health described in Chapter 1 as part of the *spiritual* aspect of health in the isosceles triangle illustration (see Fig. 1-2). They have been included in the units in this chapter in the affective domain objectives.

Values may be learned through a variety of meaningful experiences and through interaction with the environment. Thus, the sources are adults, peer cultures, the family, the church, the communication media, friends, social groups, and the school.

---

*Raths, L. E., Harmin, M., and Simon, S.: Values and teaching; working with values in the classroom, Columbus, Ohio, 1966, Charles E. Merrill Books, Inc.

Raths and others believe the focus in schools—probably starting in the intermediate grades—should be on value clarification and not on the teaching of values per se. They believe values will emerge through this process. Didactic value clarification involves a series of strategies or methods for helping students learn values. A *value* must meet these seven criteria:

Choosing
1. Choosing freely—individual should not be coerced and should have freedom of selection.
2. Choosing from alternatives—a variety of alternatives must be provided.
3. Choosing thoughtfully—consideration should be given to the consequences of each alternative.
4. Affirming—when something is cherished, it is publicly and verbally supported: doing something.

Prizing
5. Prizing and cherishing—choice has a positive tone and is held in high esteem.

Action
6. Acting on choices—life is affected through reading, spending money, and budgeting time.
7. Repeating—persistency and endurance become a pattern of life.

Ten value-rich areas identified by Raths and his associates are useful in the clarification process: money, friendship, love and sex, religion and morals, leisure, politics and social organization, work, family, maturity, and character traits.

Value clarification has a place in health education as part of both curriculum and methodology. It has particular application to the areas of mental health, drugs, human sexuality, alcohol, smoking, health care, and environment, but it is also useful in other health areas. Some of the strategies that are useful are found in Chapter 11.

Loggins* claims that the values clarification process may only superficially treat values. It cannot be assumed that students will evaluate or decide on their own values. The

*Loggins, D.: Values clarification revisited; clarifying what and how well, Health Education **7**: March/April, 1976.

conceptualization and organization of values may require cognitive elements for analysis, synthesis, and evaluation. The method does generate interest and stimulate student discussion, but Loggins is not sure about the contribution of the method of values education.

WHO IS RESPONSIBLE FOR DEVELOPING THE CURRICULUM IN HEALTH AND SAFETY?

Curriculum development and improvement has become a major function of modern education. Not too long ago the curriculum was shaped largely by experts in the various disciplines. However, in recent years the subject-matter authority has been joined by teachers, pupils, and lay citizens in planning curriculums. This does not mean that the opinions of experts are minimized or disregarded. It means simply that a curriculum can be developed to fit a certain school and community best if opportunity is provided for teachers, pupils, and lay groups to adapt the curriculum to local interests and needs.

For example, an elementary school in Florida might want to give time in the curriculum to hookworm infestation and "creeping eruption" (a skin infestation caused by dog and cat hookworms), instead of spending time on frostbite and winter sport safety. An impoverished ghetto area school in the inner city might decide to stress the problems of unwanted pregnancy and venereal disease at an earlier grade level than a school in suburbia. A rural school might emphasize the importance of water purity and sanitation, whereas an urban school might take more time for air pollution. A school whose pupils come from families where ethnic and racial backgrounds shape their daily meals would surely want to stress the place of Italian, Mexican, Oriental, Indian, and "soul" food as they apply in choosing a balanced diet.

Thus, we find real need for adapting the curriculum to best meet local problems in many areas of health and safety. Yet fundamentally the subject matter is the same for all schools and all children. It is the fringe areas and the manner of illustrating basic concepts that offer the best opportunity for adaptation.

Curriculum development is a shared responsibility. Even though the approach may differ from one community to another, the curriculum in health and safety should reflect the interests, concerns, and efforts of teachers, pupils, parents, physicians, dentists, public health specialists, law enforcement officials, civil defense authorities, school board members, fire department officials, representatives of voluntary health agencies, school nurses, principals, curriculum specialists, and school health coordinators. These people, working together at the local level, can fashion the most fundamental and functional curriculum for their local school situation while retaining the common learnings in health and safety. Often the local group will need to make only a few minor changes in a course of study that has been prepared by the state department of education, by a county school office, or perhaps by some other school district.

Again, the matter of cooperative planning and action can be very helpful. The school health council at the district level, under the direction and guidance of the health coordinator or consultant, can give considerable support to the curriculum development program. The health council usually represents the thinking of most, if not all, concerned persons and organizations. Moreover, it provides a ready-made mechanism for resolving many variances in philosophy and for implementing group decisions.

Experience in the national School Health Education Study showed that very few school districts throughout the country have the personnel resources to develop a sound, up-to-date health education curriculum on their own. If a health coordinator is not available, schools should seek guidance from state or local colleges and universities.

Most important of all is the fact that critical analysis of the curriculum in health education must be a continual process if the instructional program is to be truly functional in the lives of children. The rapid advances in the health sciences no longer permit the schools to "stand pat" for very long on content. Sequence too is affected by the increasingly frequent medical and health science developments and problems. These are in the main accurately and promptly reported in newspapers, magazines, telecasts, and other media. Often such health science reporting provides the teacher with a "teachable moment"—a time when pupils are more likely to be motivated—for a topic that had not been planned. Recent examples are many: new vaccines for measles and German measles, the venereal disease epidemic, zero population growth statistics, elimination of smallpox vaccination from the standard schedule, canned food contamination, the energy crisis, radiation hazards, new drugs being used and abused, federal legislation for health and safety, and a host of others.

The wise teacher will be flexible enough to depart from the lesson plan and take full advantage of the heightened interest of pupils when these stories "break." The unimaginative teacher will cling steadfastly to the planned sequence and, ignoring publicized fresh facts of importance, plow ahead with her unit on a less relevant topic. The choice separates the truly innovative teacher from the inferior journeyman.

HOW IS THE CURRICULUM DETERMINED?

To determine what should be taught in health education, it is necessary to identify the health interests and needs of pupils from which a scope (content) and sequence (grade levels) chart (see Table 9-2) is prepared for use in determining what units need to be constructed. Consideration must be given to the special problems of minorities. By way of illustration, American Indians have personality disorders related to ethnic identity, worries, fear, lack of self-concept and alienation, high rates of suicide, lack of safe water, alcoholism, high death rates, and tuberculosis.

Interests and needs

The following is a variety of information sources useful in determining the scope and sequence of the curriculum.

Pupil interests. Pupils learn better when they have interest in the subject matter. In essence, interest is an attitude favorable to learning. Beyond this, interest hinges on the values, desires, wants, and purposes of the pupil. As children perceive the relationship of a topic to their personal advantage and well-being, they become interested. The *active interests* are those that relate here and now to the child's daily life and world. *Latent interests* are those that the child may have had at an earlier age, but which were stifled because parents and other adults would not or could not encourage and develop them. Finally, since interests depend heavily on past experiences, there are many areas in which elementary pupils have practically no interest. It is one of the central purposes of education to amplify and diversify the interests of children. Thus, pupil interests, although vital to motivation, cannot be considered in themselves as complete indicators of the relative importance of topics in health and safety.

Yet teachers should seek out pupil interests and emphasize those already developed. This is simply good motivation. Latent health interests (for example, "What makes me grow?" "Where do I go when I sleep?" "Where do babies come from?") will have to be further developed and new interests will need to be created if health teaching is to be effective.

A 1969 report* by the Connecticut State Department of Education provides remarkable insight into the health interests, concerns, and problems of elementary school pupils. This study involved more than 5,000 students from kindergarten through the twelfth grade. It showed, among other things, that basic health interests were common to all pupils whether they lived in a city, rural, suburban, or high socioeconomic environment. The questions and comments of elementary-age children were grouped according to three levels: kindergarten through grade 2, grades 3 and 4, and grades 5 and 6.

Boys and girls in kindergarten and first and second grades showed interest in a broad variety of health problems but were unsure of what health is and had only a vague concept of it. They were more interested in not being sick than in being healthy; when not sick, they can run, play, and have fun. Most of the questions they asked were related to their health, growth, and development. Sample key interests and concerns in the various areas of health and safety are cited.

KINDERGARTEN THROUGH GRADE 2
What is good health?

"You don't have measles or mumps."
"You eat lots of vegetables and fruits and no coffee."
"You brush the dirt off of your teeth."
"You take vitamin pills."

About the body

"How does my body get made?"
"What makes you stop growing?"
"Why do men have big muscles and ladies don't?"

About aches, pains, and diseases

"How can I tell if I have a fever?"
"Does a vaccination keep you healthy?"

About family health

"My mom gets us new babies; she feeds us, picks me up when I fall, cleans me off."
"I help my mom and dad."
"I don't think I have enough love for two fathers."

About relations with peers

"You don't do anything right, you don't do it the way we do."
"He doesn't take a bath, his ears are dirty."

GRADES 3 AND 4
What is a healthy person?

"Isn't too fat or too skinny."
"Doesn't play with matches."
"Doesn't go to the hospital."
"Eats everything he should, the right vegetables, not too much fattening food or candy, has a well-balanced diet."

*Byler, R. V., Lewis, G. M., and Totman, R. J.: Teach us what we want to know, New York, 1969, Mental Health Materials Center, Inc. for the Connecticut State Department of Education.

About accidents

"The doctor is nice."

"I like the hospital."

"I was glad to come home."

About personal health and safety

"I don't want your germs."

"I didn't mean to do it. Frank was chasing me, and I ran into the street."

"A car might come along and hit him, and he'll end up in the hospital."

"How many hours should you sleep to keep healthy?"

"How does toothpaste help to keep your teeth clean?"

"Should you bite your fingernails?"

About family health

"How can you tell which is a cow or a bull?"

"They use the bull so the cows can have babies who will grow up to be milk cows."

"You can't have babies, if you're too young."

"Where does a baby come from?"

"How does it get out of the mother's stomach?"

"Do you know what abortion means?"

What would you like to study in health?

"The eyes—why do they become bloodshot?"

"Why do some people become mentally ill?"

"Why do some people go blind?"

"Why should we destroy LSD?"

About the body

"What is healthy blood?"

"How do lungs grow when we grow?"

"Why do we lose baby teeth?"

About food and nutrition

"What kinds of liquids should you drink to keep healthy?"

"How do people get fat?"

"How do vitamins help keep us strong?"

About exercise and physical education

"Does exercise help you?"

"How does exercising really take off fat?"

"What are the best exercises to do?"

About first aid and safety

"If you fall and think you are hurt, what should you do?"

"If you are way out in the woods a long way from a doctor, and someone got killed, what would you do?"

About mental health

"If you worry too much, will you get sick?"

"Why do I get so lonely?"

"How do you get mental illness?"

About problems of the entire society

"How many people in the world are healthy and how many aren't?"

"What illness do you get from smoking?"

"What is the difference between a doctor and a surgeon?"

"What do nurses do?"

About drugs, smoking, and alcohol

"Why do so many people take shots of marijuana, STP, LSD, 'snow,' and 'speed'?"

"Is marijuana a dangerous drug? How does it affect you?"

"Why do so many people smoke?"

"Why do people drink so much?"

GRADES 5 AND 6

What is a healthy person?

"He eats right and drinks milk."

"Doesn't smoke and drink."

"Goes for a checkup."

What is health?

"Health is exercising; keeping yourself fit; maintaining a strong body and preventing defects."

"Health is physical and mental."

About the body

"How does a body grow? I'd like to know *all* about the body."

"Why do we have hair?"

"Why do girls grow up faster than boys?"

"Why do girls have periods and boys don't?"

About food and nutrition

"What are the best foods for a person to eat?"

"What foods are bad for you?"

"What should we eat for a good diet?"

"What vitamins should you have and what are the effects of a lack of vitamins? This is fun to learn about."

"What makes you fat?"

About personal health

"We should know about care of the teeth and about cavities, about bathing, keeping clean, and having good breath."

About exercise and physical education

"The health plan in Connecticut should consist of a very good gym system. Have good, well-trained teachers. Have large playgrounds. Have more track meets and different sports."

About babies

"How is a baby formed?"
"How can birth control pills stop birth?"
"Why can't you have a baby when you are not married?"

About mental health

"It's the way kids get along together."
"I would like to understand my personality."
"Why do I act happy, sad, angry?"
"Why can't I control my temper?"
"I would like to help others and to understand them."

About social-emotional development

"Why do I sometimes hate my friends? What is a real friend, what can I do to make friends?"
"I am well-liked at school, but in trouble at home."
"Why can't I get along with my brother or sister?"

About drugs, alcohol, and smoking

"Why do people take drugs?"
"What do they do to you?"
"Can anyone ever break the drug habit?"
"How does it feel to go high on LSD?"
"When do people want to smoke?"
"Smoking is our greatest health problem."
"Why do they sell cigarettes?"

About environmental health

"When will air pollution, alcohol, smoking, and other things like these be cured or stopped?"
"Factories pollute the air and the water."
"Why don't people stop killing and start loving?"

Surely these provocative questions and stimulating statements confirm the adage that "out of the mouths of babes" come some of the most perceptive comments. While these are randomly selected responses of elementary school children included in the Connecticut study, they reflect some of the more important interests and concerns of children across the nation.

Pupil needs. Ideally, the entire curriculum is predicated upon the most important present and future needs of children and the society in which they live. Nowhere is this basic precept of higher significance than in the realm of health and safety. Surely the child with repeated or chronic illness cannot benefit fully from classroom activities. Nor can the boy or girl with emotional difficulties profit most from learning experiences. The child killed in an accident can, of course, only be lamented.

All education aims at fulfilling the needs of society. Elementary school health education concerns itself with fulfillment of those needs that relate to the betterment of individual, family, and community health. Certain of these needs are quite obviously manifest in vital statistics, health examinations, research on illness and absenteeism, and teacher observation of children. Others are subtly blended into the pattern and fabric of each child's physical, mental, and emotional development. Health education in our elementary schools must continue to search for and to use every valid source of information that points out the health and safety needs of pupils. All of the sources discussed here will be helpful in developing a health education curriculum that makes a real contribution toward meeting the significant needs of children.

Health and accident statistics. Most serious disease problems are pointed out by two kinds of vital statistics: mortality (death) rates and morbidity (illness) rates. These data are collected by local health departments and forwarded to the vital statistics division of the state department of health. From there the state reports are sent on to the National Office of Health Statistics of the U.S. Public Health Service. Similar data on smaller population samples are reported by the Statistical Bureau of the Metropolitan Life Insurance Company. Accidents are included in the cause-of-death classification of the National Office of Health Statistics, state departments of health, and the Statistical Bureau, but the most extensive and intensive data on accidents are provided by the National Safety Council. Since accidents are by far the leading cause of death for the elementary school population, a detailed analysis of accidental deaths and injuries by type and site, sex, and age group is of particular significance to the teacher.

These kinds of data place the teacher in a position of unique advantage. Few, if any, other subject-matter areas have the opportunity of matching curricular content against such widely available objective information reflecting human and social needs. In essence, health and accident statistics tell the curriculum specialist and the classroom teacher *what* problems pupils will face and equally important, *when* they will be most likely to face them. Tabular data in Chapters 1 and 6 provide such information on death, illness, and types of accidents for elementary school pupils.

Community health and accident problems. All classroom teachers should be alert to possibilities for vitalizing their teaching by relating subject matter to local problems and circumstances. Most of the statistical data described in previous chapters can be obtained for state and sometimes city or county situations.

Material from textbooks. There are a number of good texts for pupils in the elementary grades. The outlines, general organization, and the content of each book provide helpful guides for developing curriculums. Most publishers also provide a chart outline that serves as an overview of the basic concepts covered in each of the major areas of health and safety at each grade level, usually from grades 1 through 8. Therefore, a school using a series of up-to-date health and safety textbooks already has the basis for a grade-by-grade program. Chapter 11 gives further consideration to the place of the textbook in teaching methods.

Material from courses of study. Many state, county, and city school systems have prepared useful outlines for health education at the elementary level. Usually these curriculum guides have been developed by teachers and supervisors working together with health education consultants, representatives of the state or local medical society, dental society, health department, school

nursing staff, and other interested professional and lay groups. In many instances these publications are already available in the school, or they may be obtained by teachers or administrators on request to the appropriate publishing agency.

School health appraisals. Certainly the results of medical and dental examinations conducted as part of the school health service program should be considered a potentially profitable source of pertinent health problems. Although it is true that children over the nation are much the same in health status and development, there are often problems that appear to be especially prominent among pupils of a particular school or community.

School health examinations are concerned primarily with the detection and prompt correction of health defects, but a valid and worthwhile collateral use of the findings is in their application to the health teaching program. Then, too, alert and continual health observation of pupils by teachers will furnish abundant clues on the health problems of elementary children.

Health surveys. Data derived from health and illness surveys afford a more completely valid and reliable picture of disease and impairment than do vital statistics on reportable diseases. Health surveys serve to throw light on many important causes of disability that may be either omitted from or incompletely reported in vital statistics.* Even though they are of an essentially negative nature, these data provide excellent clues for the classroom teacher in considering prominent health and safety problems of elementary boys and girls.

Nutrition surveys. The results of nutritional appraisals of the school-age population are valuable in planning content for units on diet and nutrition. Studies that pinpoint specific dietary problems, which are not always the same for boys and girls at each grade level, can be used with marked effective-

---

*Reports of the continuing National Health Survey are available from the U.S. Public Health Service, Washington, D.C. 20025.

ness in improving nutrition education. Data of this type are available periodically from the U.S. Department of Agriculture,* the National Academy of Sciences–National Research Council,† the Council on Foods and Nutrition‡ of the American Medical Association, state departments of agriculture, professional associations in the field of nutrition, and a number of organizations concerned with food production and distribution. All these organizations, with their most recent addresses, are listed in Chapter 12.

In addition, teachers can conduct their own class surveys, though care should be taken not to embarrass individual pupils.

Analysis of social, economic, and political trends. As we learned in reviewing the needs for health education in our modern society, many developments in our country and in the world have direct or indirect bearing on the elementary school health curriculum. There is a need for including these developments as attempts are made to solve the health problems of the deprived.

Teacher-pupil sharing in selecting content. One of the most stimulating trends in modern curriculum development is that which recognizes the importance of bringing pupils into the experience of setting goals and shaping content. We cannot hope to teach most effectively unless some opportunity is provided for boys and girls to make known their interests, concerns, purposes, and values. It was pointed out earlier that there are shortcomings to the practice of selecting topics for study primarily on the basis of pupil interests. Yet, above and beyond the value of interest in pupil motivation, teachers should keep in mind the basic principle of maintaining communication with pupils. Most teachers know that much can be learned by listening to what pupils have to

say. As adults, we tend to get out of touch with children. One of the best ways to keep abreast of the shifting activities, problems, opinions, and concerns of each new class is simply to listen and observe with this purpose in mind.

SCOPE AND SEQUENCE

To determine the scope and sequence of health teaching in the elementary school program, it is necessary to consider the needs and interests of children at all age levels from the kindergarten throughout the elementary school. The material developed by the Ellensburg public schools in the state of Washington is a good illustration of how one school system provided for these needs in their scope and sequence (Table 9-2). It should be noted that recent evidence indicates learning about alcohol, tobacco, and other drugs may take place at earlier grades than shown.

Organized health instruction should be provided for at all grade levels throughout the elementary school. There are a number of important reasons why it should be offered at all levels. First, the body of knowledge concerning health and healthful living in the modern world is so extensive that it is necessary to offer it over a period of years to adequately impart the knowledge needed. Second, there is a need for a certain amount of health knowledge at all ages, even including kindergarten children. The degree of maturity of children in the elementary grades is such that they cannot be given the extensive knowledge needed for adult life. Yet it is highly important that instruction be given and that the various phases of health and healthful living be introduced to the children as rapidly as their maturity and level of intelligence will permit.

From the viewpoint of psychology it is much easier to establish proper habits of health and healthful living early in the child's life. Also, the child needs to practice good health and safety habits just as much at an early age as later. Therefore, it seems psychologically sound to teach as much as possible about health as early as possible, con-

---

*U.S. Department of Agriculture, Agricultural Research Administration, Bureau of Human Nutrition and Home Economics, Washington, D.C. 20025.

†National Academy of Sciences–National Research Council, Washington, D.C. 20025.

‡Council on Foods and Nutrition, American Medical Association, 535 North Dearborn St., Chicago, Ill. 60610.

Table 9-2. Ellensburg public school health scope and sequence

Areas	K	1	2	3	4	5	6	7	8
Alcohol							X	√	X
Anatomy and physiology	X	√	√	X	X	X	X		
Community	√	√	√		X		X		
Consumer	√	√	√		√	√	√		X
Dental	√	X	X	X	X		√		√
Disease	√	√	√	√	X		√	X	X
Drugs							X	√	X
Family	X	X	√	√	X	X	X	X	X
Health careers									√
Mental health	√	X	√	√	√	√	√	√	√
Nutrition	X	X	X	X		X			√
									First aid
Safety	X	X		X	*√	*X	*X		X
Smoking						X		X	√
Exercise, rest, and sleep						√			

X = Study in depth with relationship to the level of the learners.
√ = Unit developed and will be taught; however, depth will be left to the judgment of individual teacher.
* = Special emphasis on recreational safety to coincide with camping program.

sidering the stages of maturity of the children. An example of this is in the area of nutrition, which is a phase of the health education program at practically all grade levels. The subject of nutrition should be introduced and developed as far as the ability of the children at any particular age level permits, for nutrition is a functional part of the life of the primary-age child just as it is of an older child. If by educating children in nutrition to their capacity at the primary level we can better assure their optimum nutrition, then it is obvious that the subject should be introduced in school just as early as possible. Even though primary-age children are not mature enough to be given all the safety information they need for life, it is highly important that they know as much about safety as possible to safeguard their lives while growing up. As an example, the failure to teach elementary school children certain facts about traffic safety could result in a child's death or permanent disability.

What then can we consider to be properly included in the course of study for health and safety in our elementary schools? As we know, the needs of communities, states, and regions may differ somewhat in that some problems are specific for certain localities but not for others. Yet, in the main, the fundamental concepts are essentially the same. Content of safe and healthful living, which research and experience have shown to be necessary to a sound, productive program of health education in elementary schools, is outlined here.

Health content for the child in primary grades

What it means to be healthy
Why we need good health
How our bodies are made and how they work
How we grow
Good food for growth and health
Taking care of our feet
Rest and play for good health and growth
Seeing and hearing well
Caring for our teeth
Drugs, alcohol, and smoking
Fighting diseases that are catching
Working and playing with others
People in our town who help keep us healthy

Safety content for the child in primary grades

What it means to live safely
Why we need to act safely each day
Safety in our homes
Safety in our neighborhood
Playing safely
Safety in walking or riding to school
Preventing fires

Table 9-3. Health education for special children*

Areas	Levels†				
	I	**II**	**III**	**IV**	**V**
Safety	*Emergencies* Awareness and simple first aid Communication Report	*Traveling* Pedestrian Passenger Bicycle	*School* Classroom Building Playground	*Home* General Fire and electricity Appliances and equipment	*Recreation* Environment Use of equipment and games Bicycle and camping
Mental health	*Self-acceptance* Physical abilities and limitations Mental abilities and limitations Cultural and social differences	*Acceptance of others* Physical abilities Mental abilities and limitations Cultural and social differences	*Values* Personnel Home and school Community and national	*Adjustment to stress* School Home Community	
Family living	*Roles in family* Recognizing roles Learning roles Accepting changing roles	*Home management and maintenance* Supervised responsibilities Simple independent responsibilities Self-directed responsibilities	*Family and child care* Supervised responsibility Simple independent responsibilities Self-directed responsibilities	*Sex education* Sex organs Reproduction	
Nutrition	*Foods* Sources Types Components	*Diet* Selection of basic food Planning of daily menus Effects of components	*Preparation and preservation of foods* Cleaning and storing Preparation of food for meals Preservation of foods	*Health problems* Weight Vitality Allergies	
Body care and personal hygiene	*Cleanliness* Routine Grooming Body changes Body changes	*Respect and protection of body parts* Dental care	*Rest and exercise* Awareness of need Understanding of need Ways and means	*Proper clothing and shelter* Awareness of need Understanding Ways	
Disease and illness	*Communicable diseases* Symptoms Causes Treatment	*Sanitation* Personal Home and school Community	*Personal care* Awareness Communication Treatment	*Health services* Knowledge of community Knowledge and location of services When and how to use	

*Prepared by a group of special education teachers in Ellensburg, Washington.
†Refers to stages of learning progression. Children move from level to level upward when ready regardless of grade.

Safety in the water
Safety on the school grounds
Safety in our school buildings
People in our town who help us keep safe

Health content for the child in intermediate and upper grades

The meaning of physical, mental, and emotional health
The importance of health in living happily and usefully
The machinery of our bodies
Growing up physically (including growth problems that begin at about the fifth- or sixth-grade level)
Choosing the best foods for energy, growth, and health
Proper food and drink to protect our health
Fresh air and sunshine for everyone
Exercise, relaxation, and sleep for better health
The eyes and ears of our world
Good teeth for better health and appearance
Helping our feet support us
Caring for our skin, hair, and nails
Immunization and fighting infection
Looking and feeling best in proper clothing
Growing up socially and emotionally
Drugs, alcohol, and smoking
Wise choice of health products and services
Living healthfully in the family
Emergencies and accidents action
Working for the health of our town

Safety content for the child in intermediate and upper grades

Adventure and safety
What the accident problem means to us
Safety on our streets and highways
Safety at the beach and in the pool
Sports safety
Safety at home (including farm safety where appropriate)
Safety at school
Using firearms with care
The danger of fire
Bicycle safety
Safety as a passenger in motor vehicles
Safety in hiking and camping
Checking safety hazards in our neighborhood
People in our town who work for our safety

In general, surveys have shown that the elementary health curriculum should include units on nutrition; consumer health; growth; exercise; sleep; rest and relaxation; dental health; eyes and ears; family life and health; mental health; safety; first aid; alcohol, tobacco, and other drugs; body mechanics; structure, function, and care of the body; control of diseases; medical and dental care; community health problems; and chronic diseases. Many of these areas are covered in the illustrative units found on pp. 167-222.

Special education

Pupils in special education classrooms need to be provided learnings in health education. They have problems and interests similar to those of the so-called normal students. For those who are mentally retarded, much of what is used in the regular program in sex education can be adapted to simpler presentation. Also the use of more visual aids and repetition is necessary. For those who have cerebral palsy, special toothbrushes and prophylactic implements can be prepared for oral health. For blind students, braille materials should be created. Teachers will need to develop their own items, make adaptations, or explore community resources for assistance.

A suggested health education program usable in a classroom where there are different types of handicapped children is found in Table 9-3.

Health education curriculum for Head Start programs

Children regardless of their ages should be exposed to educational programs about health. Many habit patterns are established early in life and numerous health problems are preventable in the formative years. The school setting offers opportunities to influence the development of behaviors and to reduce problems. The Head Start programs should include curriculums in health education. The information in this chapter including the unit materials that are categorically listed as well as the activities in Chapter 11 at the primary grade levels are useful. Teachers will need to extrapolate the applicable sections and to adapt and organize them into suitable units and lessons.

However, the U.S. Office of Child Development Project Head Start prepared a curriculum guide useful to teachers. The following represents a suggested content outline adapted from that reference.*

All about me
My body (inside, outside, functions of body systems)
Who am I? (sex, race, ethnic group)
Real me (How do I feel inside? happy, sad, angry, afraid, lonely, and so forth)

Accident prevention and first aid
Home
Fire
Playground
To and from school
Dangerous strangers

Disease control
Germs
Infections
Colds
Coughs
Immunizations and their control

Dental health
Decay
Brushing and flossing
Sugar foods

Nutrition
Selection of nutritious items

Rest, sleep and exercise
Need for and adequate amounts

Who helps to take care of health
Family (parents, physician, teacher, school nurse; vision and hearing testing, and others)

THE UNIT IN HEALTH TEACHING

Few concepts in education are less understood than is the unit or the unit method. Unit teaching is basically a good way of organizing for teaching.

It is common for both prospective and inservice teachers to become confused about the definition, concept, nature, and purpose of the unit approach. This is entirely understandable when one reviews the educational

*Adapted from the Office of Child Development Project Head Start; Healthy that's me; a health education curriculum guide for Head Start, Washington, D.C., 1971, U.S. Department of Health, Education, and Welfare.

literature. It seems that each writer places his own interpretation on the unit and its use in improving instruction in the classroom. But through the fabric of a multitude of definitions is woven the common thread of organization. Both topics and learning experiences are organized in such a manner that they are related to a central theme or problem. Thus, units in health and safety are built around fundamental concepts in health and the major problems of children and society in safe and healthful living.

Most statements of unit organization and content include certain essential elements: objectives, content, teaching aids, activities, and evaluation.

Certainly the unit is far superior to teaching in a hit-or-miss fashion. Yet the most carefully planned and thoroughly detailed health unit falls short of its purpose and potential if it deals with trivia. Occasionally teachers may be led to believe that the process is more important than the learning products. When this happens, teachers may become so infatuated with the procedures and techniques of the unit approach that they fail to pay enough attention to the significance of the knowledges, attitudes, and practices they seek to develop among pupils.

The unit approach is one of the best means available for organizing more meaningful learning experiences. Beyond this, the unit helps assure a sound, logical presentation of subject matter. It represents an effective blending of psychologic and logical organization of topics and concepts.

Illustrative partial units for primary, intermediate, and upper grades

The illustrative partial units that follow, covering many of the important health content areas teachers may use in planning for health instruction, include such areas as consumer health; dental health; disease control; exercise, rest, and body control; drugs; family health; mental health; nutrition; safety and first aid; and vision and hearing. Note that they follow the basic principles previously identified and give consideration to the new definition of health, the concept approach, and values.

COMMUNITY HEALTH UNIT
Outline of content

PHYSIOLOGIC

Definitions: public health (community health), preventive medicine, preventive health care, immunity, screening tests

Community health problems: communicable diseases (venereal disease, tuberculosis, upper respiratory infections, hepatitis, measles, German measles, polio, rabies, tetanus, typhoid, mononucleosis, food infections); noncommunicable diseases (heart and circulatory disorders, cancers and leukemias, emphysema and chronic bronchitis, diabetes, arthritis, allergies, ulcers, skin conditions); blindness and other eye defects; dental problems; maternal and child health; mental health; suicide; drug abuse, including alcohol and tobacco; accidents; malnutrition; pollution, accidental pollution

PSYCHOLOGIC

Why public health? lack of public understanding of purposes and activities of community health personnel and organizations; improvement of individual, family, and group health; preventive approach; need for group efforts to prevent or correct certain health and accident problems

SOCIAL

Public health organizations: U.S. Public Health Service; state health department; local health department; World Health Organization; The American Heart Association; The American Cancer Society, Inc.; The American Lung Association (formerly the National Tuberculosis and Respiratory Disease Association); The National Society for the Prevention of Blindness; The National Association for Mental Health, Inc.; The National Foundation; The National Association of Hearing and Speech Agencies; National Clearinghouse for Drug Abuse Information; The Planned Parenthood Federation of America, Inc.; The American Social Health Association; The American National Red Cross; The American Diabetes Association, Inc.; National Sickle Cell Anemia Research Foundation; Muscular Dystrophy Association of America, Inc.; The National Safety Council

Community health programs and activities: prevention and control of diseases (communicable and chronic); infant and maternal deaths; malnutrition; mental illness; drug abuse; accidents; dental and oral defects; hearing problems; blindness and vision disorders; suicide; accidental poisoning; environmental pollution

Public health personnel: increasing need for community health personnel; career opportunities in public health (health educator, public health physician, public health dentist, public health nurse, sanitarian, environmental specialist, safety consultant, mental health counselor, hospital administrator, school nurse, and dental hygienist)

Professional societies: medical society; dental society; osteopathic association; and optometric association

SPIRITUAL

Values: value of public health in protecting, maintaining, and improving human health

Moral issues: Should citizens contribute money voluntarily to private agencies and through taxes to official organizations for the support of community health programs? Is each individual responsible for the health and safety of others?

Humanism: concern of community leaders for the health and safety of all citizens

Concepts

Concept	Application of health definition
1 Public health programs protect, maintain, and improve the health of people in a community through group effort.	Social-spiritual
2 As members of the community, children and youths are entitled to public health services and resources.	Social-spiritual

Community health concepts—cont'd

Concept	Application of health definition
3 Public health agencies and organizations function at the local, state, national, and international level.	Social
4 Community health programs are carried out by official and voluntary organizations.	Social-spiritual
5 All citizens can help improve individual, family, and community health by supporting the work of health departments and health agencies.	Social-spiritual-psychologic
6 Community health organizations conduct preventive and control programs for diseases, infant and maternal deaths, malnutrition, mental illness, drug abuse, accidents, blindness and other visual defects, hearing problems, dental neglect, poisoning, and environmental problems.	Physical-social
7 Public health departments generally are not adequately supported by tax funds.	Social
8 Through careers in the health sciences, many individuals contribute to the health of the community.	Social-spiritual-psychologic
9 The school health program is part of the overall community health program.	Social

Objectives for grades K-3

Domain	Objectives for students	Basic concepts
Cognitive	1. Explains the general purpose of public health.	1
	2. Identifies several local health agencies.	3, 4
	3. Explains why public health services should be available to everyone.	1, 2, 6
	4. Lists reasons why people should support community health programs.	5, 7
Affective	1. Displays interest in learning more about health departments and agencies.	3, 4, 6
	2. Asks questions about who pays for community health programs.	5, 7
	3. Asks questions about the work of physicians, school nurses, dentists, public health workers, and other people concerned with community health.	2, 5, 8
	4. Shows interest in the value of group effort in preventing and solving certain health problems.	1, 5, 6
Action	1. Cooperates with teachers, school nurses, and others involved in the school health program.	2, 5
	2. Assists wherever possible with school or community health efforts.	2, 5

Objectives for grades 4-6

Domain	Objectives for students	Basic concepts
Cognitive	1. Lists the major purposes of health departments.	1
	2. Cites examples of public health organizations and agencies.	3, 4
	3. Explains the chief differences between official and voluntary health agencies.	4

Community health objectives for grades 4-6—cont'd

Domain	Objectives for students	Basic concepts
	4. Understands the importance of school health and other community programs concerned with child health.	2
	5. Explains the need for community support of public health programs.	5, 7
	6. Cites examples of health careers.	8
	7. Lists health problems that may be prevented or solved by community health programs.	6
Affective	1. Displays interest in the basic philosophy of public health.	1
	2. Asks questions about the different programs and aims of official and voluntary health agencies.	3, 4
	3. Accepts the need for community health programs and personnel.	1, 2, 5
	4. Appreciates the need for financial and other public support of community health programs.	1, 5, 7
	5. Shows interest in and concern for major community health problems.	5, 6
	6. Displays interest in career possibilities in public health work.	8
Action	1. Seeks reliable sources of information regarding community health programs.	2, 5, 6
	2. Visits the health department and other local agencies when recommended as part of a community health project.	2, 5, 6
	3. Cooperates with school health projects.	2, 9

Objectives for grades 7-8

Domain	Objectives for students	Basic concepts
Cognitive	1. Understands the vital importance of public health for all communities.	1
	2. Lists reasons why community health programs are especially important for children and youths.	2
	3. Explains the nature and functions of health departments at the local, state, national, and international levels.	3
	4. Explains differences between official and voluntary agencies with regard to personnel, financing, relative emphasis on services, research, and education.	4, 5, 7
	5. Compares the need for group approach with that of private medical and dental health care.	1, 6, 8
	6. Cites the reasons for public support of community health programs.	5, 7
	7. Identifies by purpose, activities, and location major health agencies in the community.	3, 4
	8. Explains the three basic phases of the school health program.	9
Affective	1. Appreciates the social values of community health programs.	1, 5

Community health objectives for grades 7-8—cont'd

Domain	Objectives for students	Basic concepts
	2. Shows interest in the quality of local community health services.	2, 5, 7
	3. Asks questions about the most pressing needs in public health at the local, state, national, and world levels.	3, 6, 7
	4. Appreciates the purposes of the school health program.	9
	5. Offers opinions on the responsibility of government to provide effective public health programs for all citizens.	1, 3, 7
	6. Displays interest in differences between official and voluntary health agencies.	4, 5
	7. Inquires about public health career opportunities.	8
	8. Shows concern for the quality of the school health program.	9
Action	1. Cooperates whenever possible with special projects of the health department or voluntary agencies.	2, 4-6
	2. Talks with parents about the values of a good community health program.	1, 3, 5-7
	3. Takes part in school health projects.	2, 9
	4. Seeks information on needed legislation for the improvement of local, state, and federal public health programs.	1, 4, 5, 7
	5. Seeks information on educational requirements and opportunities in one or more public health careers.	8

CONSUMER HEALTH UNIT*
Outline of content
PHYSIOLOGIC

Definitions: consumer health (economics of health), health products, health services, self-diagnosis, self-medication, prevention, effects of health products, nature of various health examinations, medical care, health insurance.

PSYCHOLOGIC

Why consumer health? self-diagnosis and self-medication; advertising inducement; spiraling costs; misinformation and lack of information; vast amount of scientific information; preventive medicine concept

Why do people purchase health products and services? self-diagnosis and self-medication; less expensive treatment; improvement of health status; advertising; the need for help; condition minor in nature; ignorance of hazards; lack of information; religious beliefs; friend or peer recommendations

Why do people go to quacks? lonely; refusal of physician to listen to problem; hopeless case for treatment or cure; mysticism; the desire for pleasant, easy cure; physician's limitation in dealing with problem; psychologic problems

Budgeting for health care: estimate of yearly costs of products and services; insurance; emergencies

How to act as an intelligent health consumer: a skeptic; critical and analytical of what is read, seen, or heard regardless of source; initiator of investigation; identification of quacks and quackery, fads and frauds, or suspicious of same; knowledge about when to call or visit doctor, dentist, or other health professionals; knowledge about how to select a doctor, dentist,

---

*See also Cornacchia, H. J.: Consumer health, St. Louis, 1976, The C. V. Mosby Co.

Organizing for health teaching   171

Consumer health outline of content—cont'd
Psychologic—cont'd

and other health professionals; knowledge of what to expect from a physician, dentist, and other health professionals, and also what is expected by these individuals of patient; application of sound criteria in purchase of health products or services; reading of labels; knowledge of where to seek, how to obtain, and how to seek reliable health information; initiative taken to go to protection agencies and organizations for help.

SOCIAL

Health products

Arthritis—cures, devices

Athletics and fitness—drugs, vitamins, weight reduction, mechanical aids, spot reducers, vibrator machines, isometric versus isotonic exercises

Cancer—Krebiozen, Laetrile, Hoxey treatments and cures

Cosmetics—deodorants, hormone creams, and wrinkle removers

Dental—toothpaste, toothbrushes, Water Pik, and others

Drugs—use and misuse, aspirin, over-the-counter, and others

Hearing—hearing aids, mail order of aids

Mechanical—bust developers, rupture devices, silicones, vibrators, sea water

Nutrition—vitamins, food additives, weight control diets, organic and natural foods

Tobacco—smoking cures and filters

Vision—glasses by mail, sunglasses, and contact lenses

Others—cough and cold remedies, laxatives, preparations for hemorrhoids, skin blemish removers, allergic conditions, bad breath, hair restorers, and impotency cures

Health services

Health examinations—what, when, who does, frequency, and cost

Types of health specialists

Physicians—general practitioners, internal medicine, pediatrics, or surgery

Dentists—general practice, orthodontics, oral surgery, and others

Psychologists—general, clinical, and family counselor

Also podiatrists, pharmacists, optometrists, osteopaths and nurses

Hospitals and clinics—types, licensing, standards

Health insurance—types, services, costs

Criteria for selection of health specialists—license to practice, preparation and training, member of local health profession society in good standing, night calls, discussion of fees in advance, opinion of others, hospital affiliation

When to call health specialist—complaint or symptoms too severe to be endured; persistence of for more than few days; symptoms' repeated return; accident

Role of business in health products: self-control versus governmental control; psychology of selling; mass communication media; analysis of advertising

Protection of the consumer

Agencies and organizations

Government—FDA, FTC, Post Office, and health departments

Professional—AMA, ADA, and American Pharmaceutical Association

Voluntary—cancer, arthritis, heart, tuberculosis, Better Business Bureau

Laws—federal Food, Drug and Cosmetic Act; advertising limitations; labeling of products

Education—formal and informal, sources of information from family, friends, and school

Sources of reliable health information: reputable individuals, such as physicians or dentists; also from scientific books, magazines, and publications; questions such as, What is reputation, training, and experience of authors and sources? Is there a profit motive involved in the writing? Are the data accurate and up to date? What do other sources say about the topic or material?

Quacks and quackery

Definition—boastful pretender to medical skills; a charlatan; ignorant or dishonest practitioner

Consumer health outline of content—cont'd

Social—cont'd

> Motivational factors—money, power, prestige
>
> Identifying factors—disregard or misinterpretation of scientific evidence; acceptance of money for worthless or questionable treatments, products, or services
>
> Why some quack cures work? spontaneous remission of some diseases, placebo effect, psychosomatic effect of encouragement of patient

SPIRITUAL

Values: differing healing philosophies or cult values—medicine, osteopathy, acupuncture, herbalists, faith healers, Christian Science, Jehovah's Witnesses, and chiropractic

> What is the effect of differing values on the selection, purchase and use of health products and services?

Moral issues: Is an ethical code needed in advertising, in the business world? Is an ethical code needed in medicine, dentistry, and the health professions?

Humanism: What should be the relationship between medical practitioners and patients?

Concepts

Concept	Application of health definition
1 Health products and health services may have beneficial and harmful effects on individuals.	Physiologic
2 Self-diagnosis and self-medication and the use of quacks and quackery may be hazardous and costly to individuals.	
3 Individuals purchase and use health products and services for a variety of reasons.	Psychologic
4 Wise decisions regarding the selection, purchase, and use of health products and services necessitates individuals acting as "intelligent health consumers."	
5 The use of scientific information is necessary for the effective evaluation, selection, purchase, and use of health products and services.	
6 Appraisal, selection, purchase, and use of health products and services are influenced by one's past experiences and the environment.	Social
7 There are reliable and unreliable sources of health information.	
8 The community provides a variety of organizations, agencies, and laws to protect the health consumer.	
9 Individuals differing in values and philosophies regarding the healing and health treatment of individuals influence the selection, purchase, and use of health products and services.	Spiritual
10 Ethical considerations of involved in the selling of health products and the rendering of health services.	

Objectives for grades K-3

Domain	Objectives for students	Basic concepts
Cognitive	1. Identifies people who can help promote and protect one's health.	8
	2. Identifies people who can help when injured, ill or who prescribe medicines.	8
	3. Explains the reason for caution when taking medicines.	1, 2, 4
	4. Lists the reasons adults should help to supervise the taking of medicines.	1, 4, 8

Consumer health objectives for grades K-3—cont'd

Domain	Objectives for students	Basic concepts
	5. Concludes that medicines may be necessary at times for health.	1, 4, 7
	6. Explains the effect of mass media on the purchase and use of health products.	3-6, 8
	7. Identifies a variety of sources of health information.	4, 5, 7
Affective	1. Asks questions about the hazards involved in taking medicines without adult supervision.	1, 4, 8
	2. Is attentive to the discussion regarding the dangers involved in the consumption of unfamiliar food and liquids.	1, 3
	3. Supports the need for medicines when prescribed by physicians.	1, 2, 4, 8
	4. Is attentive to discussion about the various people who can help when a person is ill or injured.	8
	5. Displays interest in the effect of the mass media on the purchase and use of health products.	3-6, 8
Action (observable)	1. Informs parents, teachers, and others when injured or not well.	8
	2. Demonstrates limited skill in analyzing mass media advertising.	3, 4, 7, 8
	3. Seeks health information from a variety of sources.	4, 5, 7
(nonobservable or delayed)	4. Refrains from taking medicine without adult supervision.	1, 4, 8
	5. Refrains from consuming unknown foods and liquids.	1, 2, 4

Objectives for grades 4-6

Domain	Objectives for students	Basic concepts
Cognitive	1. Lists the hazards of self-diagnosis and self-medication.	2
	2. Identifies reliable sources of health information.	7
	3. Explains factors that affect the reliability of health information.	4, 5, 7
	4. Lists the types of mass media that may have an influence on the purchase and use of health products and health services.	6
	5. Is able to apply criteria in analyzing labels and advertisements of various kinds.	1, 3, 6, 8
	6. Explains the influences of friends and family on the plans to purchase and use health products and health services.	6, 8
	7. Identifies a variety of health products that are utilized in self-treatment and explains problems related to their use.	1, 2, 8
	8. Discriminates between reliable and unreliable health information and advertising.	7
	9. Cites examples of agencies and organizations that protect the consumer.	8
Affective	1. Displays interest in the need for reliable sources of health information.	5, 7

Consumer health objectives for grades 4-6—cont'd

Domain	Objectives for students	Basic concepts
	2. Asks questions in regard to the hazards of self-diagnosis and self-medication.	1, 2
	3. Accepts the need for establishing criteria for use in the selection of health products and health services.	4, 5, 7
	4. Is aware of the significance of the influence of religious beliefs, customs, superstitions, fads, and family on consumer health purchasing.	3, 6, 9
Action (observable)	1. Seeks reliable sources of health information when necessary.	5, 7
	2. Seeks appropriate health services personnel when injured or ill.	8
	3. Can analyze labels and advertisements using established criteria.	3, 4, 8
(nonobservable or delayed)	4. Avoids self-diagnosis and self-treatment.	2
	5. Utilizes established criteria when making decisions to purchase and use health products.	4, 5, 7

Objectives for grades 7-8

Domain	Objectives for students	Basic concepts
Cognitive	1. Identifies a variety of health products available and explains their effects on individuals.	1
	2. Recalls the laws that attempt to protect the health consumer.	8
	3. Explains quacks and quackery and their effects on people.	1-4
	4. Describes the nature, frequency, cost, and significance of health examinations.	2, 4, 8
	5. Identifies the various types of health specialists and services available to help individuals.	2, 4, 8
	6. Compares the healing or health treatment philosophies or cults found in society.	6, 8, 9
	7. Identifies the criteria to follow to become an "intelligent health consumer."	4
	8. Compares the role of a variety of community organizations and agencies in protecting the health consumer.	8
	9. Identifies the reasons why individuals purchase and use a variety of health products and services.	3
	10. Explains the reasons supporting a code of ethics for business establishments making health products available and for those rendering health services.	10
Affective	1. Accepts the need for reliable sources of health information.	4, 5, 7
	2. Displays interest in the need for skepticism in consumer health.	4
	3. Supports the need for laws and community organization and agencies to protect the people in consumer health.	8
	4. Is supportive of the need to understand quacks and quackery.	1, 2, 4, 5, 7

Consumer health objectives for grades 7-8—cont'd

Domain	Objectives for students	Basic concepts
	5. Is attentive to the need for health examinations.	1, 8
	6. Listens to the discussion regarding the types of health specialists available.	2, 8
	7. Asks questions about the different healing and health treatment philosophies.	6, 9
	8. Displays interest in the need for the application of a code of ethics in the business world for manufacturers, advertisers of health products, and those rendering health services.	10
Action (observable)	1. Seeks reliable sources of health information.	4, 5, 7
	2. Is skeptical regarding health information from advertising and other sources until it can be verified.	4, 5, 7
(nonobservable or delayed)	3. Utilizes the criteria for an "intelligent health consumer" when considering the purchase or use of health products and health services.	4
	4. Seeks the help of community agencies and organizations when information or assistance is needed in regard to health products and health services.	8
	5. Refrains from the purchase and use of health products that are detrimental to one's health.	1, 2

DENTAL HEALTH UNIT
Outline of content
PHYSIOLOGIC

Structure and functions of teeth

Structure—divisions—crown (top), neck, root (base); layers—enamel, dentin, cementum, pulp

Types and numbers of teeth—primary (deciduous), twenty (incisors, cuspids, molars); permanent, thirty-two (eight incisors, four cuspids, eight bicuspids, twelve molars)

Functions—chewing; speech; appearance; primary hold spaces for permanent teeth

Diseases and disorders

Dental caries—tooth decay

Causes—bacteria plus sugars = acid = decay; pathway—enamel, dentin, pulp; plaque—gluey, gelatinlike substance adhering to teeth where bacteria collect and act on food

Contributing factors—heredity, tooth structure, saliva, bacteria, sugar

Periodontal diseases

Gingivitis—inflammation of gums; pyorrhea—advanced gingivitis involving gums and bone

Symptoms—"pink" toothbrush from bleeding gums; red, swollen, tender, gums

Causes—irritation from dental calculus that results from substances secreted by bacteria in plaque; sharp edges of badly decayed teeth, worn-out fillings rubbing on gums; malocclusion, poor nutrition, systemic diseases

Prevalence—major cause for tooth loss over 35 years

Malocclusion—improper bite; effects—interferes with chewing, speech, and appearance; harder to clean

Causes—heredity, acquired factors—pressures on teeth including thumb sucking, mouth breathing, tongue twisting, lip sucking, sleep and sitting habits

Stains—(1) extrinsic—food pigments, tobacco and caffeine, metallic dusts; green stain in children—bacteria, fungi plus inorganic elements (calcium); (2) intrinsic—within tooth structure; caused by pigments in blood; imperfect tooth development

Dental health outline of content—cont'd
Physiologic—cont'd

Abscess—infection affecting blood, lymph vessels, and nerves in pulp; due to neglect of decay

Halitosis—bad breath; caused by poor dental hygiene, carious teeth, unclean mouth, periodontal disease, pyorrhea, infection, and others

Plaque—sticky, almost colorless layer of organized microcolonies of bacteria in a gelatinous substance; clings to teeth, especially near gum line

Calculus—calcified (hardened) plaque, also known as tartar; mineral deposits around gum lines that harden and are removed only by scaling

Nutrition

Need for balanced diet from basic four food groups; excess vitamins and minerals (calcium and phosphorous) not generally needed

Good "snack" food—no or minimal sugar and refined sugars; (1) potato chips, corn chips, popcorn, nuts, cheese, hard boiled eggs, raw fruits and vegetables, unsweetened fruit juices, milk; (2) detergent foods (cleanse teeth and provide exercise), raw vegetables—carrots, celery, green peppers, cauliflower, radishes; raw fruits—apples, oranges

Poor "snack" foods—candy, pastry, cookies, chocolate milk, sweetened beverages, syrups, jellies, and carbohydrate foods that are sticky and cling to teeth

PSYCHOLOGIC

Why oral health? proper tooth functioning necessary for chewing; speech; affects appearance, acceptance and rejection by peers; prevents diseases and disorders

Care of teeth and proper oral hygiene by individual

Toothbrushing—clean teeth and mouth; eliminate food particles; remove plaque; massage; prevent stains and calculus, when to brush, after eating; if not, "swish and swallow"

Toothbrush—rinse and let dry in sunlight; selection—three to four rows of bristles in straight line

Mouthwash—removes excess particles; can do with water; commercial products not effective in removing film, neutralizing acids, curing halitosis, or preventing decay; temporarily freshens and sweetens mouth; may mask disease

Flossing for plaque control with waxed or unwaxed floss between the teeth

Dentifrice—no best kind; possibly one with fluoride

Fluorides—possible use in toothpastes or powders, in tablet form, in bottled water

Periodic dental visits

Proper nutrition

Avoidance of injuries and accidents—follow safe practices; avoid detrimental habits—thumb-sucking, tongue-thrusting, chewing hard objects

SOCIAL

Problem: 90% or more of all children and youths need better oral health

Care of teeth

By dentist who examines mouth for diseases and disorders, fills cavities; provides bridges and crowns, applies topical application of fluoride, cleans and polishes teeth, replaces missing teeth, teaches dental hygiene, helps with orthodontia, and uses x-ray films, different types of fillings—silver amalgam, gold, porcelain—mouth mirror and explorer, scaler, drill, and other equipment; when to visit dentist—preferably twice yearly

By community through fluoridation of water supply (1 ppm); sodium fluoride is a chemical that becomes part of the tooth and strengthens it against decay; applied by topical application, in water, and by taking pills; favorable claims—inexpensive; reduces tooth decay significantly; reaches all people; reduces costs of repairs; unfavorable claims—forces people to drink fluoridated water against their will; dangerous to health; type of socialized medicine

Types of dentists—general practice, orthodontia; prosthetics, periodontia; pedodontia, oral surgery, and endodontia

Dental health outline of content—cont'd
Social—cont'd

How to select dentist—call local dental society for three names; call reputable hospital and ask chief of dental services for suggestions; see if dentist is member of local dental society; does postgraduate work; attends clinics and does not advertise; ask family dentist in previous community; call nearby dental school; check neighbors who are satisfied with dentist

Effects of mass media including advertising on dental health products and services

Dental health insurance

Cost of products and services for dental care

SPIRITUAL

Values: importance of dental health to self-identity; self-esteem
Moral issue: fluoridation of water supply
Humanism: responsibility of individual and community (including schools) to help needy students without funds to obtain dental health products and services

Concepts

Concept	Application of health definition
1 Positive oral health and oral health neglect have differing effects on individuals.	Physiologic
2 Most dental diseases and disorders are preventable and treatable.	
3 Differing motivations influence decisions regarding dental health.	Psychologic
4 A variety of environmental factors are important contributing causes of dental diseases and disorders and influence the purchase and use of dental health products and services.	Social
5 The community has a responsibility in the control and prevention of oral health diseases and disorders.	
6 All individuals are affected by dental health neglect.	
7 Community resources are available to assist individuals with oral health problems in varying kinds and amounts.	
8 Dental health is affected by an individual's values.	Spiritual
9 Fluoridation of the water supply is a moral issue.	
10 Equality and justice demand that dental health services and products be available to, or provided for, all individuals.	

Objectives for grades K-3

Domain	Objectives for students	Basic concepts
Cognitive	1. Explains ways to clean teeth as well as when this action should take place.	1, 2
	2. Recalls foods that help in promoting dental health.	1, 2
	3. Identifies the different teeth and their functions.	2
	4. Lists ways to prevent tooth decay or other disorders.	1, 2, 4, 7
	5. Explains the proper way to brush teeth.	1, 2
	6. States the practices that may be harmful to oral health.	4
	7. Identifies the reasons why the dentist or dental hygienist can help individuals.	2, 7
	8. Explains the procedures to follow in preparing an inexpensive dentifrice.	2
	9. Explains the proper way to floss the teeth.	1, 2

Dental health objectives for grades K-3—cont'd

Domain	Objectives for students	Basic concepts
Affective	1. Displays interest in brushing teeth properly.	1, 2
	2. Listens carefully to the ways to prevent tooth decay and other disorders.	1, 2
	3. Asks questions about teeth and their functions.	2
	4. Brings pictures to class, or is attentive to discussion of foods that may be helpful and detrimental to dental health.	1, 2, 4
	5. Talks about the need for daily health care.	1, 2, 6
	6. Accepts the dentist or dental hygienist as a friend.	2, 7
Action (observable)	1. "Swishes and swallows" when brushing the teeth is not possible.	1, 2
	2. Prepares an inexpensive dentifrice in the classroom.	2
(observable or nonobservable)	3. Eats nutritious foods, including "snack" foods.	1, 2
	4. Attempts to refrain from harmful dental health practices.	1, 2
(nonobservable, or delayed)	5. Brushes teeth properly after eating when possible.	1, 2, 4
	6. Attempts to floss teeth once daily.	1, 2, 4
	7. Uses own toothbrush and gives it proper care.	1, 2, 4
	8. Visits the dentist periodically.	2, 7

Objectives for grades 4-6

Domain	Objectives for students	Basic concepts
Cognitive	1. Explains the type, structure, functions, growth, and development of teeth.	1, 2
	2. Identifies ways in which oral health influences appearance and social relationships.	3, 4
	3. Summarizes the procedures to follow for dental health.	2, 5, 7
	4. Lists the factors that control and prevent tooth decay.	2, 5, 7
	5. Recalls the diseases and disorders that occur from oral health neglect.	1, 4, 6
	6. Explains the causes of tooth decay.	1, 2, 4
	7. Identifies the reasons for topical application of fluorides to the teeth.	1, 2, 6
	8. Recites the services that a dentist can render to an individual.	5, 7
	9. Demonstrates the proper way to floss the teeth.	1, 2
Affective	1. Accepts the responsibility for personal dental health care.	1, 3, 6-8
	2. Talks about the need for dental care including periodic dental visits.	1, 2, 7, 8
	3. Displays interest in wanting to learn more about the role of nutrition in dental health.	1, 2, 4
	4. Listens to discussion about the importance of the individual's oral health.	2, 6, 8

Dental health objectives for grades 4-6—cont'd

Domain	Objectives for students	Basic concepts
	5. Reaches the conclusion that dental health plays a role in the social acceptance and self-esteem of individuals.	2, 4, 8
	6. Supports the need for flossing the teeth as an important preventive dental health procedure.	1, 2, 6
Action (observable and nonobservable)	1. "Swishes and swallows" when brushing teeth is not possible.	2
	2. Refrains from using teeth in hazardous ways.	1, 2
	3. Eats nutritious foods and especially detergent foods.	1, 2, 4
	4. Limits the consumption of "sweets."	1, 2, 4
(nonobservable, or delayed)	5. Attempts to floss teeth daily.	1, 2
	6. Brushes teeth properly after eating when possible.	1, 2
	7. Visits the dentist periodically.	1, 2, 7
	8. Uses care in the treatment and storage of the toothbrush.	2

Objectives for grades 7-8

Domain	Objectives for students	Basic concepts
Cognitive	1. Compares the claims made for and against fluoridation.	5, 9
	2. Compares advertising claims of the product effectiveness on dental health.	4
	3. Identifies the community resources available to assist in dental health care.	7
	4. Explains the use of x-ray films in the dental care process.	1, 2, 7
	5. Lists the importance of teeth to appearance, speech, and digestion.	1, 3
	6. Lists the variety of dental specialists and the kinds of services they render.	7
	7. Compares the costs of dental services with and without proper dental care.	4, 7
	8. Identifies sources of reliable and current scientific dental health information.	4, 5, 7
Affective	1. Talks about fluoridation of the water supply as a moral issue.	9, 10
	2. Displays interest in learning about dental health and its relations to social acceptance and appearance.	3
	3. Asks questions regarding the costs of dental services with and without proper dental care.	4, 7
	4. Discusses the place of dental health in an individual's values.	8
	5. Is attentive to information presented about the variety of dental specialists and auxiliary dental personnel available in the community.	4, 7
	6. Asks questions about the benefits and hazards in the use of x-ray films by dentists.	1, 2, 7

Dental health objectives for grades 7-8—cont'd

Domain	Objectives for students	Basic concepts
Action (observable and nonobservable) (nonobservable, or delayed)	1. Is able to differentiate between reliable and unreliable dental health information.	4, 7
	2. Supports community efforts to fluoridate the water supply.	5, 6, 9, 10
	3. Supports community efforts to make dental health services and products available to needy students.	6, 10
	4. Is able to make wise decisions regarding personal dental health care.	3, 4, 8

DISEASE CONTROL UNIT
Outline of content
PHYSIOLOGIC

Definitions: disease, communicable disease, noncommunicable or chronic disease, host (focus), avenue, susceptible, acute, chronic, antigen, antibody, immunity, pathogen, vaccine, serum, antibiotic, resistance, epidemic

Types

Communicable—respiratory—colds, bronchitis, pneumonia, influenza; tuberculosis, "strep" throat; infectious hepatitis; mononucleosis; skin diseases; venereal diseases, gastrointestinal—food poisoning; childhood—measles, mumps, smallpox, chickenpox, and poliomyelitis

Causes—microorganisms-bacteria (veneral diseases, tetanus, tuberculosis, "strep" throat); viruses (colds, infectious hepatitis); fungi (ringworm); protozoa (dynsentery; malaria); parasites (worms)

Contributing causes—heredity; lack of sanitary procedures; individual susceptibility; lack of nutritious food; and exposure

Modes of transmission: air, food, water, direct contact, insects, and animals

Portals of entry—mouth, nose, breaks in skin, and other body openings

Disease process—fever, pain, infection, redness, loss of weight, bleeding, shortness of breath, and other signs and symptoms

Body defenses—skin and mucous membranes; fever; white blood cells; antibodies

Noncommunicable—heart, cancer, allergy, arthritis, diabetes, mental illness, and acne

Contributing causes—heredity; food; dysfunctioning of body organs; irritations; pressures, and a variety of other environmental factors

Effects—damage, destruction, and altered function of cells, tissues, organs, and systems; illness, disability, death

Prevention and treatment—individual—isolation, health habits; community—control of environment through laws and regulations; immunization; sanitation; water and food controls; drugs and medicines; surgery; radiation; and medical help

PSYCHOLOGIC

Effect of diseases and disorders on mental and emotional health: adjustment of self and others; success in social world

Importance of early diagnosis and treatment

Individual responsibility in disease control

Fear of disease, disability, and death

Disease and death in the family

Disease control outline of content—cont'd

SOCIAL

School and community responsibilities for prevention and control

Control procedures: laws and regulations; sanitary procedures; immunizations; availability of health department services; adequate supply of physicians and hospital and clinic facilities

Sources of help: physicians; health departments; voluntary health agencies

SPIRITUAL

Values: appreciation of healthy body; differing religious and healing philosophies toward disease

Moral issues: ethics of disease prevention and treatment on the part of individuals and the community

Humanism: attitudes toward people with disease; appreciation of healing arts; concern for others

Concepts

Concept	Application of health definition
1 Diseases can cause disability, temporary or permanent, and sometimes death.	Physical-social-spiritual
2 Communicable diseases are caused by germs and may be transmitted directly or indirectly from an infected person, or host, to someone who is not immune.	Physical-social
3 For a communicable disease to spread, there must be a host (focus of infection), an avenue or means of transmission, and a susceptible person.	Physical-social
4 Noncommunicable—sometimes called chronic—diseases are caused by hereditary factors, metabolic disorders, aging, diet, stresses, and unknown influences.	Physical
5 Acute diseases are of short duration; chronic diseases are long-lasting.	Physical
6 Elementary-school pupils should be routinely immunized against measles, polio, German measles, diphtheria, whooping cough, and tetanus.	Physical-social
7 Parents are responsible for having their children properly immunized.	Social-spiritual
8 Communicable diseases are often spread in elementary schools because of inadequate control measures at home and in school.	Physical-social-spiritual
9 Diseases occur more often among poor children and contribute to lower learning achievement for all elementary pupils.	Social-spiritual
10 Adequate medical care and public health services are necessary for control of disease in a community.	Social-spiritual

Objectives for grades K-3

Domain	Objectives for students	Basic concepts
Cognitive	1. Tells why it is important to avoid disease.	1, 9
	2. Explains the reasons for covering coughs and sneezes in the classroom.	2, 3, 8
	3. Lists the ways a communicable disease may be spread.	2, 3, 8

Disease control objectives for grades K-3—cont'd

Domain	Objectives for students	Basic concepts
	4. Identifies some communicable diseases fairly common among children.	2, 3, 8
	5. Tells why it is necessary to be immunized against certain diseases.	2, 3, 6
Affective	1. Displays interest in preventing and controlling disease.	1, 8
	2. Asks questions about different kinds of diseases.	2, 4
	3. Is aware of spread of "catching diseases" among children.	2, 3, 6, 8
	4. Accepts the value of immunizations.	3, 6
	5. Appreciates the effect of illness on learning.	9
Action	1. Covers coughs and sneezes, and follows other sanitary practices in school.	2, 8
	2. Cooperates in school or community immunization program.	6, 7
	3. Remains at home when ill with a communicable disease.	8
	4. Talks about reasons why poor people are sick more often than others.	9

Objectives for grades 4-6

Domain	Objectives for students	Basic concepts
Cognitive	1. Lists the major disease causes of death for all Americans and for children of elementary school age.	1
	2. Explains the differences between communicable and chronic diseases.	1-5
	3. Cites the differences between a vaccine and a serum.	2, 6
	4. Compares acute diseases with chronic diseases.	5
	5. Gives reasons for higher rates of disease among poverty groups.	4, 7, 9, 10
	6. Lists the communicable diseases against which elementary pupils should be immunized.	6
	7. Explains causes, prevention, and medical care for major chronic diseases.	1, 4, 10
Affective	1. Is attentive to information presented on methods for individuals, families, and communities to control diseases.	1, 3, 4, 9, 10
	2. Accepts the responsibility for taking steps to avoid spreading disease to others.	3, 6, 8
	3. Appreciates the responsibility of parents to have children immunized against certain diseases.	6, 7
	4. Supports local, state, and federal efforts to control communicable and chronic diseases.	1, 10
	5. Displays interest in government plans for health care of older people and other Americans.	1, 9, 10

Disease control objectives for grades 4-6—cont'd

Domain	Objectives for students	Basic concepts
Action	1. Follows personal and family practices to prevent disease.	1, 8
	2. Seeks medical care when symptoms of illness are present.	1, 10
	3. Cooperates with school policy by keeping immunizations up to date and staying home when ill.	3, 6, 8, 10
	4. Reports symptoms of illness to parents, teacher, or school nurse when feeling ill.	3, 8, 10

Objectives for grades 7-8*

Domain	Objectives for students	Basic concepts
Cognitive	1. Explains specific causes, preventive measures, and community control of heart diseases, cancers, stroke, and other major diseases.	1, 4, 9, 10
	2. Cites differences between communicable and non-communicable and acute and chronic diseases.	1, 2, 4, 5
	3. Lists recent medical and health science advances that have helped control disease.	1, 10
	4. Illustrates ways that individuals, families, and communities can help control disease.	1, 8, 10
Affective	1. Appreciates the fact that some diseases can be controlled more easily than others.	1, 4, 5, 10
	2. Displays interest in plans to provide better medical and hospital care for all Americans.	1, 9, 10
	3. Realizes the importance of immunizations for self-protection and the protection of others.	3, 6, 7
	4. Supports government and other research efforts to improve preventive and control measures for disease.	1, 10
	5. Accepts responsibility for having periodic medical checkups.	1, 10
Action	1. Has regular medical checkups.	1, 10
	2. Has all routinely recommended immunizations.	3, 6, 8
	3. Follows personal and family practices to prevent disease.	1, 8
	4. Avoids smoking, drinking, drug use, and other practices that may cause illness.	1, 9
	5. Avoids or minimizes physical, chemical, or emotional stresses that may cause disease.	1, 4

DRUG UNIT
Outline of content
PHARMACOLOGIC

Definitions: drug, drug use, misuse, and abuse, addiction, dependency, habituation, tolerance, toxicity, slang terms

Identification of abused drugs: technical help needed

---

*Special attention may be given to heart disease and risk-taking factors and cancer.

Drug unit outline of content—cont'd
Pharmacologic—cont'd

> Classification of drugs
> > Legal and illegal
> > > Legal—over the counter and prescription
> > > Illegal—marijuana, heroin, LSD, and others
> > Pharmacologic
> > > Stimulants—amphetamines, tobacco, coffee, cocaine
> > > Depressants (sedatives-hypnotics)—alcohol, barbiturates, inhalants, marijuana
> > > Psychedelics—LSD, psilocybin, peyote, STP
> > > Narcotic—heroin, morphine, opium, codeine, methadone
> > > Tranquilizers—Thorazine, Compazine, Serpasil
> > > Over-the-counter—aspirin, antihistamines, cough medicines, diet pills, sleeping pills
> > Common or trade name (brand) and generic (chemical) identity

PHYSIOLOGIC

The nervous system
Drug effects: dose response, biologic variability, potency, tolerance
Medical uses: dependent on drug of use
Abuse potential: physical and psychologic dependence, tolerance
Effects: short-term and long-term dependence on drugs of use
Duration of action: dependent on drug of use
Method of administration: pills, capsules, injections, sniffing, liquid, smoking, or chewing

PSYCHOLOGIC

Why people use, misuse, and abuse drugs: curiosity, personal conflicts—insecurity, escape, boredom, rebelliousness; kicks; peer pressures; search for identity; rejection of culture including schools; television; commercial exploitation
Characteristics of potential drug abusers: high-risk youths are those with behavioral problems at school with mild conduct disorders; lack of self-confidence; maybe self-centered and self-indulgent
Alternatives to drugs: athletics and recreational activities; counseling and group therapy in personal development; improved communications; social service participation; political service activities; intellectual motivation—reading discussion, creative games; participation in creative art activities; philosophic discussions on ethics, morality, values; spiritual involvement; survival training

SOCIAL

Patterns of drug use and abuse: classification of users and abusers
Nature and extent of drug use and abuse: legal and illegal; youth, adults
Factors affecting drug use and abuse
> Conflicts in reality—escape, values
> Economics—business and communication media
> Social and political climate
> Youth life-styles—counter-culture, youth identity, adolescent revolt
Role of home, school, community: prevention, control, treatment, and rehabilitation
Rehabilitation and treatment: multimodality concept
> Crisis intervention
> Detoxification
> After care
> > Pharmaceutical—Cyclazocine, methadone
> > Psychiatric—individual counseling in psychiatric hospital
> > Psychosocial—Syanon, Daytop Village, and others
> > Religious—Teen Challenge, AA
Courts and the law: laws; enforcement procedures and problems; criminal justice process

Drug unit outline of content—cont'd
Social—cont'd

Community resources: federal, state, and local governmental agencies—FTC, FDA, OE, NIMH; private sources; mass media and the business world; education; laws and enforcement; facilities—crisis centers, clinics, hotlines, ongoing groups, self-help groups; drug abuse council or committee

Identification of drug abusers

Observations of signs and symptoms

General and specific—change in attendance, discipline, and performance; unusual activity or inactivity; deterioration of personal appearance and health habits; unpredictable outbreaks of temper

Characteristics of potential users

Tell-tale evidence

Peer identification, self-identification, clinical test

SPIRITUAL

Values: developing a value system; self-identity and self-concept

Moral issues: implications of use and abuse of drugs on self, home, and community; drug use by students and adults; commercial interests; the mass media; the sale of drugs; the justice of laws controlling drugs

Humanism: individual and community responsibilities for drug abusers; the job market for rehabilitated drug abusers or drug abusers in industry

Concepts

Concept	Application of health definition
1 Drugs differ in kind and degree; they have multiple uses with a variety of effects on individuals.	Pharmacologic
2 Proper use of drugs may be beneficial to individuals, the family, and the community.	
3 Improper use of drugs may result in health and safety problems to individuals, the family, and the community.	
4 Numerous factors and forces influence the availability as well as the use and misuse of legal and illegal drugs by individuals and the community.	Psychologic-social
5 The individual, the family, and the community have interrelated and reciprocal responsibilities to help control the availability, to prevent the misuse and abuse, and to assist individuals who become misusers and abusers of drugs in society.	Social
6 The use and misuse of drugs by individuals involve moral principles and issues and are related to one's sense of values as well as to the humane and just treatment of all people in society.	Spiritual

Objectives for grades K-3

Domain	Objectives for students	Basic concepts
Cognitive	1. Identifies drugs commonly used.	1
	2. Illustrates ways common drugs are used by individuals.	1
	3. Lists beneficial effects of drugs.	2
	4. Identifies substances that can be harmful or misused.	3
	5. Lists responsible people who can help when medicines are needed.	2, 3

Drug unit objectives for grades K-3—cont'd

Domain	Objectives for students	Basic concepts
	6. Explains why medicines should be taken under supervision of parent as prescribed or recommended by a physician or dentist.	4
	7. States conditions under which individuals show lack of responsibility when using medicine.	5
	8. Cites ways in which individual shows respect for drugs.	5
Affective	1. Is aware of differences between alcohol and other drugs and of their usage by individuals.	1, 4
	2. Displays interest in learning about the beneficial as well as harmful effects of drugs.	2, 3
	3. Desires to use drugs in useful and responsible ways.	4, 5
	4. Shows interest in discovering people who can help when medicines are needed.	5
Action (nonobservable, or delayed)	1. Uses only substances that aid in proper responsible supervision.	3
	2. Takes medicines and drugs only under responsible supervision.	3
	3. Refuses to accept substances from strangers.	3-5
	4. Limits or refrains from use of drugs, except medicines prescribed and recommended, until grown up.	3, 5

Objectives for grades 4-6

Domain	Objectives for students	Basic concepts
Cognitive	1. Identifies varieties of drugs used by individuals.	1
	2. Lists reasons for drugs in society.	3
	3. Explains medical uses of commonly used drugs.	2
	4. Explains physiologic effects of some of the commonly used drugs.	1
	5. Lists reasons persons react differently to chemicals contained in drugs.	1
	6. Cites examples of misuse and abuse of drugs.	3, 4
	7. Identifies difficulties or possible problems from misuse and abuse of drugs.	3
	8. Explains why misuse and abuse of drugs may start early in life.	4
	9. Lists ways society tries to protect individuals from abuse of drugs.	4
	10. Identifies ways to protect self against misuse and abuse of drugs.	3, 4
	11. Starts to analyze information about drugs on television, in newspapers and magazines.	4, 5
Affective	1. Displays interest in learning about varieties of drugs and their effects on the body.	1-3
	2. Asks questions about problems involved with misuse or abuse of drugs.	3, 5
	3. Seeks further information about community efforts to help people who misuse and abuse drugs.	5

Drug unit objectives for grades 4-6—cont'd

Domain	Objectives for students	Basic concepts
	4. Discusses ways to protect self against misuse and abuse of drugs.	5, 6
	5. Expresses desire to use drugs responsibly and usefully.	2, 6
Action (nonobservable, or delayed)	1. Uses only substances that aid in proper growth and development.	2
	2. Takes medicine and drugs only under responsible supervision.	3
	3. Limits or refrains from use of drugs, except medicines prescribed or recommended, until grown up.	3
	4. Refuses to use illegal drugs.	3, 6
	5. Starts to develop own practices and habit patterns to protect self against abuse of drugs.	3, 4

Objectives for grades 7-8

Domain	Objectives for students	Basic concepts
Cognitive	1. Recalls varieties of drugs used by people.	1
	2. Describes how medicines can be used to benefit individual.	2
	3. Lists variety of individual and social factors that influence misuse and abuse of drugs.	4
	4. Interprets role of business and advertising in sale of drugs.	4, 5
	5. Identifies differing effects of variety of drugs on the body.	1, 4
	6. Compares benefits of smoking, drinking, and using drugs with possible detrimental effects.	2, 3
	7. Identifies reasons why people do and do not use, misuse, and abuse drugs.	4
	8. Illustrates ways to cope with social and emotional pressures of life other than through use of drugs.	4, 5
	9. States procedures used by community to control availability, sale, and use of drugs.	5
	10. Discusses need for development of a value system.	6
	11. Recalls signs and symptoms of drug misusers and abusers.	1
Affective	1. Is attentive to information presented on varieties of drugs used by people, their benefits, their hazards, and their differing physiologic effects.	1-3
	2. Shows interest in comparisons of benefits and detrimental effects of alcohol, tobacco, and drugs on individuals and society.	2, 3
	3. Gives opinions regarding role of business and advertising in sale and availability of drugs.	2, 3, 5
	4. Asks questions about alternatives to drug use.	4, 5
	5. Displays interest in developing a value system.	6
	6. Is aware and discusses long-term results from frequent and regular misuse and abuse of drugs.	4, 5

Drug unit objectives for grades 7-8—cont'd

Domain	Objectives for students	Basic concepts
Action (nonobservable, or delayed)	1. Make judgments about drugs and drug users after reviewing all aspects of problem.	4-6
	2. Seeks to discover one's own identity and purposes in life.	6
	3. Participates in a school-education-information program.	5
	4. Seeks help from school personnel if having a drug problem.	4, 5
	5. Refrains from regular use of drugs that may lead to dependency, disease, or disability.	3-6
	6. Avoids use of drugs that may affect ability to think clearly and react normally.	3-6
	7. Refuses to use illegal drugs.	3-6

EXERCISE, REST, RELAXATION, AND BODY CONTROL UNIT
Outline of content
PHYSIOLOGIC

Definitions: physical fitness, physiology, physiology of exercise, body mechanics, muscular system, cardiovascular system, strength, speed, endurance, posture, rest, sleep

Exercise
 Muscles—types—skeletal (external body control), heart, and smooth (internal organs—blood vessels, glands, others)
 Characteristic—contractility when stimulated by nerves
 Skeletal muscles:
  Structure—attached to bones of body
  Locations—back, chest, abdominal wall, arms and legs
  Functions—movement of body (exercise), maintenance of posture, production of body heat
 Kinds of exercise—many forms; light or heavy, including walking, running, bicycling, hiking, sports, recreational activities
  Effects—muscle tone, strength, size and control of skeletal muscles; aid in individual's meeting demands of daily activity; help in creation of reserves for emergencies and safety; aid in cardiovascular, respiratory, and nervous system functioning; improvement of posture; stamina, endurance; relief from tension; fun and pleasure; aid in mental health; control of body weight; one factor involved in heart disease

Rest, relaxation, and sleep
 Requirements—need for a balance of work, play, rest, relaxation, and sleep daily; sleep requirements—8 to 10 hours daily for children and adolescents
 Fatigue—types—physical, mental or emotional
  Causes—intense of prolonged physical activity; psychologic factors—nervousness, boredom, worry, tensions and stress, emotions, noise; infections and disease conditions
  Effects—less attention, drowsy, irritability, lowered resistance to fatigue, less alert to possible hazards—more accident prone, less ability to perform effectively
 Procedures for relaxation—sleep, rest, exercise, change of activity, music, art, and other pleasurable activities

Body control
 Dependent on proper exercise, practice of bodily movements, adequate rest, relaxation and sleep, nutrition, and other environmental factors
 Poor posture because of lack of, or improper, exercise, rest, and sleep; poor habits of sitting, standing, reclining, or walking; improper nutrition; ill-fitting clothes and shoes

Exercise, rest, relaxation, and body control outline of content—cont'd

PSYCHOLOGIC

Importance of relaxation in helping endure stress
Importance of exercise, rest, and sleep to the individual
Selection of activities to fulfill individual needs
Competition and its psychologic effects on children and youths
Games and sports and their provision for success experiences and self-reliance opportunities

SOCIAL

Role of school, home, and community: providing facilities and opportunities for exercise, rest, and relaxation
School curriculum: its inclusion of an education program to help students with postural or exercise problems or to fulfill pupil needs
Social interaction: through games, sport, dance, or other forms of exercise and activity
Improvement of teacher-pupil relationships

SPIRITUAL

Values: appreciation of physical fitness, rest, sleep, relaxation, and posture to health and effective living; appreciation of differing attitudes of individuals toward exercise and physical activity
Moral issues: fair play and good sportsmanship in games and sports
Humanism: teacher-pupil relations in an informal atmosphere through play experiences; guidance by providing for the differing physical abilities of pupils

Concepts

Concept	Application of health definition
1 Physical fitness is one aspect of total health and requires regular vigorous exercise.	Physical
2 Regular exercise produces good muscle tone and efficient circulation and helps maintain desirably body weight.	Physical-social
3 Everyone needs a balance of exercise and rest for optimal health.	Physical-psychologic
4 Sports and dance provide opportunity for healthful exercise and pleasant social interaction.	Physical-social-psychologic
5 Sound body dynamics improves efficiency and appearance.	Physical-social-psychologic

Objectives for grades K-3

Domain	Objectives for students	Basic concepts
Cognitive	1. Tells why exercise, rest, and relaxation are important for good health.	1-4
	2. Identifies ways to relax.	3
	3. Recalls pleasant experiences in games or dance activities.	4
	4. Identifies the values of good posture and sound body mechanics.	5
	5. Explains the importance of rest, relaxation, and sleep to optimal health.	3
Affective	1. Appreciates value of exercise, rest, and relaxation in maintaining good health and growth.	1, 2
	2. Desires to learn and play games regularly.	1, 2, 4
	3. Shows interest in individual and group games and dances.	1, 2, 4

Exercise, rest, relaxation, and body control objectives for grades K-3—cont'd

Domain	Objectives for students	Basic concepts
	4. Shows interest in using own body most efficiently.	5
	5. Is aware of the daily need for rest, relaxation, and sleep.	3
Action	1. Takes an active part in games and dances at school and after school.	1, 2, 4
	2. Practices good body dynamics in daily activities.	5
	3. Sleeps 8 to 10 hours each night and rests occasionally during the day.	3
	4. Demonstrates good sportsmanship and a spirit of cooperation in games and dances.	4

Objectives for grades 4-6

Domain	Objectives for students	Basic concepts
Cognitive	1. Explains physiologic reasons for regular, vigorous exercise.	1, 2
	2. Understands emotional health values of sports and dance.	4
	3. Can demonstrate the basics of functional body movement.	5
	4. Lists reasons for adequate rest, relaxation, and sleep.	3
	5. Identifies ways to relax at home and school.	3
Affective	1. Appreciates the values of physical fitness as a part of total good health.	1, 2, 4
	2. Asks questions about the physiologic and mental benefits of exercise.	1, 2, 4
	3. Desires to learn more about basic skills, strategy, and rules of sports.	4
	4. Is attentive to information on the importance of rest, relaxation, and sleep.	3
	5. Appreciates the esthetic and physiologic values of efficient body movement.	5
Action	1. Takes an active part in games and dance activities at school.	1, 2, 4
	2. Participates in sports after school and on weekends.	1, 2, 4
	3. Sleeps 8 to 10 hours each night and rests when fatigued during the day.	3
	4. Demonstrates good sportsmanship in sports and dance activities.	4
	5. Practices good body dynamics in daily activities.	5
	6. Takes time daily to participate in some type of relaxation activity.	3

Objectives for grades 7-8

Domain	Objectives for students	Basic concepts
Cognitive	1. Explains specific changes in muscular and circulatory systems during exercise.	1, 2
	2. Describes mental health values of sports and dance.	4

Exercise, rest, relaxation, and body control objectives for grades 7-8—cont'd

Domain	Objectives for students	Basic concepts
	3. Understands the kinesiology of fundamental body movements as in standing, sitting, walking, lifting, pushing, and pulling.	5
	4. Cites the physical and mental values of proper sleep, relaxation, and rest.	3
	5. Lists health values of regular exercise.	1, 2, 4
Affective	1. Believes that physical fitness is one of the values in the good life.	1-5
	2. Appreciates the physiologic and emotional values of regular exercise.	1, 2, 4
	3. Desires to learn more about basic skills, strategy, and rules of sports.	4
	4. Appreciates the physical and mental values of adequate rest, relaxation, and sleep.	3
	5. Believes that one's appearance and efficiency are enhanced by sound body dynamics.	5
Action	1. Participates regularly in sports, dance, or other forms of physical exercise.	1, 2, 4
	2. Sleeps 8 to 10 hours each night and rests when fatigued during the day.	3
	3. Demonstrates cooperation, leadership, and good sportsmanship in sports or dance activities.	4
	4. Maintains desirable muscle development and figure control through exercise.	1, 2
	5. Follows principles of sound body dynamics in daily activities.	5
	6. Relaxes daily using a satisfactory method.	3

FAMILY HEALTH UNIT
Outline of content
PHYSIOLOGIC

Life: purpose and order, a life cycle or pattern of growth, all living things from living things
  Characteristics—a beginning, changes, and death; reproduction; need for food, water, air, protection; movement; response to light, sound, cold, pain, danger
  Differences—form, structure, functions, life cycle, pattern of growth, dependency and needs, methods of reproduction
  Types—plant, animal, and human; plant reproduction—budding, runners, seeds, pollination; animal reproduction—asexually—cell division or fission; sexually—internally with males and females, and externally as in some fish who lay eggs
Human life: man—unique; rational; decision maker; possessor of freedom, self-awareness, consciousness, and dignity; controller of actions; similarities and differences—heredity, race, size, intellect, ethnic background
Human growth and development
  Definitions—"growing up," puberty, maturity
    Puberty—special growth stage reaching physical adulthood; girls reach this stage 1½ years earlier than boys
    Maturity—growth stage in which the person is more cooperative; has positive sex attitudes; is not easily hurt, is not dominated by moods, is able to meet problems constructively, is able to meet responsibilities, is able to make wise decisions
  Cause—action of endocrine glands and their hormones

Family health outline of content—cont'd
Physiologic—cont'd

Results—a variety of physical, emotional, and social changes

Physical—size and shape changes; appearance of secondary sex characteristics; boys—muscle development; hair on face, chest, and pubic areas; seminal emissions; appearance of sex drive; girls—hair under arms and pubic areas; breasts, widening of hips; menstrual cycle; appearance of sex drive

Emotional—physical attraction; fears and emotions with possible moodiness

Social—increase in boy-girl relations; need for friends

Role of heredity—physical characteristics; chromosomes and genes

Human reproduction

Start of life—union of male (sperm) and female (ovum) cells; need for father and mother

Reproductive organs

Male—external—penis, scrotum, testicles, pubic hair; internal—urethra, bladder, prostate, seminal vesicles, vas deferens, epididymis

Female—external—pubic hair, labia majora and minora, urethral opening, clitoris, vaginal opening, hymen; internal—vagina, cervix, uterus, oviduct, ovaries, bladder

Other concepts—fertilization, conception, implantation, fetus growth, birth, menstruation, birth control

PSYCHOLOGIC

Understanding self: strengths and weaknesses; personality; worth; ability to succeed, but ability to accept failure; understanding and control of emotions; experience of joy through self-fulfillment; wholesome relations with others; decision making by problem solving process; good use of abilities

Sex drive—normal reaction; perpetuation of mankind; provides pleasure

Sex behavior in adolescence—interest in one's body and sex normal; question of sex before marriage; sex deviation—homosexuality, exhibitionism, rape

Factors influencing sex drive—biologic makeup; early childhood experiences; parental attitudes; environmental influences

Purpose of family—satisfaction of physical and psychologic needs; stability and security important for good mental health; guidance of individuals to adulthood

SOCIAL

The family

Nature—size; structure, or composition; culture or ethnic; religion; changes

Types—two parents; one parent; no parents, guardian; step-parents; mixed ethnic

Needs—physical, psychologic, and emotional

Functions—different roles because of different types of families and geographic location, but inclusion of sharing and transmission of feelings, ideas, heritage, and income; security by fulfilling needs; aid in education; growth and development; affection, worthy use of leisure time

Role of individual family members—assumption of responsibilities; cooperation in functioning of home; respect of others' rights; consideration; acceptance of differences; trying to understand members; not making unreasonable demands; working together; helping in different ways including financial support; use of constructive ways to solve differences

Status in family of oldest child—only child; only boy in group of girls; only girl in group of boys

Family influence on ability of members to make adjustments in society dependent on—cultural background of parents; family dwelling and location; health practices of members; economic status; type of structure; values

Problems and conflicts—parents; siblings; grandparents; money; use of car; discourtesy; failure to assume responsibilities at home, school, or elsewhere; use of drugs; choice and selection of friends; use of time

Family health outline of content—cont'd
Social—cont'd

Boy-girl relations

Development—building of friendships; popularity; qualities boys and girls are seeking

Purpose—sense of belonging; affection; getting along with opposite sex; enjoyment; learning of social behavior

Dating—types; purposes; responsibilities; choosing a date; dating behavior and society's moral code; drinking and drugs

Steady dating—why; advantages and disadvantages; parents' attitudes and reactions

Values of sex in marriage—legal; emotional; social; medical; spiritual

Family planning

Love

SPIRITUAL

Values: finding a purpose and meaningfulness in life; a philosophy of life; importance of friendships; interpersonal relationships with adults and peers; influence on personality development; relation to acquisition and use of money

Moral issues: premarital sex; failure to assume home responsibilities; relations with others, including parents

Concepts

Concept	Application of health definition
1 All living things come from living things.	Physiologic
2 Individuals in some ways are like all individuals, in some ways like some individuals, and in some ways like no other individual.	
3 The sex drive and reproduction are normal functions of humans.	Psychologic
4 Maturity is dependent on a variety of physical, social, and emotional factors.	
5 The family, with its unique features that are subject to change, is the basic unit in American society.	Social
6 Individuals influence and are influenced by the family and its members.	
7 Boy-girl relationships are important preludes to family life and family relations.	
8 Values and moral issues affect attitudes and behaviors regarding the family and sex.	Spiritual

Objectives for grades K-3

Domain	Objectives for students	Basic concepts
Cognitive	1. Identifies the differences that exist between boys and girls.	2
	2. Concludes the human baby grows and develops inside the mother.	1, 2
	3. Recites the correct vocabulary for body parts and body functions.	1, 2
	4. Lists the responsibilities to be completed at home and at school.	5, 6
	5. Explains how humans reproduce.	1
	6. Compares how families differ in their composition and functions.	5
	7. Recalls that living things come from living things.	1
	8. Explains the way parents and family members help individuals.	4-6, 8

Family health objectives for grades K-3—cont'd

Domain	Objectives for students	Basic concepts
	9. Identifies the rights of others in need of respect.	2, 4-8
	10. Describes the role and responsibilities of family members.	5
Affective	1. Displays interest in learning about the differences between boys and girls.	2
	2. Asks questions about the growth of the baby inside the mother.	1, 2
	3. Is interested in wanting to learn the correct vocabulary for body parts and body functions.	1, 2
	4. Believes there are responsibilities individuals must give their attention to at school and at home.	5, 6
	5. Is attentive to the discussion regarding human reproduction.	1, 2
	6. Talks about the differing compositions and functions of families.	5, 6
	7. Accepts the conclusion that living things come from living things.	1
	8. Believes that parents and family members may be helpful to individuals.	4-6, 8
	9. Is supportive of the need to respect the rights of others.	2, 5-8
	10. Is attentive to the discussion about the role and responsibilities of family members.	5
Action (observable) (observable and non-observable)	1. Uses the correct vocabulary for body parts and body functions.	1, 2
	2. Assumes responsibilities at school and at home.	5, 6
	3. Tries to respect the rights of others, including their right to privacy.	5, 6

Objectives for grades 4-6

Domain	Objectives for students	Basic concepts
Cognitive	1. Identifies the responsibilities that need attention as a family member.	5, 6
	2. Lists the rights of others in need of respect.	2, 4-8
	3. Is familiar with the terminology utilized in describing the human reproductive process.	1
	4. Summarizes the meaning of puberty and its effect upon growth and development.	1-4
	5. Explains the responsibilities of all members of a family.	5, 6
	6. Recalls that sex is a basic life function.	1-4
	7. Identifies the role of heredity in the growth and development of individuals.	2-4, 7
	8. Lists the variety of characteristics displayed by the family.	5, 6
Affective	1. Believes that it is necessary as a family member to assume home responsibilities.	5, 6

Family health objectives for grades 4-6—cont'd

Domain	Objectives for students	Basic concepts
	2. Supports the concept that the rights of others must be respected.	2, 4-8
	3. Is interested in learning the terminology necessary to describe the human reproductive process.	1
	4. Listens to the discussion about puberty and its effect on growth and development.	1-4
	5. Displays interest in the responsibilities of all family members.	5, 6
	6. Accepts sex as a basic life function.	1-3
	7. Asks questions regarding the role of heredity on the growth and development of individuals.	1, 2, 4
	8. Accepts the basic life function of menstruation as an important phenomenon.	2, 3
	9. Believes it is necessary to cooperate with other family members to achieve a happy family unit.	5, 6
	10. Is aware that families display a variety of characteristics.	5
Action (nonobservable)	1. Assumes responsibilities at home as a family member.	5, 6
(observable, nonobservable, or delayed)	2. Tries to cooperate with family members to achieve a happy family unit.	5, 6
	3. Makes efforts to consistently respect the rights of others.	2, 4-8
(observable, and non-observable)	4. Is able to discuss human reproduction using appropriate terminology without embarrassment.	1

Objectives for grades 7-8

Domain	Objectives for students	Basic concepts
Cognitive	1. Explains the sex drive and its effect on individuals.	1-4, 7
	2. Identifies factors that may influence one's sex drive.	3, 4, 6-8
	3. Differentiates between physical, emotional, and social maturity.	4
	4. Summarizes the human reproductive process from conception through birth.	1-3
	5. Concludes that the family is the basic unit of American society and is familiar with its changing roles.	5
	6. Identifies the importance of boy-girl relationships and the qualities boys and girls seek in one another.	7
	7. Prepares criteria for behavior on dates.	3, 4, 7, 8
	8. Compares the advantages and disadvantages of steady dating.	7, 8
	9. Discusses sexual behavior in adolescence and before marriage.	3-5, 8
	10. Explains the meaning of love.	7

Family health objectives for grades 7-8—cont'd

Domain	Objectives for students	Basic concepts
	11. Identifies the social, economic, and cultural influences on family life.	5, 6, 8
	12. Selects values or a value system having meaning in life.	8
	13. Is familiar with the problem solving process to help make decisions about the family and sex behavior.	4, 5, 8
	14. Concludes there are moral issues involved in premarital sex, acceptance of responsibilities in the home, and others.	3-5, 8
	15. Describes the concept and purpose of family planning.	3-5, 7, 8
Affective	1. Accepts sex as a natural drive and function of individuals that is accompanied by related responsibilities.	1-4, 7
	2. Believes that maturity in life is essential for successful living.	4
	3. Displays interest in the human reproductive process from conception through birth.	1-3
	4. Is sensitive to the acceptance of the family as the basic unit of American society and its changing roles.	5
	5. Is aware of the need to develop boy-girl relationships and procedures for building friendships.	7
	6. Asks questions regarding the advantages and disadvantages of steady dating.	7, 8
	7. Is interested in discussing and preparing criteria for behavior on dates.	3, 4, 7, 8
	8. Displays a readiness to want to discuss sexual behavior in adolescence and before marriage.	3, 4, 7, 8
	9. Accepts the meaning of love to be more inclusive than physical attraction.	7
	10. Is aware of the variety of social, economic, and cultural influences on family life.	5, 6
	11. Believes that individuals need to determine the values that help them develop a philosophy of life.	8
	12. Supports the problem solving process as a useful method in making decisions about sex and family behavior.	4, 6
	13. Is sensitive to the moral issues involved in premarital sex relations, acceptance of responsibilities in the home, and others.	3-5, 8
	14. Is aware of the importance of family planning.	3-5, 7, 8
Action (observable and nonobservable)	1. Attempts to act as a physically, emotionally, and socially mature individual.	4
(nonobservable)	2. Tries to become a contributing and effective member of the family.	5, 6
(nonobservable, or	3. Demonstrates the ability to achieve a balance between expression, behavior, and the sex drive.	1-4, 7, 8

Family health objectives for grades 7-8—cont'd

Domain	Objectives for students	Basic concepts
delayed)	4. Develops wholesome relationships with members of the opposite sex.	7
	5. Behaves in socially accepted ways with members of the opposite sex.	7
	6. Attempts to develop values or a value system that will give life meaningfulness.	8
	7. Utilizes the problem solving process to help make decisions about the family and sex behavior.	3, 4, 6

MENTAL HEALTH UNIT*
Outline of content
PHYSIOLOGIC

Definitions: Mental health—adjustment to self and society; faces realities of life; functions effectively

Mental illness—varying degrees of emotional disturbance; in severe forms—psychoses, neuroses, personality disorders

Death†—physiologic, social, and psychologic aspects and concepts, causes, and effects

Growth and development of individual: factors influencing

Heredity—nervous system and endocrine glands; effect on thinking, feeling, acting

Environment—economically rich or deprived; stresses and pressure of parents, peers, of teacher; physical atmosphere—housing, climate

Interrelationship of biologic and environmental influences—heredity sets limits; environment determines level of attainment; stress situations may cause biologic reactions and anxiety; pleasant environment brings feelings of calmness and tranquility

PSYCHOLOGIC

Mentally healthy individual: pursuer of reasonable goals; self-respect; knowledge of being liked and loved; sense of security; ability to think and act rationally; distinguishes between facts and feelings; maintenance of integrity in work and play; ability to work in group; respect for rights of others; faces realities of life; acceptance of responsibilities

Needs of individuals: physical—food, air, water, rest and sleep, housing, clothing, freedom from disease

Psychologic—affection, security, acceptance as an individual, achievement, independence, authority, self-respect, success

Mature personality: a clear self-concept‡

Definition of personality—involving total physical, social, mental, and emotional aspects of individual including interests, size, shape, dress; the way the individual walks, talks, thinks, feels; ability to get along with people

Understanding of own strengths, weaknesses, and academic, intellectual, and physical potentials

---

*See Chapter 7.

†Death education has been introduced into school curriculums. It is believed to be a part of mental health. References at the end of the chapter provide selected readings. Chapter 12 contains suggested activities.

‡Stenner and Katzenmeyer claim that children during the early school years who have positive self-concepts are confident of their ability to meet everyday problems and demands and are at ease in their relationships with other people. These children tend to be independent and reliable and are relatively free from anxiety, nervousness, excessive worry, tiredness, and loneliness. They are seldom considered behavior problems. They tend to be above average in reading and mathematics. They view school as a happy, worthwhile place.

Mental health outline of content—cont'd
Psychologic—cont'd

Understanding of emotions' role in development
Types—anger, fear, love, hate, jealousy, happiness, prejudice, sorrow, joy
Effects—helpful or harmful
Relief from effects by talk with someone, play, work, hobbies
Influence on personal health—sleep and rest; eating; posture; physical activity
Control—sense of humor; ability to accept criticism, disappointment, failure, and unhappiness in normal fashion
Understanding of the physical growth changes taking place
Ability to make adjustments, develop coping skills
Solving of problems and making decisions after weighing alternatives and consequences about study, work, sex, parent relations, peer relations
Establishment of realistic goals within potentials; achievable to reduce stress
Assumption and carrying out of responsibilities at home, school, and community
Ability to handle stress
Nature—tensions or pressures build attempting to carry out responsibilities, to achieve goals, or to solve problems resulting in anxieties, fears, worries and other emotional responses; degree dependent on factors involved
Causes—competition, desire to succeed, failure, sibling rivalry, parent expectations, school demands
Values and limits—some individuals work better under slight stress; may be motivational; may interfere with normal response
Relief from—modification of goals; activity change; balance of work and play; assumption of responsibilities; talking it out; taking one thing at a time; working off
Risk taking—positive and negative; includes financial gambles and monetary, bodily harm and physical injury, ethical, self-esteem, and social
Coping with death and dying; bereavement and grief
Adjustment mechanisms: result from inability to adequately solve problems; individual resorts to other procedures to gain satisfaction, such as rationalization, projection, identification; misuse results in maladjusted behavior
Causes of mental illness: multiplicity of complex environmental factors
Physical and chemical—infections, nutritional deficiencies, accidents, gland deficiencies, alcohol, anemia, physical defects
Psychologic—social relations, love and marriage, family conflicts, sibling conflicts; sex adjustments, religious conflicts, parental attitudes and personality, school and peer experiences
Emotional maladjustment or mental illness: mental illness is a matter of degree and kind; for some individuals, mild emotional disturbances; for others, severe mental health problems manifested in a variety of symptomatic behaviors
Death: meaningfulness and relation to birth and life, to individuals, animals, and pets; bereavement and grief—stages of grief, need for others, need to be alone, helping others grieve; coping mechanisms—denial, anger, bargaining, depression, acceptance; feelings—perception of death; suicide—causes, signs, and symptoms

SOCIAL

Building of satisfying human relations: effective interaction with adults, peers, and opposite sex
Acquisition and retention of friends: sharing possessions and time; development of trust and fair play; respect of people as individuals; willingness to work with people; courteous and considerate; ability to give as well as to take
Choice of friends: need to establish criteria
Influence of people: rewards; threats; authority; expertness
Warm, safe, and secure home and school climate
Alternative life-styles

Mental health outline of content—cont'd
Social—cont'd

Successful group functioning involving respect and acceptance of all members; participation of all members; acceptance of responsibilities by each member; need for authority; a must to have constructive ways to resolve differences

Recognition of worth: realization that all individuals have differing human worths; ability to give consideration to rights of others; value of individual differences including race, religion or ethnic origin

Community resource available to help with problems: school—nurse, teacher, counselor; home—parents; church—clergymen; community—physicians, psychiatrists, organizations and agencies, public health departments

Death: death rituals and funerals—cultural and ethnic differences; communication with terminally ill; costs; suicide—sources of help

SPIRITUAL

Values: the individual needs to attempt to define own values or value system; the individual's acceptance of differing values and value system of others

Moral issue: basic principles to use in the development and retention of relationships with others

Humanism: recognition that all individuals should receive equal and just treatment regardless of socioeconomic status, religious, cultural, or ethnic backgrounds

Death: right to life; euthanasia

Concepts

Concept	Application of health definition
1 Mental health is influenced by biologic and environmental factors.	Physiologic
2 Each individual is like all others, like some others, and like no others.	
3 Understanding and acceptance of the concept of one's self is important in mental health.	Psychologic
4 All individuals have dignity and worth.	
5 Individuals should be able to face the realities of life with emotional maturity.	
6 Stress can be beneficial and detrimental to individuals.	
7 The ability to get along with others is important in mental health.	Social
8 The community has a variety of sources available to help individuals with mental and emotional problems and difficulties.	
9 Values help to provide meaningfulness to life.	Spiritual

Objectives for grades K-3

Domain	Objectives for students	Basic concepts
Cognitive	1. Explains the reasons why sharing and taking turns are necessary.	7
	2. Lists ways to respect the feelings, rights, and property of individuals.	4, 7
	3. Lists ways of making and keeping friends.	7
	4. Identifies basic emotions.	5-7
	5. Discusses ways emotions may be helpful and harmful and their effects on personal worth.	5-7
	6. Recalls possible ways to sublimate or control emotional reactions.	1, 3, 5-7
	7. Recites ways to assume responsibilities in school and at home.	7

Mental health objectives for grades K-3—cont'd

Domain	Objectives for students	Basic concepts
	8. Identifies ways to have success and to be independent at school.	3, 5
	9. Explains ways to prevent hurting someone or causing hard feelings.	1, 4, 5, 7
	10. Explains life and death in terms of loss of pets and animals.	5
Affective	1. Is interested in sharing and taking turns.	7
	2. Talks about the feelings, rights, and property of individuals.	4, 7
	3. Is attentive to discussion regarding emotions and their effects on individuals.	1, 5-7
	4. Asks questions regarding ways to prevent hurting people or causing hard feelings.	1, 4, 5, 7
	5. Accepts the need for successful and independent school experiences.	3, 4
	6. Displays interest in wanting and learning how to make and retain friends.	7
	7. Supports the need to assume responsibilities in school and at home.	7
	8. Realizes that living things must die.	5
Action (observable)	1. Participates in sharing and taking turns.	7
	2. Experiences success and independence in a variety of ways in school.	3, 4
(observable, nonobservable, and delayed)	3. Is able to acquire friends and to maintain them.	4, 7
	4. Respects the feelings, rights, and property of others.	4, 7
	5. Attempts to control emotions.	1, 5-7
	6. Is able to express feelings in a mature fashion.	1, 5-7
	7. Refrains from behavior that will hurt someone or cause hard feelings.	1, 4, 5
	8. Assumes responsibilities expected in school and at home.	7

Objectives for grades 4-6

Domain	Objectives for students	Basic concepts
Cognitive	1. Identifies adults who are receptive to talking over problems.	8
	2. Identifies adults who are available to help with problems.	8
	3. Lists the rules necessary for classroom behavior.	1, 7
	4. Identifies the characteristics in which individuals are alike, different, or unique.	1, 2
	5. Identifies goals that are within the possibility of achievement by the individual.	3, 5
	6. Describes ways emotions can be controlled.	1, 3, 5-7
	7. Explains the reasons for treating all individuals with dignity and respect.	4
	8. Discusses the biologic and environmental factors affecting mental health.	1

Mental health objectives for grades 4-6—cont'd

Domain	Objectives for students	Basic concepts
	9. Lists situations when stress may occur and discusses helpfulness or harmfulness.	1, 6
	10. Recalls the scientific principles needed to solve problems.	5
	11. Illustrates ways to be able to work productively as an individual in small groups.	3, 4, 7
	12. Recalls a variety of interesting leisure time activities.	1, 3, 8
	13. Identifies ways individuals try to adjust to demands of daily living.	5
	14. Explains the role of the brain, nervous system, and endocrine glands in mental health.	7
	15. Explains risk-taking behavior.	6
	16. Discusses life and death, meaning and causes.	5
Affective	1. Believes a variety of individuals are willing and available to help solve problems.	8
	2. Accepts the realization that there are adults willing to help students with problems.	8
	3. Is attentive to the preparation of rules for classroom behavior.	1, 7
	4. Talks about the significance of establishing realistic goals.	3, 5
	5. Displays interest in characteristics that identify individuals as alike, different, or unique persons.	1, 2
	6. Believes emotions need to be controlled.	1, 3, 5-7
	7. Is attentive to the importance of treating all individuals with dignity and respect.	4
	8. Asks questions regarding the biologic and environmental factors affecting mental health.	1
	9. Believes stress situations may be helpful and harmful.	1, 6
	10. Supports the need to try to solve problems using scientific principles.	5
	11. Displays interest in being able to work productively as an individual and in small groups.	3, 4, 7
	12. Enjoys and is interested in participating in a variety of leisure time activities.	1, 3, 8
	13. Believes that risk-taking behavior may be hazardous.	6
	14. Realizes that grief is part of death and must cope with loss of loved ones.	5
Action (observable) (observable, nonobservable, and delayed)	1. Participates in the formulation of rules for classroom behavior.	1, 7
	2. Seeks help when facing unsolvable problems.	8
	3. Talks over problems with trusted adults.	8
	4. Attempts to establish realistic goals.	3, 5
	5. Treats all individuals with dignity and respect.	4
	6. Attempts to control emotions.	1, 3, 5-7
	7. Attempts to avoid or reduce stressful situations.	1, 6
	8. Tries to solve problems using scientific principles.	5

Mental health objectives for grades 4-6—cont'd

Domain	Objectives for students	Basic concepts
	9. Is able to work productively as an individual and in groups.	3, 4, 7
	10. Participates in a variety of interesting leisure time activities.	1, 3, 8

Objectives for grades 7-8

Domain	Objectives for students	Basic concepts
Cognitive	1. Describes the values believed to be important to self.	9
	2. Explains the interrelationships between biologic and environmental influences on mental health.	1
	3. Identifies the characteristics of the mentally healthy individual.	3, 5
	4. States the strengths, weaknesses, and potential abilities of the self.	1, 2, 3
	5. Describes the growth and developmental changes taking place in the individual.	1, 2
	6. Concludes an individual's personality is comprised of a variety of components and is unique.	2
	7. Discusses the procedures necessary and problems faced in attempting to improve relationships with parents and teachers.	7
	8. Compares the helpful and harmful aspects of friends and friendships.	7
	9. Explains the scientific principles usable in solving problems.	5
	10. Translates all the evidence needed to make decisions.	5
	11. Interprets the effect of peer pressures on individual behavior.	6
	12. Indicates ways stress produced by peer pressures can be handled.	6
	13. Identifies the types and symptoms of maladjustive behavior and the community sources and services available.	1, 8
	14. Discusses positive and negative aspects of risk-taking behavior.	6
	15. Identifies awareness of death and life.	5
	16. Lists ways to cope with death.	5
	17. Analyzes suicide in terms of causes, signs and symptoms and sources of help.	5
Affective	1. Believes that establishing values or a value system is necessary to find meaningfulness in life.	9
	2. Is attentive to discussion about the interrelationships between biologic and environmental influences on mental health.	1
	3. Displays interest in the characteristics of the mentally healthy individual.	3, 5
	4. Is supportive of the need to constantly improve individual abilities.	2, 3, 5

Mental health objectives for grades 7-8—cont'd

Domain	Objectives for students	Basic concepts
	5. Asks questions regarding the growth and developmental changes taking place in the individual.	1, 2
	6. Is interested in identifying one's personality characteristics and its uniqueness.	2, 3
	7. Believes that parent and teacher relationships are important.	7
	8. Accepts the fact that friends can be helpful as well as harmful to individuals.	5, 7
	9. Supports the need to solve problems using scientific principles.	5
	10. Listens to the idea that decisions cannot be made without careful consideration.	5
	11. Displays interest in learning the effect of peer pressures on behavior.	2, 3, 5, 6
	12. Believes that stress created by peers may not always be beneficial.	6
	13. Asks questions regarding the types and symptoms of maladjustive behavior and the treatment sources and services available in the community.	1, 8
	14. Realizes the positive and negative aspects of risk-taking behavior.	6
	15. Asks questions regarding funerals, rituals, and bereavement.	5
	16. Is attentive to discussion about euthanasia.	5
Action (observable, nonobservable, and delayed)	1. Tries to develop a set of values or a value system.	9
	2. Attempts to improve the strengths, weaknesses, and potential abilities of the self.	3-5
	3. Endeavors to improve parent and teacher relationships.	7
	4. Chooses friends after careful consideration of a variety of factors.	2, 5, 7
	5. Solves problems using scientific principles.	5
	6. Tries to make decisions after viewing all the alternatives and consequences.	5
	7. Attempts not to be unduly influenced by stress created by peers.	2, 3, 5, 6
	8. Seeks help when maladjustive symptoms of a persistent nature appear.	8
	9. Attempts to help others in times of death of loved ones.	5

NUTRITION UNIT
Outline of content
PHYSIOLOGIC

Definitions: food, nutrition, calorie

Purposes of food: energy, tissue building, protection and maintenance of bodily functions

Nutrients needed: reasons; good sources of proteins and fats; daily recommended allowances by age, sex, size, activity

Food needed: Basic 4 food groups; daily recommended allowances by age, sex, activity

Planning for meals or sample meals: breakfast, lunch, dinner, snacks, camping, picnics, sports, children, aged, pregnancy, parties

Nutrition outline of content—cont'd
Physiologic—cont'd

Diet and weight control: desirable weights—age, sex, size; identification of overweight and obesity; food intake; role of exercise; reducing fads and fallacies; sources of help; reliable and unreliable sources of information

Body processing of foods: digestion; absorption; utilization

Effects on the body: performance—mental, nervous stability, motor, disease; body structure and size—teeth, bones, soft tissues; length of life; energy needs—internal and external body activities

Disorders and diseases: appendicitis, constipation, allergies, diabetes, cancer, food poisoning, heart disease (genetic and environmental risk factors)

PSYCHOLOGIC

Food = Power: security; prestige and status; symbol of hospitality and friendship

Effect and outlet for emotions: joy, sorrow, conflict, comfort, fear, worry, anxiety

Motivations for modifying food habits

Specific—weight reduction; weight control; lower blood pressure; pregnancy; sports; looks and personality; old age

General—good health; longer life

SOCIAL

Eating patterns and preferences: influencing factors including cultural, ethnic, religious, racial and social customs and traditions—Italian, Mexican, Chinese, Indian, black; economic factors; age, sex, size; sensory reactions to food—texture, color, odor, taste, looks; social climate and atmosphere including companionship; education influences—TV, radio, newspapers, magazines, school, family, community, friends, neighbors

Sanitation and safety: home, school, community (restaurants); laws; protective agencies

Preparation, processing, preservation, and storage: procedures—canning, frozen, dehydrated, powdered, refrigerated, pasteurized, irradiated, adulterated

Consumer protection: laws—additives, advertising, safety, adulteration, pasteurization, sanitation, food production, processing; agencies—FDA, FTC, health departments

Fads and fallacies: misconceptions, weight control, "soul," natural and organic foods

Selection and purchase of foods: wise economic expenditures

Problems of hunger in society: role of individual and community

SPIRITUAL

Values: value of food in human life; importance of food for health of individuals

Moral issues: Does society have the obligation to feed the hungry and the poor? Should the hungry and the poor receive food?

Humanism: How should people treat individuals who are hungry and in need of food?

Concepts

Concept	Application of health definition
1 Foods differ in kind, sources, and nutritive value and serve a variety of purposes for individuals.	Physiologic
2 Individuals require the same nutrients but in varying amounts throughout life.	
3 The selection of nutritious foods contained in a balanced diet are necessary for the proper growth, good health, and everyday functioning of the individual.	
4 Lack of nutritious food resulting from a variety of factors may be detrimental to the health of individuals.	

Nutrition unit concepts—cont'd

Concept	Application of health definition
5 Differing motivations influence the types and amounts of food consumed by individuals.	Psychologic
6 Foods help to satisfy the emotional needs of individuals.	
7 Cultural, social, economic, and educational factors affect an individual's food selections.	Social
8 Production, processing, storage, preparation, and dispensing of foods influence their nutritional value, safety, and consumption.	
9 The social atmosphere present at meals, or when food is consumed, may have positive and negative effects on individuals.	
10 Food should be made available to all individuals regardless of their cultural, social, economic, or educational status.	Spiritual

Objectives for grades K-3

Domain	Objectives for students	Basic concepts
Cognitive	1. Identifies the Basic 4 food groups.	1-3
	2. Recalls the importance of milk in the daily diet.	1-3
	3. Explains the purposes of food and relates to the Basic 4 food groups.	1, 3
	4. Lists nutritious snack foods.	3
	5. Is able to limitedly plan nutritious breakfasts, lunches, and dinners from the Basic 4 food groups.	1, 3
	6. Recalls the sources of foods from plants and animals.	1
	7. Explains the reasons for sanitary practices in the preparing, serving, and eating of foods.	9
	8. Identifies the cultural and social differences in foods consumed by people.	8
Affective	1. Is attentive to discussions about the Basic 4 food groups.	1, 3
	2. Displays interest in eating a variety of foods.	1, 3
	3. Raises questions regarding the sources of food from plants and animals.	1
	4. Accepts the importance of tasting new and different foods.	1, 3
	5. Listens to the discussion for socially acceptable behavior at mealtime.	10
	6. Talks about cultural and social differences in foods consumed by people.	8
Action (observable)	1. Eats breakfast before attending school or while at school.	3
	2. Eats nutritious snack foods.	1, 3
	3. Acts in a socially acceptable manner at mealtime.	10
	4. Follows sanitary practices in the preparing, handling, and eating of foods.	9
(nonobservable and delayed)	5. Eats well-balanced meals selected from the Basic 4 food groups.	1, 3
	6. Demonstrates willingness to try and eat a variety of foods, including new ones.	1, 3
	7. Takes only the amount of food that can be eaten.	8

Nutrition unit—cont'd
Objectives for grades 4-6

Domain	Objectives for students	Basic concepts
Cognitive	1. Recalls the Basic 4 food groups.	1-3
	2. Identifies the nutrients found in foods as well as the foods in which they are found.	1
	3. Is able to plan nutritious meals with some degree of efficiency.	1, 3
	4. Identifies the reasons why individuals need the same nutrients but in varying amounts throughout life.	2
	5. Recalls how the body processes foods in terms of digestion, absorption, and utilization.	2, 3
	6. Compares the foods and eating practices of various community, ethnic, religious, racial and cultural groups of people to the Basic 4 food groups.	7
	7. Explains the relationships of poorly balanced diets and lack of food to diseases and disorders.	4
	8. Lists factors that affect choices of foods by individuals.	5
	9. Compares the nutritive values of highly advertised foods to the Basic 4 food groups and to the nutrients needed by individuals.	1, 2, 7
	10. Identifies reliable sources of nutrition information.	7
Affective	1. Listens to discussions about the importance of nutritious foods for growth and health.	1-3
	2. Displays interest in the selection of nutritious foods.	1, 3
	3. Accepts the fact that new and different foods can add interest to eating.	1-3
	4. Questions the value of highly advertised foods.	1, 3
	5. Reacts to class discussions by raising questions regarding how foods satisfy differing emotional needs of individuals.	6
	6. Raises questions regarding reasons individuals require different types and amounts of food.	2
	7. Displays interest in learning more about the relationships of food to disease and disorders.	4
	8. Is attentive to discussions regarding the cultural and ethnic patterns and eating practices of individuals.	7
	9. Supports the need to locate and use reliable sources of nutrition information.	7
Action (observable)	1. Eats nutritious foods at mealtime and at snacktime.	1, 3
	2. Eats breakfast before attending school or while at school.	3
	3. Follows sanitary practices in the preparation, serving, storing, and eating of food.	8
(nonobservable, or delayed)	4. Eats a variety of foods and is willing to try new ones.	1, 3
	5. Use reliable sources for nutrition information.	7

Nutrition unit—cont'd
Objectives for grades 7-8

Domain	Objectives for students	Basic concepts
Cognitive	1. Explains how it is possible to obtain all the essential nutrients by eating a balanced diet selected from a variety of foods.	1, 3
	2. Describes diseases and disorders that may be associated with nutritional practices.	4
	3. Lists the dangers to growth, health, and body functioning through the consumption of improper foods or poor eating habits.	4
	4. Identifies the differing motivations that bring about changes in food consumption habits, such as sports, weight control, length of life.	5
	5. Analyzes TV and other commercials about food and their nutritive value.	1, 3, 5, 7
	6. Identifies federal, state, and local agencies and their functions in the control of the purity and quality of foods.	8
	7. Explains how weight can be controlled in many individuals through proper diet and exercise.	2
	8. Summarizes the current food fads and misconceptions.	5, 7
	9. Illustrates the differing effects of food and lack of food on the body.	4
	10. Compares the cultural or ethnic food patterns of community groups to the basic four food groups.	1, 7
	11. Concludes that all people need food and that efforts should be made to assure that it is available when needed.	10
	12. Examines food consumption at breakfast, lunch, dinner, and snacktime and compares with Basic 4 food groups.	1, 3
	13. Identifies the genetic and environmental risk factors related to heart disease.	4
	14. Lists reliable sources of nutrition information.	7
Affective	1. Displays interest in attempting to help individuals in need of food.	10
	2. Accepts the importance of weight control through proper diet and exercise.	2
	3. Accepts and understands the cultural and ethnic differences in foods consumed by individuals.	7
	4. Asks questions in regard to agencies and their functions that have responsibility for the control of the purity and quality of foods.	8
	5. Is attentive to discussions regarding current food fads and misconceptions.	5, 7
	6. Displays interest in the differing motivations for food habits.	5
	7. Talks about food as a socializing agent by participating in discussions.	7, 9
	8. Is supportive of the concept that a balanced diet	1, 3

Nutrition unit objectives for grades 7-8—cont'd

Domain	Objectives for students	Basic concepts
	selected from a variety of foods is necessary for proper growth and health.	
	9. Believes that advertising about foods and food products must be carefully analyzed in terms of nutritional value.	1, 3, 5, 7
	10. Realizes the role of nutrition as a risk factor in heart disease.	4
	11. Accepts the importance of the use of reliable sources of nutrition information.	7
Action (observable)	1. Eats breakfast before attending school or while at school.	3
	2. Eats nutritious foods at mealtime and snacktime.	1, 3
(nonobservable, or delayed)	3. Periodically provides assistance by helping needy individuals obtain food.	10
	4. Attempts to keep weight and intake of foods under control through the wise selection and consumption of nutritious items.	2, 3
	5. Refrains, or attempts to encourage parents to refrain, from purchasing highly advertised foods unless they have been analyzed for nutritional value.	1, 3, 5, 7
	6. Reduces food intake that is related to heart disease.	4
	7. Uses reliable sources of nutrition information.	7

SAFETY AND FIRST AID UNIT*
Outline of content
PHYSIOLOGIC

Definitions: injury, sudden illness, hemorrhage, respiration, concussion, fracture, shock, abrasion, laceration, resuscitation, burn classifications, poisons, sprain, strain, contusion, heat stroke and heat exhaustion, "g" levels, defensive driving

Effects of accidents: disability and death

Areas: home; school; community; fire and electric; bicycle; farm; sports and recreation; firearms; winter and summer

PSYCHOLOGIC

Individual responsibility for safety
Accident proneness
Emotional factors in accidents and emergencies
Alcohol and other drugs in accidents
Emotional effects of accidents and emergencies on first aiders
Emotional influence in shock
Attitude toward mouth-to-mouth resuscitation
Importance of safe practices

SOCIAL

Accident costs in money, disability, and death responsibility: safe construction of motor vehicles, highways and information signs, toys, household appliances, farm and ranch equipment, houses and hotels, schools, business and industrial plants, children's clothing, and industrial equipment

---

*See Chapter 6.

Safety and first aid outline of content—cont'd
Social—cont'd

    Accident insurance and legal liability

        Dangerous strangers
        Responsibility for community emergency care programs
        Sources of aid in accidents and emergencies

    SPIRITUAL

Values: importance of safety and health for all
Moral issues: protection of life and health of others in school, home, and other places
Humanism: responsibility of individual and community to prevent accidents and provide emergency care

Concepts

Concept	Application of health definition
1 Accident hazards and unsafe conditions exist in all environments.	Physical
2 An individual's safety depends on own ability to adjust to own environment.	Physical
3 Accidents are the leading cause of death and injury among elementary-school pupils.	Physical
4 Combinations of factors and forces contribute to the occurrence of accidents.	Psychologic-social
5 Individuals, families, and community groups should be prepared to act effectively in the event of injury or sudden illness.	Social
6 Everyone has an obligation to reduce accident hazards in the environment.	Social
7 Safety and emergency care procedures are based on appreciation of the value and quality of life.	Spiritual

Objectives for grades K-3

Domain	Objectives for students	Basic concepts
Cognitive	1. Identifies accident hazards in own immediate environment.	1, 2, 6
	2. Explains the reasons for protecting people from accidents.	1-3
	3. Lists ways of avoiding accidents.	2, 4
	4. Cites examples of disrespect for safety procedures in motor vehicle, home, school, and public activities.	4, 6, 7
	5. Explains why first aid is important.	5, 7
	6. Identifies ways to care for minor injuries.	5, 7
	7. Cites best methods for getting help in emergencies.	5, 7
	8. Lists most common kinds of accidents among kindergarten to third grade pupils.	3, 4
Affective	1. Asks questions about hazards in the environment.	1, 2, 6
	2. Shows interest in the causes of accidents.	2, 4, 6
	3. Reacts to class discussions on loss of life and health by accidents.	2, 3, 6
	4. Expresses a desire to do something about the accident problem.	1, 3, 6
	5. Is attentive to information presented on simple first-aid measures and procedures for obtaining expert assistance.	5, 7

Safety and first aid objectives for grades K-3—cont'd

Domain	Objectives for students	Basic concepts
	6. Displays interest in helping others who may be sick or hurt.	5, 7
Action	1. Follows safe practices in classroom, lunchroom, hallways, and playground.	1-6
	2. Acts in a safe manner enroute to and from school—in bus or car, as pedestrian, or cycling.	1-4, 6
	3. Seeks aid from school personnel for injury or sudden illness.	5
	4. Helps other pupils when they are hurt or sick.	5, 7
	5. Improves safe practices at home and in his immediate environment.	1-4, 6
	6. Provides care for minor injuries.	5

Objectives for grades 4-6

Domain	Objectives for students	Basic concepts
Cognitive	1. Identifies the four classes of accidents: motor vehicle, home, public, and occupational.	1, 2
	2. Lists new environmental accident hazards resulting from technologic advances.	1, 2, 4
	3. Explains ways to reduce potential for accidents.	1, 2, 4, 6
	4. Tells how mental upsets may help cause accidents.	1, 4
	5. Lists the steps in first aid to help someone who has been injured or become ill.	5, 7
	6. Explains the most common emergency care procedures.	5
Affective	1. Asks questions about specific potential causes for various types of accidents.	1-4, 6
	2. Shows interest in environmental improvement to remove hazards.	1-4, 6
	3. Displays an appreciation of the accident toll on children, youths, and adults.	3, 7
	4. Is aware of the indifference and ignorance of the public with regard to safety.	2, 4, 7
	5. Inquires about ways to improve safety conditions in and around the school.	1, 3, 6, 7
	6. Expresses desire to become competent in first aid methods.	5, 7
	7. Shows concern for need to improve emergency care programs.	5, 7
Action	1. Acts in a safe manner in school and in the community.	1-4, 6
	2. Starts to develop habits of helping others in preventing accidents.	3, 6, 7
	3. Assists safety patrol or other school personnel when occasion arises.	3, 6, 7
	4. Seeks information on underlying causes of accidents.	4, 6
	5. Administers first aid for minor injuries.	5, 7
	6. Secures information on the community's emergency aid program.	5, 7

Safety and first aid unit—cont'd
Objectives for grades 7-8

Domain	Objectives for students	Basic concepts
Cognitive	1. Lists deaths and injuries by age groups for the four major classes of accidents.	1, 2
	2. Explains the ways in which modern environment can threaten own safety.	1, 2, 4, 7
	3. Contrasts of pleasures and dangers of motorcycling, aquatic sports (scuba and skin diving, surfing, and water skiing), snow skiing, and other locally popular sport activities.	1, 4, 6
	4. Identifies reliable sources of safety information.	1, 3, 6
	5. Identifies safety organizations at the national, state, and local level.	1, 6
	6. Explains and illustrates specific major first-aid procedures.	5
	7. Lists reasons for needed improvements in community emergency care programs.	5, 7
	8. Lists school and community resources that can render assistance in emergencies.	5
Affective	1. Displays interest in doing own part to reduce hazards.	2, 6
	2. Accepts the need for improving environmental conditions and human behavior.	1, 2, 4, 6, 7
	3. Supports the concept that safety is everyone's responsibility.	6, 7
	4. Believes that improved safety measures could reduce deaths and injuries among elementary-age children and youths.	2, 3, 7
	5. Supports the work of the National Safety Council and other organizations in accident prevention.	6, 7
	6. Is aware of the need for better first-aid training for youth and adults.	5, 7
	7. Believes that there is an urgent need to improve community programs for emergency care.	5, 7
	8. Realizes there are school and community resources that provide assistance in emergencies.	5
Action	1. Attempts to act in a consistently safe manner under all conditions.	1, 2, 6
	2. Shows leadership in helping others avoid accidents.	2, 3, 6
	3. Demonstrates acceptance of the values of safe behavior.	2, 7
	4. Seeks solutions to accident problems in a scientific manner.	2, 4, 6
	5. Demonstrates leadership in school, home, or community emergency care program.	1, 5, 7
	6. Utilizes school and community resources in emergencies.	5-7
	7. Effectively carries out sound first-aid measures if and when an emergency occurs.	5, 7

SAFETY-FIRE UNIT*
Outline of content
PHYSIOLOGIC

Effects

Harmful—three million fires, 300,000 injuries (50,000 hospitalized), 8,800 deaths, $4 billion property damage yearly

Beneficial—warmth, cook food, manufacture products, scientific research, others

Leading causes of fire: electrical, smoking and matches, heating and cooking equipment, incendiary, children and matches, open flames, flammable liquids, lightning, chimneys and flues, and spontaneous ignition

Types of fires: slow-burning, flash, explosion

Classes of fires: combustibles (A); flammable liquids, grease, and oil (B); electrical (C); and metals (D)

Fire essentials: heat, fuel, oxygen

Where fires start in homes in rank order: living room, den or family room, basement, kitchen, bedroom, bathroom

Fabric flammability: cotton, linen, and silk burn more easily; tight-weave materials and those treated with flame-resistant substance and also nylon, acrylic or polyester materials are more difficult to ignite; nylon, and so on, when ignited melts and causes severe burns

Control of fires: remove fuel (turn off electricity, dispose of wood, trash, and so forth), remove heat (cool), remove oxygen (smother)

PSYCHOLOGIC

Risk-taking behavior hazards: injuries, deaths, property damage

Prevention behaviors

Before fires occur

Public places—hotels, theaters, restaurants, and others—identify escape exits and plan for escape; schools—participate in fire drills

Homes

Escape plans, periodic inspection of hazards, installation of smoke and flame detectors

Safety procedures

General—good housekeeping—trash removal, as well as clutter in basements, attics and other places, safe storage of flammable materials, remove damaged wires

Specific

Matches—close matchbook before striking, extinguish completely, do not play with

Outside fires—burn trash only when permitted, do not burn unless with adult, do not use flammable liquid to start and rekindle, among others

Lightning—stay indoors; be away from metal objects, such as wire fences; if outside avoid trees and small sheds, get away from water

Flammable liquids—do not use for home dry cleaning

Electrical appliances—turn off when not in use, do not use if fuse blown, keep away from objects that can burn, inspect regularly

Electricity—do not overload circuits, remove broken or bare wires, replace blown fuses

Clothing—wear sturdy jeans, tight-fitting jerseys, blouses without frills, jersey pajamas, tight-fitting or short-sleeve clothes

Baby-sitter—know all exits, escape plan, emergency telephone number; do not leave children alone

Holidays—do not use fireworks, use flashlight rather than candles on Halloween, do not use paper decorations, keep Christmas trees moist and in water and turn off lights when not at home or nearby

---

*National Fire Protection Association is in the process of developing and launching a fire prevention and safety program in American schools.

Safety-fire outline of content—cont'd
Psychologic—cont'd

> After fires occur
>> General—survival, escape, alarm, rescue, first aid
>> Specific
>>> Home or building—follow escape plan
>>> Report of fire—telephone, alarm box
>>> When trapped—*crawl low* and get out of room, check door before opening and if hot fill cracks, signal for help in window with light-colored cloth or use telephone
>>> First aid—burns, asphyxiation, summon medical aid
>>> Clothing—drop to ground and roll

SOCIAL

Fire department: sole responsibility to fight fires, services usually available 24 hours daily, telephones readily available
Fire alarm boxes: purpose to summon fire fighters quickly, false alarms delay saving of lives and property
Fire codes, regulations, and laws

SPIRITUAL

Values: importance of fire prevention and safety to prevent injuries and death and protect property
Moral issue: protection of people and property is a responsibility of all individuals

Concepts

Concept	Application of health definition
1 Fire has both beneficial and harmful effects.	Physical
2 Risk-taking behavior is the result of a variety of motivations.	Psychologic
3 Individuals, families, and communities can prevent fires, save lives, and prevent injury and loss of property.	Psychologic-social
4 Fire fighters are friends and necessary community helpers who render necessary services.	Social
5 Fire codes, regulations, and laws are necessary for the protection of individuals and property	Social
6 Individuals have responsibility to protect their own lives and property as well as their neighbors'.	Spiritual

Objectives for grades K-3

Domain	Objectives for students	Basic concepts
Cognitive	1. Identifies the benefits and harmful effects of fire.	1-3, 6
	2. Describes the actions to take in a fire drill.	3-6
	3. Demonstrates the proper stop, drop, and roll technique when clothes are on fire.	3, 6
	4. Describes the crawling low method to exit from a a smoke-filled room.	3, 6
	5. Lists the procedures to follow when smoke or fire is discovered in a building.	3, 6
	6. Explains the reasons for reporting fire and smoke conditions immediately.	1, 3, 4, 6
	7. States reason to look for two exits from every building.	1, 3, 5, 6
	8. Lists the dangers of playing with or using matches properly.	1-3, 6

Safety-fire objectives for grades K-3—cont'd

Domain	Objectives for students	Basic concepts
	9. Recalls the dangers and safety procedures around heat producing appliances.	1-3, 6
	10. Lists the types of electrical hazards in homes.	1, 3, 5, 6
	11. Recites the need for fire-safe holidays.	1-3, 6
	12. Recalls the way combustibles can be ignited.	1-3, 6
Affective	1. Values fire and smoke drills as necessary for fire safety.	3, 5, 6
	2. Supports the need to use the stop, drop, and roll technique when clothes are on fire.	3, 6
	3. Is interested in learning the crawling low procedure to exit from a smoke-filled room.	3, 6
	4. Values the need for prompt action when smoke or fire is discovered.	1, 3, 4, 6
	5. Realizes why fire and smoke conditions should be reported immediately.	1, 3, 6
	6. Realizes the importance of identifying and being able to locate two exits at all times.	3, 6
	7. Wishes to protect self and others from the hazards of improper use of matches.	1-3, 6
	8. Is interested in learning about fire safety around lighted stoves, heaters, and small appliances.	1-3, 6
	9. Wishes to keep family members fire safe when camping, picnicking, or cooking outdoors.	1-3, 5, 6
	10. Recognizes that electrical hazards may result in fire, injury, death and loss of property.	1-3, 6
	11. Believes in identifying and removing fire hazards.	1, 3, 4, 6
	12. Supports the need for fire-safe holidays.	1-3, 6
	13. Realizes the hazard of inserting objects into electrical outlets.	3, 6
Action (observable)	1. Participates in fire and smoke drills at schools.	3, 5, 6
(observable and non-observable)	2. Participates in the planning of a home evacuation plan.	3, 4, 6
	3. Immediately reports fire, heat, or smoke conditions to a responsible adult.	3, 4, 6
	4. Refrains from playing with or improperly using matches in home, school, or outdoors.	1-3, 6
	5. Refrains from playing near stoves, heaters, or fireplaces.	1-3, 6
	6. Reports electrical hazards to responsible adults.	1, 3, 4, 6
(nonobservable)	7. Is able to crawl low to exit from a smoke-filled room.	3, 6
	8. Prepares evacuation plan for multistoried building when necessary.	3, 6
	9. Applies cold water on minor burns if no adult is present.	3, 6
	10. Seeks help for severe burns.	3, 6
	11. Practices and encourages family members to practice fire safety when camping, picnicking, or cooking outdoors.	1-3, 5, 6
	12. Practices and encourages fire safety on holidays and special occasions.	1, 3, 6

Safety-fire unit—cont'd
Objectives for grades 4-6

Domain	Objectives for students	Basic concepts
Cognitive	1. Describes the actions to take in fire drills.	3-6
	2. Demonstrates the proper way to stop, drop, and roll when clothes are on fire.	3, 6
	3. Identifies hazardous types of clothing.	3, 6
	4. States reason for crawling low in a smoke-filled room.	1, 3
	5. Lists procedures to follow when smoke or fire is discovered.	1, 3, 4, 6
	6. Explains reasons for reporting fire and smoke conditions immediately.	1, 3, 4, 6
	7. Describes the purpose of two exits from buildings.	3, 4, 6
	8. Identifies the first-aid procedures for burns.	3, 6
	9. Explains the procedures for fire safety when serving as a baby-sitter.	1, 3, 6
	10. States the reason for remaining clear of fire fighters while fires are in progress.	4
	11. Recites the reasons for refusing to turn in false fire alarms.	2, 4
	12. Lists the dangers of playing with or using matches improperly.	1-3, 6
	13. Identifies fire safety behavior around lighted stoves, heaters, and small appliances.	1-3, 6
	14. Recalls how to safely store flammable liquids.	1-3, 5, 6
	15. Explains the ways to extinguish outdoor fires.	1, 3, 6
	16. Identifies the types of electrical hazards in homes.	3, 6
	17. States the reasons for conducting periodic home hazard inspections.	2, 3, 6
	18. Recalls the need to use gasoline in well-ventilated places outside of buildings.	2, 3, 6
Affective	1. Values fire and smoke drills for fire safety.	3-6
	2. Values the need to use the stop, drop, and roll technique when clothes are on fire.	3, 6
	3. Is interested in learning the crawling low technique to exit from a smoke-filled room.	3, 6
	4. Realizes the importance for prompt action when smoke or fire is discovered.	1-4, 6
	5. Appreciates the importance of locating two exits from buildings.	3, 4, 6
	6. Realizes the need for immediate attention to burns.	3, 6
	7. Supports the need to refrain from interfering with fire fighters while fires are in progress.	4
	8. Believes that false fire alarms are dangerous.	4
	9. Wishes to protect self and others from the misuse of matches and lighted objects.	1-3, 6
	10. Realizes the hazards when around lighted stoves, heaters and small appliances.	1-3, 6
	11. Recognizes the hazards of improperly stored flammable liquids.	1-3, 5, 6
	12. Supports the need to extinguish outdoor fires properly.	1, 3, 5, 6

Safety-fire objectives for grades 4-6—cont'd

Domain	Objectives for students	Basic concepts
	13. Believes in the importance of the use of nonflammable substances inside homes and buildings.	1-3, 6
Action (observable) (observable and non-servable)	1. Helps teachers in the conduct of fire drills.	3, 6
	2. Helps family in the preparation and the following of a home evacuation plan.	3, 6
	3. Immediately reports fire, heat, or smoke observed to a responsible adult after leaving a building.	1, 3, 4, 6
	4. Refrains from improperly using matches and helps to store them properly.	1-3, 6
	5. Practices and encourages others to practice fire safety when outdoors.	1-3, 5, 6,
	6. Assists in regular inspection of buildings and grounds.	3, 6
(nonobservable)	7. Performs accurately the stop, drop, and roll technique when clothes are on fire.	3, 6
	8. Properly performs the crawling procedure to exit from a smoke-filled room.	1, 3, 6
	9. Establishes an evacuation plan in case of fire in a multistoried building.	3, 5, 6
	10. Applies cold water to a minor burn if no adult is present or seeks help with a severe burn.	3, 6
	11. Aids fire fighters on arrival regarding location of fire and whether persons are in building.	4, 5
	12. Refrains from turning in false fire alarms.	4, 5
	13. Helps to maintain storage of flammable liquids in proper containers.	1-3, 5, 6
	14. Encourages safe smoking habits in buildings, outdoors, and other places.	2, 3, 6
	15. Persuades others to use gasoline and other volatile substances in well-ventilated places.	1-3, 6

Objectives for grades 7-8

Domain	Objectives for students	Basic concepts
Cognitive	1. Identifies reasons for fire drills.	3-6
	2. Demonstrates proper technique for stop, drop, and roll technique when clothes are on fire.	3, 6
	3. Identifies reason to crawl low to exit from smoke-filled room.	1, 3, 6
	4. Lists procedures to follow when smoke or fire is discovered.	1, 3, 4, 6
	5. Explains reasons for reporting fire and smoke conditions discovered immediately.	1, 3, 4, 6
	6. Demonstrates first aid for use with burn victims.	3, 6
	7. Describes procedure to plan a baby-sitter safety plan.	3, 6
	8. States the importance of remaining clear of fire fighters while fires are in progress.	4
	9. Lists the hazards of false fire alarms.	4
	10. Lists the hazards of the improper use of matches.	1-3, 6

Safety-fire objectives for grades 7-8—cont'd

Domain	Objectives for students	Basic concepts
	11. Recalls the dangers and safety procedures when around cooking, heating, and other heat-producing appliances.	1-3, 6
	12. Describes the flammability dangers from volatile substances.	1-3, 6
	13. Identifies the safety procedures for use in outdoor fires.	1-3, 5, 6
	14. Explains the purposes of fuses and the safe way to replace them.	1, 3, 6
	15. Lists procedures used in the conduct of regular inspection of buildings for fire hazards.	3, 6
	16. Lists the procedures to follow for fire-safe holidays.	3, 6
	17. Recalls the need for safe smoking habits in buildings, outdoors, and in automobiles.	1, 3, 5, 6
	18. Explains the types, costs and operation of fire and smoke detectors.	3, 5, 6
	19. Describes the significance of the use of the UL label on electrical appliances and equipment.	3, 5, 6
	20. States the reason for licensed or certified personnel performing electrical repairs and maintenance.	3, 5, 6
Affective	1. Supports the need for fire drills and accepts responsibility for sharing in their conduct.	3-6
	2. Values the need to use the stop, drop, and roll technique when clothing is on fire.	3, 6
	3. Is interested in learning the crawling low method to exit from a smoke-filled building.	3, 6
	4. Values the need for prompt action when smoke or fire is discovered.	1, 3, 4, 6
	5. Is interested in learning the first aid for burn victims.	3, 6
	6. Believes it is necessary to help children to escape from fire when serving as a baby-sitter.	3, 6
	7. Supports the need to refrain from interfering with fire fighters while fires in progress.	4
	8. Believes that false fire alarms should not be turned in.	4
	9. Realizes the importance of using matches safely.	1-3, 6
	10. Willingly accepts the responsibility to protect children when around heat-producing equipment.	1-3, 6
	11. Recognizes the hazards of improperly used and stored flammable liquids.	1-3, 6
	12. Desires to practice fire safety outdoors.	2, 3, 5, 6
	13. Realizes the need for fuses and circuit breakers to protect from electrical overloads.	3, 5, 6
	14. Values the importance of periodic building inspections for fire hazards.	3, 6
	15. Supports the need for fire-safe holidays and special occasions.	3, 5, 6

Safety-fire objectives for grades 7-8—cont'd

Domain	Objectives for students	Basic concepts
	16. Recognizes the high risk of smoking in bed and the improper disposal of smoking materials.	2, 3, 6
	17. Supports the need for fire and smoke detectors.	3, 5, 6
	18. Is interested in learning the importance of the UL label.	3, 5, 6
	19. Recognizes the need for the repair and maintenance of electrical equipment by licensed or certified personnel.	3, 5, 6
	20. Is aware that lightning may cause fires and personal injury.	1, 3, 5, 6
Action (observable)	1. Willingly participates in fire and smoke drills at school and assumes responsibility to help conduct same.	3-6
(observable and non-observable)	2. Participates in helping family and others develop and follow a home escape plan.	3, 6
	3. Prepares evacuation plan in case of fire for use in multistoried building.	3, 5, 6
	4. Conducts or assists in periodic building fire safety inspections.	3, 6
(nonobservable)	5. Performs stop, drop, and roll technique when clothes are on fire.	3, 6
	6. Performs crawling low procedure to exit from smoke-filled room.	3, 6
	7. Immediately reports observed fire, heat or smoke after leaving a building to responsible adult or fire department.	1, 3, 4, 6
	8. Administers first aid for minor burns and shock and seeks medical help for major burns.	3, 6
	9. Plans safety procedures with parents when baby-sitting.	3, 6
	10. Assists fire fighters regarding location of fires and persons in burning buildings.	3, 4, 6
	11. Refrains from turning in false fire alarms.	3, 4, 6
	12. Refrains and discourages others from the improper use of matches.	1-3, 6
	13. Helps keep children away from heat-producing equipment and appliances.	3, 6
	14. Aids in the proper use and storage of flammable liquids.	1, 3, 6
	15. Assists with the removal of electrical hazards in the home.	3, 6
	16. Encourages safe smoking habits in buildings, outdoors, and automobiles.	1, 3, 6
	17. Persuades others to install fire and smoke detectors and to purchase electrical equipment with the UL label.	1, 3, 5, 6
	18. Encourages adults to install lightning protection on buildings where appropriate.	1, 3, 6

VISION AND HEARING UNIT*
Outline of content
PHYSIOLOGIC

Definitions: hyperopia, myopia, astigmatism, amblyopia, glaucoma, color blindness, night blindness, strabismus, conjunctivitis, ophthalmologist, optometrist, optician, otitis media, otitis externa, conduction deafness, nerve deafness

Structure and function of eyes and ears
- Eye structure—cornea, iris, lens, retina, optic nerve
- Eye function—vision, appearance
- Ear structure—outer ear, middle ear, inner ear, auditory nerve
- Ear function—hearing

Refractive errors; eye diseases and ear disorders
Signs and symptoms of problems (see Chapter 4)

PSYCHOLOGIC

Emotional problems: due to strabismus, nearsightedness and farsightedness, partial or complete blindness, partial or complete deafness, learning difficulties
Purposes of testing and care of vision and hearing

SOCIAL

Selection of eye specialist
Selection of physician for earache or hearing problem
Choice of glasses, contact lenses, or hearing aid if needed
Periodic eye and ear examinations or screening tests—types, frequency

SPIRITUAL

Values: importance of eye and ear health to self-image
Moral issues: provision of eye and ear care by government funding or private sources; protection of worker's vision and hearing in certain industries
Humanism: attitudes toward blind and deaf people; responsibility to help blind and deaf persons

---

*See Chapter 4.

Concepts

Concept	Application of health definition
1 Vision and hearing are the two most important senses for life and health.	Physical
2 Vision should be clear, sharp, and bright, with good distinction of color.	Physical
3 Common eye disorders include nearsightedness, farsightedness, and astigmatism.	Physical
4 One in five elementary pupils has a visual problem requiring professional care.	Physical-social
5 Visual disorders may cause learning difficulties or psychologic problems.	Psychologic-social
6 Good hearing depends on efficient function of the outer, middle, and inner ear as well as the auditory nerve.	Physical
7 Most hearing loss in childhood is a result of middle ear infection.	Physical

Vision and hearing concepts—cont'd

Concept	Application of health definition
8 Nerve deafness may be caused by long-term exposure to loud noise, birth defects, certain diseases or medicines, head injury, or heredity.	Physical-social
9 One in twenty elementary school pupils have a hearing problem requiring professional care.	Physical-social
10 Hearing disorders may cause learning difficulties or psychologic problems.	Psychologic-social
11 During the elementary schools years, parents have the primary responsibility for correction of hearing or vision problems in pupils.	Spiritual
12 Prompt professional care can correct or improve most disorders of vision and hearing.	Physical-spiritual

Objectives for grades K-3

Domain	Objectives for students	Basic concepts
Cognitive	1. Tells why good eyesight and hearing are important.	1
	2. Explains the reasons for having vision and hearing tests.	2-4, 7, 9, 12
	3. Identifies the main parts of the eye and ear.	1, 2, 6
	4. Lists ways that good sight and hearing can help learning.	5, 10
	5. Discusses factors that may impair vision or hearing.	3, 7, 8
	6. Recalls any experiences of visual difficulty or earache.	3, 7
Affective	1. Is aware of the importance of good vision and hearing.	1
	2. Accepts the need for vision and hearing tests.	4, 9, 12
	3. Displays interests in how the eyes and ears function.	2, 6
	4. Listens carefully to the ways to protect vision and hearing.	1, 5, 10
	5. Shows interest in finding professional specialists in eye and ear health.	11, 12
Action	1. Participates cooperatively when vision or hearing tests are given at school.	4, 5, 9, 10
	2. Tells about any personal seeing or hearing difficulty.	4, 9, 12
	3. Uses textbooks and other printed materials in a proper, efficient manner.	2, 5
	4. Does not habitually ask the teacher or others to repeat what they have said.	6, 10

Objectives for grades 4-6

Domain	Objectives for students	Basic concepts
Cognitive	1. Explains the basic structure and function of eyes and ears.	1, 2, 6
	2. Identifies ways to protect vision and hearing.	1, 3, 7, 8
	3. Cites major causes of visual and hearing disorders.	3, 4, 7-9
	4. Illustrates how middle ear infection can cause hearing loss.	6, 7

Vision and hearing objectives for grades 4-6—cont'd

Domain	Objectives for students	Basic concepts
	5. Describes effect of glare on visual acuity and eye fatigue.	2
	6. Explains important effects of color blindness and night blindness.	1, 2
	7. Explains the importance of regular eye and ear checkups and follow-up for corrections.	4, 9, 11, 12
Affective	1. Understands and appreciates the critical value of good vision and hearing.	1, 5, 6
	2. Accepts responsibility along with parents for care of eyes and ears.	1, 4, 9, 11, 12
	3. Displays interest in the effects of heredity on eye and ear disorders.	3, 8
	4. Appreciates the role of teachers, school nurses, and health specialists in the prevention and correction of eye and ear defects.	4, 5, 9-12
	5. Believes that healthy vision and hearing are necessary for a good education.	5, 10
Action	1. Takes an active, cooperative part when vision or hearing tests are given at school.	4, 5, 9, 10
	2. Protects his own eyes and avoids endangering the eyes of others in sports and other physical activities.	1
	3. Reports any personal problem of seeing or hearing to the teacher, school nurse, or other professional person.	4, 9, 12
	4. Avoids probing ears with sharp objects, looking directly at sun, or other practices that can be harmful.	1
	5. Does not habitually ask the teacher or others to repeat what they have said.	6, 10
	6. Avoids exposure to excessively loud rock music or other high decibel noise.	1, 8

Objectives for grades 7-8

Domain	Objectives for students	Basic concepts
Cognitive	1. Explains major errors of refraction in terms of altered structure and function and professional care.	3, 12
	2. Cites causes, prevention, and reasons for professional care of middle ear infection.	7, 12
	3. Lists types of environmental noise that can damage hearing.	8
	4. Analyzes differences between and among ophthalmologists, optometrists, and opticians.	12
	5. Describes possible effects on studying and learning of eye and ear disorders.	5, 10
	6. Describes possible emotional effects of eye and ear disorders.	5, 10
	7. Compares advantages and disadvantages of glasses and contact lenses.	12
	8. Cites dangers of delayed treatment for amblyopia (lazy eye) and glaucoma.	12

Vision and hearing objectives for grades 7-8—cont'd

Domain	Objectives for students	Basic concepts
Affective	1. Understands and appreciates the critical value of good vision and hearing.	1, 5, 6
	2. Accepts responsibility for protecting and caring for own eyes and ears.	1, 4, 9
	3. Recognizes the responsibility of parents to seek professional care for children with eye or ear problems.	1, 4, 9, 11
	4. Inquires about the relative merits of various types of eye and ear specialists.	4, 9, 12
	5. Discusses the problem of providing medical care for the poor who have eye or ear problems.	1, 12
	6. Recognizes and appreciates the growing problem of noise pollution in the environment.	1, 8
Action	1. Takes an active, cooperative part when vision or hearing tests are given at school.	4, 5, 9, 10
	2. Protects own eyes and avoids endangering the eyes of others in sports, laboratory work, and other physical activities.	1
	3. Is able to make wise decisions regarding personal eye and ear care.	1
	4. Supports school and community efforts to protect and improve eye and ear health.	1, 4, 9, 11, 12
	5. Seeks reliable information on eye and ear health.	1, 3, 7, 8
	6. Consistently wears glasses or hearing aid if prescribed.	1, 5, 10
	7. Avoids exposure to excessively loud rock music or other high decibel noise.	1, 8

HOW DOES THE TEACHER PLAN?

The classroom teacher plan of organization in the elementary school simplifies the problem of organizing the framework for a health teaching program. The usual recommendations are that classroom teachers assume the responsibility for teaching health to the children in their rooms. Even though health specialists who might take the responsibility for teaching health in the various grades are available, it is usually not recommended that they do so unless the specialist has had specific training and experience in elementary school teaching methods. Ordinarily, the classroom teacher can have better success in the teaching of health to her pupils than the health specialist.

Two things the teacher must do well are (1) plan health instruction for the school year and (2) develop appropriate lesson plans.

Yearly plan

An example of how a teacher might plan for health teaching for the school year, using the illustrative units previously described, is shown in Table 9-4.

Lesson plan

Regardless of the length of a health teaching unit most teachers make some provision for daily lesson planning. In other words, it is essential that the unit be broken down on a day-to-day basis. This does not imply that a lesson will cover only one class period. It is possible that a lesson will cover less than one class period or extend into more than one class period. The important consideration to keep in mind is that the continuity preserved from one class period to another should be such that the objectives of the health teaching unit are realized. This im-

Table 9-4. Second grade teacher plans for health education, Ellensburg, Washington, public schools

Month	Area	Concepts	Learning activities	Teaching aids	Integration
September	Mental health	New experiences may give satisfaction. Home, school, church, and community can be warm, safe places.	Have children act as "big brother" or "big sister" to new students. Encourage drawings about things they love, how it feels when hurt or scared, how to be helpful. Encourage art work to relieve tensions. Discuss leaders and followers, forgiveness, and other topics. Dramatize putting self in other's shoes. Films	Films: We play and share together Courtesy at school Laidlaw text: Second and third grade	Language arts: Write short experiences. Music: Listen to quiet music if tense. Physical education: Suggest activities to relax. Social studies: Discover community helpers.
October	Dental health	Daily care promotes dental health. Dentists help maintain healthy teeth. Community resources provide for dental care.	Demonstrate, using model, brushing teeth. Make toothpowder in class. Show films and filmstrips and discuss them. Survey for number of dental visits. Have vocabulary bingo game. Write creative story about detergent foods.	Films: The beaver tale Learning to brush Salt and baking soda Toothbrush dental kit Pictures: Detergent foods and other foods	Mathematics: Count teeth; subtract missing teeth. Social studies: Characterize dentist as community helper. Art: Make detergent-food mobile.
November	Family health	Families help each other in the community.	Make pictures of the family. Tell experiences. List ways neighbors can be helpful. Arrange bulletin board about good neighborhood. Keep home duty chart.	Laidlaw text Record: Community helpers, Bowman Family fun with familiar music	Language arts: Employ creative dramatics. Music: Play records and songs. Art: Draw pictures.
January	Consumer and community health	Doctors and dentists who help us are our friends. Hazards of the environment can cause discomfort and problems. Many people keep water and air safe. Individuals can improve their surroundings.	Use atomizers to show how odors disperse. Show films and filmstrips. Make notebook on community helpers' relation to environment. Dramatize how children help at home. Locate on map local family and health agencies. Decorate flannelboard with creative story with characters. Leave food out, covered and uncovered, to relate to improper storage.	Film: Magic touch Filmstrip: Dentist School nurse Record: Community helpers Personal pictures Map of community	Social studies: Relate to community helpers unit. Language arts: Encourage reports or notebooks. Art: Make mural of community helpers.

Continued.

Table 9-4. Second grade teacher plans for health education, Ellensburg, Washington, public schools—cont'd

Month	Area	Concepts	Learning activities	Teaching aids	Integration
February	Nutrition	There are many kinds of foods. Some foods may be better than others for you.	Try new foods at tasting party. Experiment with white rat. Make vegetable soup. Make grocery store; use food models and shop for nutritious foods. Make clay or paper maché fruit. Select Basic 4 foods, using magazine pictures.	Film: Eat for health Filmstrip: The food we eat Transparencies: See unit Food models of cardboard cutouts Laidlaw text	Art: Draw basic four food groups; prepare mural. Mathematics: Sell items in grocery store and add costs. Science: Experiment with white rat. Social studies: Take trip to store.
March	Anatomy-physiology	Good posture helps prevent fatigue, enables the body to work better, and makes use more attractive.	Use horizontal ladder for proper alignment. Use plumbline to check posture. Decorate bulletin board with stick figures or pipe cleaners. Show film and discuss.	Film: Beginning good posture Filmstrip: Let's stand tall	Physical education: Relate to apparatus activities. Art: Make silhouettes and individual pictures. Language arts: Show and tell
April	Disease control	Good health habits help to keep us well. When ill, certain practices help us get well. We depend on others for good health.	Use poster to illustrate ways to protect others. Stage choral reading and speaking. Use chart to show ways germs are transmitted. Write reports. Grow germs on cloth in warm and cool places. Dramatize going to doctor for help. Experiment with potato and agar in petri dish.	Films: Common cold; Soapy the germ fighter Milne: We are six (Wheezie and Sneezie)	Language arts: Relate to experiences when sick, affects of care, creative stories. Science: Experiment with potatoes and agar.
May	Family health	An egg grows into a baby.	Discuss charts of mammal reproduction. Prepare chart on life cycle of animal reproduction. Hatch egg in incubator. Chart and discuss fish egg development Make mural of animals caring for own babies. Show films and filmstrips.	Eye Gate charts of mammal reproduction series and fish egg development Films: Baby animals; animals growing up Filmstrip: The zoo trip	Science: Hatch egg; relate to insect unit. Art: Prepare mural.

plies that in daily lesson planning the teacher should have a clear perspective of the total learning that is expected from the unit. In this respect it becomes necessary for the teacher to determine whether procedures in daily lesson planning are such that they are related to the inclusive teaching unit. With these factors in mind the following criteria are suggested for lesson planning:

1. Does lesson planning ensure definite objectives for the lesson?
2. Does lesson planning ensure proper continuity of one lesson with another?
3. Does lesson planning ensure proper selection and organization of learning activities?
4. Does lesson planning give attention to the most desirable teaching procedures?
5. Does lesson planning ensure provision for individual differences of pupils?
6. Does lesson planning provide for sufficient flexibility with regard to the total teaching unit?
7. Does lesson planning provide for suitable evaluation of the outcomes of teaching?

QUESTIONS FOR DISCUSSION

1. Who should be responsible for curriculum development in the school?
2. What are the basic principles upon which the health curriculum should be based?
3. Why is both formal and informal health education necessary in schools?
4. What is the meaning and significance of the inclusion of values in the curriculum?
5. What is the meaning of the concept approach, and how can it be applied to health education?
6. Who should be responsible for the development of the health and safety education curriculum?
7. How is the curriculum in health education determined?
8. To what extent would you use the health interests of children as shown by the Connecticut study?
9. What are some of the sources of helpful information in determining health content for elementary pupils?
10. What are the procedures to be followed in determining the health education curriculum for elementary schools?
11. What is the fundamental purpose of the unit in health teaching?
12. What is the meaning of the phrase "scope and sequence"?

13. What are the common, essential elements of a good *teaching* unit?
14. What should be the nature of the health education curriculum for students in special education and Head Start programs?
15. What must the teacher do to plan for health instruction?
16. How can the broad concept of health (wholistic) identified in Chapter 1 be utilized in the development of the health education curriculum?
17. What content should be included in the curriculum for death education and fire safety in schools?

SUGGESTED CLASS ACTIVITIES

1. Prepare a proposal for a school administrator in which you point out the values of a planned course of study and list the topics you think should be covered in each grade, 1 to 8.
2. Conduct a panel discussion-debate on the relative merits of basing the curriculum on pupil needs and pupil interests.
3. Survey the literature for several authoritative outlines of teaching units and list those elements or steps that are common to all the outlines reviewed.
4. Plan a yearly health education program for the grade you plan to teach (also see Chapters 10 to 12).
5. Develop a lesson using one concept from one of the illustrative partial units in this chapter.
6. Develop a health teaching unit for a specific grade (also see Chapters 10 to 12).
7. Develop a safety teaching unit for a specific grade (also see Chapters 10 to 12).
8. Develop a curriculum for the grade level you plan to teach using the illustrative partial units in the chapter (also see Chapters 10 to 12).
9. From one of the teaching units in this chapter, prepare a lesson plan and teach a demonstration lesson to your school health class.

REFERENCES

Allen, R. E., and Holyoak, O. J.: Evaluation of the conceptual approach to teaching health education: a second look, Journal of School Health **43**: May, 1973.

American Educational Research Association, Committee on Curriculum: Curriculum planning and development, Review of Educational Research **30**: June, 1960.

Anderson, C. L.: School health practice, ed. 5, St. Louis, 1972, The C. V. Mosby Co.

Bouchard, R. P.: Behavioral objectives; a change agent for improved instruction, paper presented at the annual meeting of the Association for Supervision and Curriculum Development, Atlantic City, N.J., March, 1968.

Byler, R. V., Lewis, G. M., and Tottman, R. J.: Teach us what we want to know, New York, 1969, Mental Health Materials Center, Inc.

Corey, J. E.: Dietary factors and atherosclerosis; prevention should begin early, Journal of School Health **44:** Nov., 1974.

Corliss, L. M.: A report of the Denver research project on health interests of children, Journal of School Health **32:** Nov., 1962.

Cornacchia, H. J.: How we developed our elementary health education curriculum, Journal of Health, Physical Education, and Recreation **29:** April, 1958.

Cornacchia, H. J.: Consumer health, St. Louis, 1976, The C. V. Mosby Co.

Dearth, F.: Construction and utilization of visual aids in dental health education, Thorofare, N.J., 1974, Charles B. Slack, Inc.

Fodor, J. T.: A conceptual approach to curriculum development in venereal disease education, Journal of School Health **43:** May, 1973.

Fodor, J. T., Gmur, B. C., and Sutton, W. C.: Framework for health instruction in California public schools (adapted by California State Board of Education), Sacramento, Calif., 1970, California State Department of Education.

Goodlad, J. I., Stoephasius, R., and Klein, M. F.: The changing school curriculum, New York, 1966, Fund for the Advancement of Education.

Havighurst, R. J.: The values of youth. In Issues in American education, New York, 1970, Oxford University Press.

Hoyman, H. S.: Health ethics and relevant issues, Journal of School Health **42:** Nov., 1972.

Hoyman, H.: A synthetic health curriculum design in ecologic perspective, Journal of School Health **47:** Jan., 1977.

Irwin, L. W., Merrill, C. D., and Staton, W. M.: Concepts of healthful living of functional vlaue in the general education of elementary school pupils, Research Quarterly **24:** Dec., 1953.

Joint Committee on Health Problems in Education of the National Education Association and the American Medical Association (Moss, B. R., Southworth, W. H., and Reichart, J. L., editors): Health education, Washington, D.C., 1961, The National Education Association.

La Salle, D., and Greer, G.: Health instruction for today's schools, Englewood Cliffs, N.J., 1963, Prentice-Hall, Inc.

Lieberman, E. J., editor: Mental health; the public health challenge, Washington, D.C., 1975, American Public Health Association.

Loggins, D.: Values clarification revisited; clarifying what and how well, Health Education **7:** March/April, 1976.

Mayshark, C.: Health education. In Encyclopedia of educational research, New York, 1968, Macmillan, Inc.

Murphy, M. L.: Values and health problems, Journal of School Health **43:** Jan., 1973.

Oberteuffer, D., Harrelson, O. A., and Pollock, M. B.: School health education, New York, 1972, Harper & Row, Publishers, Inc.

Pollock, M. B.: Curriculum planning; a gamesmanship approach, Journal of School Health **39:** Oct., 1969.

School Health Education Study, Inc.: Health education; a conceptual approach, St. Paul, Minn., 1967, 3M Education Press.

Sliepcevich, E. M.: Curriculum development; a macroscopic or microscopic view? The National Elementary Principal **48:** Nov., 1968.

Stenner, A. J., and Katzenmeyer, W. G.: Self-concept development in young people, Phi Delta Kappan **58:** Dec., 1976.

Tyler, L. L.: A selected guide to curriculum literature: an annotated bibliography, Washington, D.C., 1970, The National Education Association.

Tyler, R.: Basic principles of curriculum and instruction, Chicago, 1969, University of Chicago Press.

Valett, R. E.: Humanistic education; developing the total person, St. Louis, 1977, The C. V. Mosby Co.

Werden, P. K.: Health education for Indian students, Journal of School Health **44:** June, 1974.

Willgoose, C. E.: Health education in the elementary school, Philadelphia, 1972, W. B. Saunders Co.

Willgoose, C. E.: Saving the curriculum in health education, Journal of School Health **43:** March, 1973.

SELECTED DEATH REFERENCES

Farberow, N. E., and others: Research in suicide. In Resnik, H. L. P., and Hawthorne, B. C., editors: Suicide prevention in the 70's, Washington, D.C., 1973, U.S. Department of Health, Education, and Welfare Publication HSM 72-9054, U.S. Government Printing Office.

Feifel, D., editor: New meanings of death, New York, 1977, McGraw-Hill Book Co.

Frederick, C. J.: Crisis intervention and emergency mental health. In Johnson, W. R., editor: Health in action, New York, 1977, Holt, Rinehart & Winston.

Frederick, C. J.: Suicide in the United States, Health Education **8:** Nov./Dec., 1977.

Gray, V. R.: Dealing with dying, Nursing, June, 1973.

Hafen, B. Q.: Death and dying, Health Education **8:** Nov./Dec., 1977.

Hart, E. J.: Philosophical views of death, Health Education **8:** Nov./Dec., 1977.

Hendin, D.: Death as a fact of life, New York, 1973, Warner Paperback Library.

Kastenbaum, R.: Death, society, and human experience, St. Louis, 1977, The C. V. Mosby Co.

Kübler-Ross, E.: On death and dying, New York, 1969, Macmillan, Inc.

Kübler-Ross, E.: Death; the final stages of growth, Englewood Cliffs, N.J., 1975, Prentice-Hall, Inc.

Switzer, D. K.: The Dynamics of Grief, Nashville, Tenn., 1970, Abingdon Press.

PART FIVE

Methods and materials in health education

10 Behavior modification in health education

Health education frequently has been attacked for its failure to help individuals develop practices and habits that prevent illness and maintain and promote good health. It often has been guilty of solely providing information of a physiologic nature. However, the problem of how to modify or whether to try to modify the health behavior of people has not been adequately resolved. Human health behavior is a complex process that may be resistant to change but is influenced by a variety of factors previously identified in the concept of health (see Chapter 1) that include physiologic, psychologic, social/cultural, and spiritual components (wholistic health*). Home atmosphere, racial, ethnic, or cultural background, peer influences, adequacy of housing and food intake, affection received, achievements, self-respect, and bias and prejudice have specific impact on children and youth. The needs, motivations, beliefs, values, experiences, and the environment of people affect the health habit patterns they develop. They enable people to make responsible health decisions and to cope with or adjust to problems they face in the society in which they live. These factors are in need of recognition and utilization if educational programs are to aid individuals to achieve high levels of wellness.

It is the purpose of this chapter to provide understanding in regard to behavior modification that will: (1) help teachers to become better informed in regard to the learning process necessary for successful teaching in health education, and (2) demonstrate the application of essential principles of learning to be used in the selection of methods/techniques (see Chapter 11) for effective instructional programs.

WHAT IS BEHAVIOR MODIFICATION?

Health behavior modification refers to the changing of health knowledges, attitudes, and practices acquired by individuals. It is an internal process that is influenced by personal needs and environmental exposures. It is not something done to pupils but rather involves educational procedures or methods used to help individuals adapt, adjust, solve problems, or cope with situations in regard to their health. Health education should attempt to aid students to make intelligent and responsible decisions.

The question of the extent to which educators should try to modify health behavior is a moot one. Should the use of alcohol or tobacco be condemned or condoned? Should all individuals exercise at regular intervals and in the same manner? Should the use of contraceptives be promoted? Should pupils reduce the consumption of foods containing high levels of sugar and cholesterol? Should the flossing and brushing of teeth be universally advocated? Hochbaum* states that in controversial aspects of health behavior, no attempt should be made to make modifications in line with rigid criteria (not to drink, not to smoke). He believes that students should be helped to develop skills and motivation that will enable them to arrive at rational decisions. Smith and Ojemann have identified a four-step model for decision

---

*Wholistic health is a term in vogue that refers to the health of the total person and not merely the physiologic aspects.

*Hochbaum, G. M.: Behavior modification, School Health Review 2: Sept., 1971.

making that is worthy of consideration:*

1. Examine the motivating forces operating in a give situation; identify the needs individuals are trying to satisfy through their behavior.
2. Devise and examine the probable intermediate and remote effects of possible alternative ways of satisfying these motivations.
3. Apply your personal standard to the proposed course of action to determine if the effects of the action are compatible.
4. Decide either for or against the selected behavior at this point in time.

WHAT IS LEARNING?

Learning is a complex process that is dependent on factors taking place both inside and outside the individual. It refers to the physical, intellectual, and emotional changes that occur in human organisms as a result of their interaction with the environment. It is the growth and development process that goes on within individuals as a result of their participation in a variety of experiences, feelings, attitudes, and interests. The health-educated pupil, having been exposed to a variety of health opportunities and activities, is better able to promote and maintain good health.

It should be made clear that the process of learning happens within the individual but is influenced by the teacher through the methods and techniques (see Chapter 11) used in teaching. Knowledge of the nature and conditions of learning is basic to an understanding of the teaching process in the health instruction program.

HOW DO CHILDREN LEARN?

The exact nature of learning is not known. However, the process does involve a series of rewards and punishments of both a desirable and undesirable nature. Positive reinforcers may include money, candy, privileges, grades, peer approval, praise, attention, and self-interest. Negative reinforcers

---

*Smith, L. V., and Ojemann, R. H.: A decision making model, School Health Review **5:** Jan./Feb., 1974.

that result in the elimination of behavior may include loud sounds, disapproval, punishment, poor grades, and use of unpleasant substances. It is believed that learning takes place most efficiently and effectively when someone wants to learn something. This person is then said to be motivated to action—to be goal-directed. A diagram best illustrates the learning process as it probably occurs (Fig. 10-1).

The process of learning may be illustrated by the example of the teacher who desires to have a student learn procedures that will help to prevent and control communicable disease. The goal having been set and the student ready to learn, the teacher provides a variety of activities that will aid in achieving the goal. These experiences may include reading about germs, discussing the hazards of respiratory infections, washing hands before lunch, and looking at bacteria under a microscope. The extent to which emotional tension, or conflict, is created in the pupil will depend on a number of factors, such as the intensity of the motivation, the difficulty encountered in reaching a solution, the amount of work required to be completed, and the desire for a good grade. If the activities provide satisfying experiences in learning for the child, the goal will be reached and the pupil will return to a state of equilibrium. Should the goal not be reached, the pupil may react by making such excuses as, "There was too much work to do," "The teacher didn't help me enough," or "I didn't understand what to do."

Learning occurs when a learner encounters experiences in his environment. However, teacher guidance can motivate this learning and reduce the errors a pupil may make in the learning process by controlling, manipulating, and selecting the appropriate activities.

WHAT IS THE CONCEPTUAL APPROACH TO HEALTH EDUCATION?

The current approach to teaching health is through the emphasis on concepts. Today, it is important to help students develop big

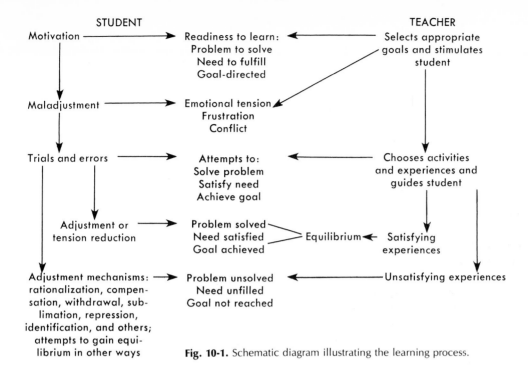

STUDENT

TEACHER

Motivation ——————→ Readiness to learn: ←——————— Selects appropriate
Problem to solve   goals and stimulates
Need to fulfill   student
Goal-directed

Maladjustment ——————→ Emotional tension
Frustration
Conflict

Trials and errors ——————→ Attempts to: ←——————— Chooses activities
Solve problem   and experiences and
Satisfy need   guides student
Achieve goal

Adjustment or ——————→ Problem solved
tension reduction   Need satisfied ——→ Equilibrium ←— Satisfying
Goal achieved   experiences

Adjustment mechanisms: ——→ Problem unsolved ←——————— Unsatisfying experiences
rationalization, compen-   Need unfilled
sation, withdrawal, sub-   Goal not reached
limation, repression,
identification, and others;
attempts to gain equi-
librium in other ways

Fig. 10-1. Schematic diagram illustrating the learning process.

ideas or reach conclusions about health that will enable them to take positive action and to make wise decisions regarding their own, their families', and their community's health. Teachers must be aware of these generalizations and help students to achieve them. Such concepts as smoking may be harmful to the human body, drugs are mood modifiers, certain foods are needed for proper growth and development, and there are ways to protect ourselves from disease help teachers to determine more relevant and effective health education goals (see illustrative units in Chapter 9).

WHAT ARE THE GOALS OF HEALTH EDUCATION?

Knowledge of the objectives of health education is important to the learning and teaching processes. Goals give direction to the learning that enables pupils to acquire the concepts needed for healthful living. It is necessary therefore that teachers clearly understand the purposes of health education for the most effective teaching. Precisely defined health objectives have particular meaning,

since learning should be centered on behavior outcomes as well as on factual achievements. Learning should lead students to the acquisition of health education concepts.

The present aim of health education is to develop practices and attitudes of safe and healthful living through the understanding of scientific health information. Individuals should be able to make intelligent decisions about the physical, mental, and social aspects of health. Health behaviors are therefore related to and dependent on the cognitive learning acquired by pupils. It is important that children obtain correct understanding about health. Attitudes also affect health habits.

The precise interrelationships of knowledge and attitudes to practices are not known today except that they are interdependent. Present evidence, however, indicates that the possession of understanding by itself does not necessarily result in good health habits. Knowing how to brush the teeth does not mean that this practice will be followed. Knowing that some snacktime foods are more nutritious than others is no assurance that they will be eaten. Knowing that immunizations protect against diseases does not always result in these preventive measures being obtained. Knowing the physiologic effects of drugs does not necessarily reduce their usage. There are also data that support appreciation and feelings as the means of bridging the gap between the "knowing" and the "doing" in health. Some authorities therefore believe that stress must be placed on the attitudinal effects of knowledge in health teaching. In any event, attitudes are significant in health education; and although knowing may not always lead to doing, there will be no doing without knowing.

Consideration must be given to the fact that behavioral and attitudinal changes in health do not necessarily take place immediately after teaching. Cultural, social, and other values and beliefs that pupils bring from home and community are extremely difficult to change within short periods of time. However, some behavior changes may be observable in the classroom and are subject to measurement; those occurring in the home and elsewhere outside of school may not be seen and may be extremely difficult to assess. It should be recognized that the impact of health learning frequently takes time to have its effect upon children. Despite these difficulties, health education must provide correct understanding if appropriate health behaviors are to be acquired by pupils.

Good health behavior is significant only in terms of its effect on the lives of pupils. Good health therefore should be a means to an end and not an end in itself. Being healthy should enable children to obtain a better education, to be happier, to have fun, to be able to play for longer periods of time without undue fatigue, to be more productive in the world, and to be better citizens in the community. When good health is an end in itself, pupils are likely to become overly concerned about their health and become health neurotics.

Teachers should be aware of the fact that all students may not be able to acquire the same health levels because of hereditary and environmental factors. Children who are blind or deaf may never have these senses restored. Pupils who are paralyzed from poliomyelitis may never be able to walk as others do. Boys and girls with uncorrectable heart defects may never have the stamina to play in strenuous games. Students without food may be hungry and malnourished. Despite these handicaps, students need to maintain the best health status possible for themselves within their own limitations. Numerous illustrations of handicapped people leading well-adjusted, happy, and productive lives are found in society. The goals in health education therefore may need to be modified to fit the individual differences of children.

Inspection of the specific outcomes of health education that teachers seek to achieve reveals them to be categorized into the following:
1. Practices, habits, skills—action domain
2. Attitudes, feelings, ideals, interests, appreciations—affective domain
3. Knowledge, understanding, information —cognitive domain

Illustrations of these goals in health education that reflect the psychologic, social, and spiritual as well as the physiologic aspects of health (see Chapter 9) include the following:

Practices—action domain

The pupil:
1. Eats the proper foods for growth.
2. Obtains adequate sleep, rest, and exercise.
3. Acts safely.
4. Critically analyzes and evaluates health advertising and publicity.
5. Uses community health resources effectively.
6. Takes proper care of teeth.
7. Faces the realities of life.
8. Obtains proper immunizations.
9. Refrains from the use and abuse of drugs.
10. Refrains from the use of tobacco.
11. Attempts to develop a value system.

Attitudes—affective domain

The pupil:
1. Appreciates the dangers to self and others of communicable diseases.

2. Supports the need to have a concept of self.
3. Realizes that health departments and other community health organizations are needed in society.
4. Appreciates the need for periodic health examinations.
5. Is aware of the health hazards of the use of tobacco.
6. Is interested in providing for the rights of others.

Knowledge—cognitive domain

The pupil:
1. Explains how to protect himself against disease.
2. Identifies the procedures to follow when ill.
3. Recalls how to care for the skin, feet, ears, and eyes.
4. Summarizes how growth and development occurs.
5. Demonstrates how to administer first aid.
6. Identifies the physiologic, sociologic, and psychologic effects of drugs on individuals.
7. Discusses ways emotions may be helpful and harmful.

The health objectives listed are not all inclusive, nor are they appropriate for all grades (see Chapter 9). It is necessary to study the needs and interests of children in individual schools and school districts to determine the total program and the grade placement.

The *decision-making process* must receive attention by teachers. Pupils are growing and developing organisms that are being exposed constantly to environmental influences affecting health and about which decisions must be made. Young people must have the opportunity to make their own decisions and not be expected to follow the dictates of the teacher. However, such decisions must be based on complete awareness of the consequences. To make wise decisions, it is important that students be exposed to all the possible alternatives for action. Such teacher consideration is vital to health teaching because it aids in the establishment of credibility; it allows for the free choice of action; it prepares students to think and act for themselves. It is teaching for the future. By way of illustration, young people find cigarettes available in their communities and are constantly being persuaded to use them. If these individuals are to be able to determine intelligently whether to smoke or not to smoke, they must learn the positive as well as the negative effects of smoking on the human organism. Merely condemning cigarettes may create distrust among students who talk to peers and adults and obtain conflicting evidence regarding the beneficial or detrimental aspects. This is not to imply the use of tobacco is not hazardous but rather to emphasize that wise decisions will come about when the total spectrum of tobacco's effects are provided.

HOW CAN TEACHERS RELATE KNOWLEDGE TO BEHAVIOR IN THE INSTRUCTION PROGRAM?

The importance of health practices and habits points out the need for the use of teaching procedures that will help bridge the gap between the knowledge and behaviors that preserve and maintain health. Unfortunately the precise methods are not known today. However, there is significant evidence that indicates that attitudes play an important role in student health behaviors. It is believed that the acquisition of feelings, interests, and appreciation will lessen the time needed to convert the basic understanding that pupils receive into desirable practices.

An attitude refers to a mind set to action; it is an internal readiness to perform or behave. Therefore, what pupils believe, feel, or value affects what they do. Children who feel they are not susceptible to diseases may not think it necessary to be immunized against these diseases. Pupils who do not believe that excessive sugar consumption might lead to dental decay may not attempt to eat nutritious snack-time foods. Boys and girls who do not realize the dangers of jaywalking may not cross streets at the proper places. Young people may need to be helped to develop an interest in the concept of self. Effective learning in health education therefore must give consideration to including teaching methods that will attempt to develop appropriate student health attitudes as well as proper understanding.

A health education program that tries to stress the development of health attitudes is difficult to achieve, particularly since children are coming to school with ideals, interests, values, and feelings developed and influenced by their home and community experiences. For example, in arithmetic or spelling the child may come to school lacking any information. Yet in matters relating to health and safety the child may not only lack scientifically sound information but also, more important, may have strong beliefs affirmed by family and community that are false and perhaps even dangerous. Getting pupils to take responsibility for their own lives, whereby they seek to protect and maintain good health, takes much teaching skill and thoughtful planning. It involves initiative, ingenuity, creativeness, and fortitude on the part of teachers who aspire to reach this goal.

The applied principles of learning that follow, as well as the specific methods and materials found in succeeding chapters, should provide guidelines and specific teaching aids that will help teachers to enable pupils to acquire the behaviors necessary for healthful living.

WHY ARE PRINCIPLES OF LEARNING IMPORTANT IN HEALTH?

Knowledge of the principles of learning is important to teachers in health instruction programs because:
1. Learning is a complex process.
2. Behavior-centered emphasis in learning compounds the complexity of the learning process; attitudes are difficult to assess, and many practices are nonobservable in the classroom.
3. Understanding about motivation and behavior is necessary for effective teaching.
4. Teaching methods and learning are interrelated.

WHAT ARE THE PRINCIPLES OF LEARNING?
Motivation is essential to learning

Health behavior is determined by individuals' motives and beliefs or values about various courses of action open to them. Since all behavior is motivated, the extent to which health behavior of individuals can be understood, predicted, or controlled depends on the ability of teachers to identify these motives and beliefs and to use them in their health teaching.

Positively, motives refer to those drives, needs, urges, or inner compulsions that stimulate individuals to want certain things. They are classified as the following:
1. Physiologic needs, such as food, water, sleep, rest, air, sunshine, and exercise
2. Psychologic needs, such as security, love, achievement, independence, responsibility, and authority

Motives may also be considered in a negative sense, such as barriers that individuals must overcome.

Values are the strong beliefs or attitudinal concerns that have influence on positive or negative motives. The use of alcohol and tobacco, the significance of immunization, periodic visits to physicians, daily exercise, playing safely, and support for health departments depend on individual beliefs of the importance of these action on their lives. People have to feel that their practices will enable them to play longer, have more fun, and be more productive citizens.

Values are acquired from a variety of sources including the family, social groups, television and other mass media, adults admired by children, and peer cultures in school. When they are consistent with the goals of health education, they will reinforce learning, but when they are in conflict, learning may be limited or restricted. They are not completely resistant to change despite the cultural and social factors that may have influenced their formation. The earlier in the lives of children that attempts are made to acquire proper health behaviors, the greater are the possibilities that these practices will be highly valued by pupils. The school therefore has both a responsibility and an opportunity to modify beliefs and attitudes as well as to develop new ones that will promote and maintain good health.

PRINCIPLES OF MOTIVATION. Several principles of motivation based on current research provide some important information about health behavior:

Preventive health action is determined by the degree to which a person sees a health problem as threatening in terms of the following:

1. Its probability of susceptibility or occurrence. Will smoking cause lung cancer?

2. Its seriousness, severity, or urgency of the consequences. Is dental caries sufficiently important to warrant attention? Will an infection be painful?

3. Its benefits or courses of action open that will reduce or remove the threat to the individual's health. What health practices should individuals follow, and will these practices be beneficial? Are vision screening and hearing tests important, and will they reveal important findings? How much will it cost?

Individual motives and beliefs about various courses of action are often in conflict with each other, and behavior emerges as the conflicts are resolved. The kinds of conflicts referred to include the following:

1. When two motives compete with each other for dominance, the one of greater importance or the more highly valued one will become dominant. A family may spend what little money it has for food, shelter, and necessities rather than on medical or dental visitations. A child who must wear glasses because of poor eyesight may not wear them because the peer group at school disapproves of this practice. A pupil will smoke cigarettes because of gaining social acceptance by this behavior.

2. If a pupil is motivated to act in a healthful manner (sees a course of action open), but the action is unpleasant, painful, time-consuming, or inconvenient, the pupil may not complete the action.

3. A pupil may not accept a teacher's beliefs or opinions that there are ways to prevent or help a specific health condition and therefore does not see an effective way (course of action) to resolve the problem. A child with a boil on her leg may have been advised to visit a doctor but fails to do so be-

cause she may not believe the condition is serious or because she does not see how this action can help her. She may try self-medication, but as the infection grows worse she may find that her concerns and fears increase because she is not sure what action she should take. An adult who is told he might have incurable cancer may not wish to believe the authority who gave him the diagnosis and may resort to magic and mysticism to find a solution. Later, his fears may become so great that he is no longer able to think rationally because his own attempts to find a solution were not effective.

Health-related motives may sometimes lead to behavior unrelated to health, and conversely some behavior that has the appearance of being health related may in fact be determined by motives unrelated to health. A hungry child may not reveal his hunger to a teacher and may be untruthful when asked whether he has eaten any food. An illustration of the converse part of this principle is one in which a child may submit to poliomyelitis immunization because other children in her class are receiving it.

It should be evident that teachers play an important role in health instruction programs by motivating children to seek appropriate health goals as well as by helping boys and girls to acquire beliefs and values related to these motives. Teachers must provide pupils with experiences and activities that will improve their values of good health so that they will be better prepared to resolve conflicts in motives when they occur.

Fear can lead to rational as well as irrational behavior. It serves to protect, and it can be destructive to individuals. The fear of cancer may help students to refrain from smoking. The fear of becoming overweight may lead pupils to reduce food intake. However, a teenager with a genital sore or infection may be afraid to learn that venereal disease has been contracted and may not have the condition checked by a physician.

Risk-taking is normal and necessary and demands selectivity on the part of individuals after determination of benefit and harm. Everything people do involves risks of varying degrees. The decision to take them is dependent on whether the rewards outweigh the penalties. Crossing the street safely or eating food in a restaurant or lunchroom involves risk. However, they are minimum in comparison to the advantages. Surgery is hazardous, but if the chances of survival are increased, the benefits predominate in the decision. The dangers of using heroin or driving an automobile when under the influence of alcohol may be greater than the pleasures derived. Young people need to be taught to compare the advantages and disadvantages of risk-taking behavior in order to make responsible decisions.

SUBPRINCIPLES OF MOTIVATION. The subprinciples of motivation that follow will point out additional aspects valuable in both the learning and teaching processes.

Cultural and social factors may be barriers to learning. The traditions and practices in the home, at play, in social groups, with adults, in the peer culture at school, and in the total environment in which children live affect and influence the values, prejudices, and perceptions that pupils bring to class. There is a relationship between the socioeconomic status of families and the amount of money spent for health services and products. Families that rank highest generally spend more of their income on health services. Some families may not have funds to purchase glasses, toothbrushes, or food, or to provide health examinations for children. Some parents may not be concerned with immunizations or dental care. The nutritional and dress habits of certain ethnic and racial groups may differ somewhat from those advocated in school. Working parents may not be able to adequately supervise the eating habits and behaviors of their children. Certain religious groups may not believe in health examinations and appraisals, treatment, services, or fluoridation of the water supply.

Teachers should be cognizant of these cultural and social factors and realize that they may have an effect on the health education program. They may support the health instruction program, or they may adversely affect it.

Size of objects, use of color, and movement in instructional materials may aid in attracting attention and developing interest in learning. The principle concerning size, color, and movement emphasizes the importance of using a variety of teaching aids in the health instruction program. These materials aid in gaining attention, increasing interest, and helping to make teaching more effective, therefore making learning more concrete and specific.

The use of a variety of films, filmstrips, tape recorders, television and radio programs, phonograph records, exhibits, flannelboards, magnetic boards, objects, specimens, graphs, and charts will stimulate interest in the learning experiences provided by the teacher.

The use of such models as the human torso, heart, eyes, ears, and teeth serve as valuable teaching tools. Exhibits of the contents of first-aid kits or the hazardous objects found in the home help to create interest in the area of safety. Use of food models and flannelboards will increase attention when the Basic 4 in nutrition are being taught.

Chapter 12 provides detailed information about teaching aids usable in the health instruction program.

Extrinsic motivation is less effective than intrinsic motivation. Should children perform good health habits because of some material reward they will receive or because of the inherent values of the practices performed? Should teachers award gold stars to children who come to school with clean handkerchiefs, when they have brushed their teeth, and for other such reasons? Is it advisable to present a special scroll to classrooms that report 100% attendance of their pupils? Should pupils receive candy or toys as rewards for visits to dentists or doctors? The external stimuli described may obtain the health action desired, but the results are usually of temporary duration. The procedures described are questionable practices because:

1. Some parents do not give their children clean handkerchiefs to bring to school.

2. Some parents do not buy toothbrushes for their offspring, nor do they take them to physicians.

3. Pupils not able to have clean handkerchiefs or not having brushed their teeth may be embarrassed when special note of these practices occurs in class. The mental health implications may be of greater importance than the rewards themselves.

4. Children who are ill may infect others in school.

Teachers should motivate children to good health practices through the use of meaningful experiences and other approaches that develop intrinsic values for good health rather than through the use of artificial stimuli. This kind of health teaching will more likely provide the lasting behaviors desired. Further illustrations of this point will be found in other principles of learning.

Moderate tension facilitates learning, but severe tension may inhibit learning. Teachers often question the degree to which they should pressure children into desirable health behaviors and practices. The illustrations that follow provide examples that give some guidance.

The cause of a child's dislike for or never having tried celery and carrot sticks may be related to some unpleasant home experience involving pressure or punishment. This same pupil, however, is more likely to try these foods in the classroom during a tasting party where the pressures of group approval are not quite as severe and there is an accompanying pleasant experience.

The teacher who is consistently sarcastic, rude, and unfair, or who expects absolute quiet at all times, who does not ever have a sense of humor or permit pupil planning or decisions in the classroom undoubtedly provides a mental health environment that is less conducive to learning. Whereas the teacher who is generally courteous and fair and who frequently uses democratic procedures in class presents a more permissive atmosphere that probably provides a better balance of tension that will facilitate learning.

The fear approach in health in which the teacher exhorts and admonishes children by using the statement, "If you don't do this, here's what will happen," may create tensions that will inhibit the acquisition of the desired health behaviors. The teacher who strongly urges poliomyelitis shots because failure to do so will bring on the dreaded disease and paralysis may create such great tensions that fewer pupils participate in the program. Although children may be afraid of having a needle injected into the skin, they are more likely to obtain these immunizations if some understanding of their nature and values is provided in a positive manner and if their classmates are obtaining them.

Learning is generally greater when praise is used more often than blame or reproof, when success occurs more often than failure. Success and praise reinforce learning, but constant frustration and failure adversely affect learning. The importance of the application of this statement to the mental health of children is extremely significant to classroom teachers. It emphasizes the need for teachers to recognize improvement based on individual standards rather than on general levels of achievement. Pupils with poor vision, defective hearing, or other physical ailments may need special praise or opportunities for success experiences in the classroom or on the playground.

Achievement standards should be individual. From a mental health viewpoint, the expectation level of children toward the health goals established should be constant with their powers of accomplishment. A few specific illustrations of the application of this principle to a behavior-centered health education program are the following:

1. Children's need for sleep may vary in amount.
2. The brushing of teeth after meals may not be possible in those homes that do not provide toothbrushes or dentifrices.
3. Some children may be allergic or diabetic and should not be expected to drink milk or to eat all the foods prepared by the cafeteria at lunch.

Knowledge of results is a strong incentive to learning. The principle of knowledge as a strong incentive to learning refers to evaluation of the instructional program in terms of the achievement of the health education goals discussed earlier. Teachers as well as pupils want to know whether they are progressing toward the attainment of these purposes. They will want to know whether the practices, attitudes, and knowledge of healthful living have been acquired. This assessment of learning serves as a stimulus as well as an aid in redirecting the learning when necessary. Through the use of paper and pencil tests, demonstrations, observations, surveys, and other such techniques, some of the following questions may be answered:

1. Are children receiving the appropriate immunizations?
2. Do children know what to do when injured or ill at school?
3. Can children identify hazardous play areas?
4. Do children know how to administer simple first aid?
5. Are children getting adequate sleep, rest, and exercise?

A more complete discussion of evaluation can be found in Chapter 13.

Maturation and readiness of the child affects learning

Heredity, or the constitution of the pupil, sets the limits of learning of that individual by determining the individual's native intelligence and other capacities as well as physical and mental disabilities. However, maturation, or the physiologic growth and development of the pupil, determines whether the pupil is mentally, physically, socially, or emotionally ready to learn. It provides a state of readiness important in health education as well as in all learning.

In dental health 6- and 7-year-old children may have difficulty accurately learning the proper toothbrushing technique. This coordination involves use of the small muscles of the fingers and hands, and pupils may not be ready to learn this difficult procedure as completely or as accurately as desired. Although the brush is a fairly large implement, expertness of performance will

take time and may be delayed until the child physically matures. Nevertheless, the brushing habit needs to be started early, and teachers should introduce this motor skill in school.

In the area of safety, children may not be ready to learn to manipulate sharp-pointed implements, to use apparatus safely, to operate bicycles safely, or to perform other motor skills. Teachers need to be aware of these pupil limitations in their education programs.

The taking of heights and weights in school is a time when pupils are ready to learn about their individual physical and emotional growth patterns. Pupils will be able to better understand their constitutional limitations in weight, height, size, and shape at this time.

The menstrual process generally begins in girls in the fifth and sixth grades, and an educational program is appropriate when this growth change appears.

Adolescence is a time when students are interested in the growth changes taking place in their bodies.

In the early grades especially, pupils are not completely ready to learn to be social individuals. However, it becomes necessary for children to learn to get along with others, to respect authority, and to cooperate in school if they are to grow into emotionally healthy individuals.

Experiences and the environment affect learning

Despite the variety of health behaviors that children bring to schools, provisions must be made for learning experiences and environmental conditions that are conducive to good health. Teachers and other personnel have responsibilities to control the daily activities and conditions under which pupils learn. Some of the health experiences and conditions that should be included are the following:

1. The curriculum should include opportunities for children to learn how to live healthfully and safely.
2. Nutritious snack-time foods should be

sold at lunchtime or used at parties and social gatherings, rather than candy, cakes, and soft drinks that may not be conducive to good dental health.

3. Provision of a hot lunch at noon may help to develop good nutrition habits.
4. Playgrounds, classrooms, halls, and other places should be free of hazardous conditions and should be safe areas for learning.
5. Classrooms, halls, and playgrounds should be maintained in a neat, clean, and sanitary fashion.
6. Lavatories should provide soap and water for use when necessary.
7. Teachers should be free of communicable diseases and in good physical and mental health.
8. Adequate lighting, heating, and ventilation should be provided.
9. A democratic atmosphere in the classroom and the school will result in greater learning than an autocratic atmosphere where discipline is severe or nonexistent.

Guidance is necessary for the most effective learning

Health instruction must be a part of the school curriculum if the greatest health learning is to occur. An organized education program is necessary if children are to learn how to play fairly and how to get along with others, understand fears, know how to prevent and control diseases, know what to do when injured, realize the importance of adequate sleep and rest, and numerous other health practices and attitudes. Inclusion of this program means that schools must make teachers available to teach the subject area and must also provide materials that will enable them to carry out this teaching responsibility. These items should include teachers' guides or units that have been developed around pupils' health problems as well as a variety of teaching aids and materials.

The teacher aids children in the health instruction program by motivating them to learn, by selecting the goals to be achieved, by determining the content to teach, and by choosing and arranging the experience or activities to be used. Teachers help children to wash their hands properly, to brush their teeth properly, to assume responsibilities, to have success experiences, and to ride bicycles safely by using a variety of experiences and techniques including dramatizations, demonstrations, experiments, and discussions.

The teacher serves to facilitate learning by controlling motivation, distributing the learning at appropriate intervals, and organizing the learning process. Use of the learning principles found in this chapter will aid in this organization process.

Learning is a self-active process

The behavior-centered emphasis of health education makes the active participation of the learner particularly important and appropriate. Merely telling pupils "you should eat the proper foods," "you should take the safest route home," or "you should play fairly" will not achieve the desired health behaviors. Bridging the gap between knowledge and practices is more likely to come through pupil participation. Children must feel, see, discuss, act out, manipulate, and even taste things if the attitudes that affect good health practices are to be developed. The teacher has the important role of determining the nature of the experiences to be used in the learning process. Whenever possible, children should have two, three, or more of their senses involved in learning. It is believed that the greater the pupil participation, the greater will be the possibility of developing the appropriate behaviors.

To illustrate the application of this principle, the following specific activities are listed:

1. Have children learn about good snacktime foods by conducting a tasting party in which pupils eat appropriate nutritious foods.
2. Have children learn the proper way to brush their teeth by actually performing the exact procedure in class. Merely demonstrating this technique will not be satisfactory.

3. Have children make a survey of the unsafe conditions in the school and help to develop solutions for their elimination.
4. Take the class on a field trip and actually follow the safest way to the home of one class member.
5. Teach fair play, honesty, getting along with others, or waiting turns by including them in a softball game, a tag game, or as part of apparatus play.
6. Have pupils collect and analyze a variety of advertisements relating to health products.

Most effective learning occurs when there are good personal relationships between the pupil and the teacher

The dominant factor in any learning situation is the combination of personal and social relationships that exist between the pupils and the teacher in the classroom. Learning should take place in a democratic setting with the opportunity for free expression and participation by all children. Consideration must be given to the fair, just, and humane treatment of all pupils, regardless of race or ethnic background. The school and classroom should provide a warm, comfortable, and friendly environment. The teacher should be understanding and permissive but must also provide guidance and security. The emotional climate that pervades a school is extremely important to the effectiveness of the learning process.

Teachers should realize that their personal values, beliefs, prejudices, enthusiasms, and perceptions of health are brought to the classroom. They may affect the human relationship's atmosphere should they be in conflict with those of their pupils, their peer groups, or their families. They may influence the health behavior of children in a way that is contrary to best practice. Illustrations of these differences include the following:

1. Cleanliness and appropriate clothing
2. Amount of sugar consumed and significance to dental health
3. Appropriate foods for parties and snack times

4. Food faddism—use of vitamins and other food supplements
5. Food aversions—spinach, milk, liver
6. Fluoridation of the water supply
7. Use of alcohol and tobacco
8. Exercise and play
9. Choice of medical practitioner or health adviser

Teachers who make conscious efforts to avoid permitting their prejudices to influence pupils' health and who are willing to objectively permit children to look at scientific evidence do not necessarily have to compromise their own beliefs and values. This approach should enable teachers to maintain the good relations previously established.

Much learning is soon forgotten, and only a fraction of what was once learned is ultimately remembered

Studies reveal the greatest forgetting by pupils occurs when emphasis in learning is placed on the recall of factual material; evidence shows that meaningful information related to attitudes and practices is more easily learned and is remembered more completely and for longer periods of time. Understanding and knowledge should be provided in a context other than that of unrelated, isolated, factual information. Mere memorization or regurgitation of the names of the teeth, the digestion of foods, or the body systems will not be remembered unless the facts are more closely associated with the attitudes and habits of healthful living. They should lead to the acquisition of big ideas or generalizations, to concepts of health.

This principle emphasizes the need to stress the psychologic approach over the logical or structure-and-function approach to teaching. It indicates the importance of the greater use of problem solving in the health instruction program. It demonstrates the importance of learning centered around health needs and problems of pupils. Here are several illustrations to demonstrate this principle:

1. Pupils' appreciations of the possible hazards of using tobacco and narcotics must be

more meaningfully related to the ingredients of tobacco and the names of the various narcotic drugs. Pupils must feel that these substances may affect their performances in athletics, in recreation, and in school as well as their growth and health.

2. Pupils' interests in immunizations against diseases and the prevention of infections' spread will be greater if the diseases considered are those they or their parents may acquire or have acquired.

3. Pupils' appreciation for eating the proper foods will be increased if the lack of vitamins, minerals, and other substances is related to their own or their families' food needs or deficiency diseases.

Well-organized, meaningful material is more easily learned and is remembered longer than meaningless or nonsense material

The content of the health education program should be based on the needs and interests of pupils if it is to be meaningful. Various studies indicate the following areas to be representative of these needs and interests: cleanliness and grooming; community health; consumer health; dental health; control and prevention of disease; care of the eyes, ears, and feet; exercise and fitness; family health; growth and development; mental health; nutrition; rest; sleep and fatigue; safety; alcohol, tobacco, and drugs. Learning organized around these areas will result in the most effective health behaviors.

Schools should have teacher guides to health education containing units of instruction focused around the health areas identified in the previous paragraph. These manuals should define the learning that should take place at the various grade levels. They should provide a sequence of learning that avoids excessive overlapping and duplication of content.

Teachers should capitalize on incidents that occur at school or in the home and use these "teachable moments" (see Chapter 11) in their instruction programs, thus making health education practical as well as functional. Such incidents as the following are

usable:

1. The class is going to use the playground apparatus.
2. The nurse is coming to do the vision screening.
3. Fire Prevention Week is emphasized in the community.
4. A child reports a visit to the dentist.
5. Children wash their hands before lunch and after going to the lavatory.

The ability to solve problems, to reason, and to do reflective thinking involves training and must be learned

Reasoning ability does not appear suddenly, but rather it develops gradually with age and experience. Differences in the reasoning ability of children and adults are differences in degree and not in kind. Children should be taught how to think rather than what to think. In the primary grades this process can be done more simply using questions that challenge pupils' thoughts.

The many quacks, charlatans, and pseudomedical people who live in our communities together with the millions of dollars spent yearly on unnecessary drugs, vitamins, and patent medicines make it necessary that children begin to be able to do reflective thinking in health as they do in other phases of learning. Children and adults need to know whether health facts they are hearing are valid and to know reliable health information sources.

Illustrations of problems that teachers may use for children to solve may include the following:

1. What should you do when injured?
2. What should you do when you are ill?
3. Who can help you when you are ill or injured?
4. How can you make friends?
5. What kinds of clothing should you wear to protect your body?
6. How does the health department protect the health of the people?
7. Should we believe what we read and hear about health products?
8. What hazards in the home may cause accidents?

9. Where can you get help if you have venereal disease?

The learning process must specifically include teaching for transfer of training or learning if this transfer is to occur

Health knowledge that carries over into or transfers to pupil activities outside of school is the most significant kind of learning. Transfer does not happen by chance but rather by design. Teachers must include teaching for carryover in their planning if school health activities are to occur in the home and community.

The most effective transfer of learning happens when the learning in school is as near real-life situations as possible. Learning, therefore, must be lifelike to obtain the greatest transfer.

When teaching pupils about safety at street corners, it may be necessary either to go to the corner itself and perform the safe behavior or to simulate a street corner on the school grounds using traffic lights, small cars, and other props with the children participating in a role-playing activity.

To obtain the greatest safety in the home, it may be necessary for children to survey the hazards therein and to suggest ways to reduce or remove these hazards.

To expect children to eat balanced meals at home, it may be advisable to provide such meals in schools at noontime.

To expect children to reduce their consumption of sugars and sweets, it will be necessary to curtail, or remove, their availability in schools, at lunchtime, at snacktime, during parties, and during other social occasions in school. However, some health educators believe that foods containing sugars should be available but controlled as an educational means of teaching children their proper use.

The use of repetition and reinforcement is necessary in learning

Health learnings must be repeated and reinforced if they are to have the greatest effect on the health behavior of individuals and if they are to be useful in the children's daily lives. A brief exposure in a classroom, or elsewhere, to a discussion, demonstration, or report of the safest way home from school, the safe way to act on the bus, the use of hand signals when riding a bicycle, the importance of eating the proper foods, the hazards of smoking, what to do when someone is injured, or the proper way to brush teeth does not assure that these actions will be followed consistently for any length of time. Activities used to achieve health and safety objectives must be used on several occasions either during the unit, during the semester, or during the entire school year.

In psychologic terms, this type of learning is frequently referred to as spaced learning— a repetition of what has been taught after intervals of time have elapsed. These time intervals may occur during or at the end of a lesson, in the middle or end of a unit, or during the semester, or there might be longer spacing. To illustrate, when teaching the proper technique for brushing the teeth during a unit on dental health, a demonstration of the correct procedure might have to be made again during the lesson and followed by the pupils actually performing the correct technique. The entire sequence, or some modification, may have to be repeated one time or more during the unit and possibly reviewed during the semester. Had this learning occurred in the first or second grade, it may be advisable and necessary to repeat or reinforce it in the third or fourth grades and possibly again in the fifth, sixth, or seventh grades.

The extent and degree of repetition will vary and will be dependent on any or all of the following:

1. The individual differences in pupil abilities
2. The health values pupils bring to the classroom
3. The nature of the health environment in the home and in the community
4. The parental cooperation and assistance

SUMMARY

The chapters that follow will be of specific help to teachers in the planning and teaching of health education in their schools. However, when selecting and using methods and materials for the instruction program, teachers should be concerned with the behavior-centered emphasis and the principles of learning. A summary of these principles for quick reference follows:

1. Motivation
   a. Principles
   b. Subprinciples
      (1) Cultural and social factors
      (2) Size of objects, color, and movement
      (3) Extrinsic versus intrinsic
      (4) Moderate versus severe tension
      (5) Praise versus blame
      (6) Individual achievement standards
      (7) Knowledge of results
2. Maturation and readiness
3. Experiences and environment
4. Guidance
5. Self-active process
6. Good personal relationships
7. Much learning forgotten
8. Meaningful material
9. Problem solving
10. Transfer of training or learning
11. Repetition and reinforcement

QUESTIONS FOR DISCUSSION

1. What is the meaning of the term "behavior modification"?
2. What is believed to be the process of how children learn? Apply this to health education.
3. What is the role of the teacher in the learning process in health education?
4. Why must the teacher be familiar with the goals of health education?
5. What are the goals of health education?
6. What is the aim of health education? Discuss its relationship to pupils and their individual differences.
7. What are the general as well as specific objectives that the teacher should achieve in health education?
8. What is meant by the term "bridging the gap" between health knowledge and health behavior?
9. Why are the principles of learning important in health teaching?
10. What are the principles of learning that will help the teacher in the health instruction program and provide specific illustrations of their application to health education?
11. What are the principles of motivation that have an effect on learning in health education?
12. What is the significance of pupil values and beliefs in health education?
13. Why are good personal relationships important and necessary for effective health teaching?

14. What are several illustrations of ways the teacher can make health learning a self-active process?
15. What is the meaning of the term "decision-making process" when applied to health education?
16. What is the significance of fear and risk taking in behavior modification in health education?

SUGGESTED CLASS ACTIVITIES

1. Discuss the process of learning and prepare illustrations that apply to health education.
2. Discuss the interrelationships between the learning and teaching processes.
3. Have a committee review several school district teachers' guides in health education and report on the objectives found therein.
4. Have reports on illustrations of motivation in health education.
5. Invite a school health supervisor, director, consultant, or coordinator to discuss the objectives of health education established in the district.
6. Discuss the principles of learning and illustrate their application to health education.
7. Have reports on interviews with in-service elementary school teachers regarding the use of any, or all, of the principles of learning in the health instruction program.
8. Have pupils complete a self-test of true-false questions about the principles of learning and follow with a discussion.
9. Prepare a list of the cultural and social factors that have an effect on health education.
10. Prepare a checklist of the principles of learning and have pupils obtain ratings and reasons for choices of the most important ones from in-service elementary school teachers.
11. Prepare lists of questions by grade levels and by areas that could be usable in teaching children how to solve health problems.
12. Take one health area, such as nutrition, and have pupils illustrate applications of the principles of learning in health teaching.
13. Conduct a health demonstration lesson and have pupils evaluate it in terms of the variety of principles of learning used.
14. Using specific health illustrations, have students identify where and how fear and risk taking affected behavior modification.

REFERENCES

Bernard, H. W.: Psychology of learning and teaching, ed. 3, 1972, Oregon State System of Higher Education.

Carroll, H. A.: Motivation and learning; their significance in a mental-health program for education. In National Society for the Study of Education: Mental health in modern medicine, forty-fourth yearbook, Part II, Chicago, 1955, University of Chicago Press.

Cassell, R. N.: The psychology of instruction, Boston, 1957, Christopher Publishing House.

Clarke, K. S.: Values and risk-taking behavior; the concept of calculated risk, Health Education **6:** Nov./Dec., 1975.

Derryberry, M.: Health education in transition, American Journal of Public Health **47:** Nov., 1957.

Eastern States Health Education Council: Psychological dynamics of health education, New York, 1951, Columbia University Press.

Fodor, J. T., and Dalis, G. T.: Health instruction; theory and application, ed. 2, Philadelphia, 1974, Lea & Febiger.

Fransen, F. J., and Landholm, J.: Changing behavior by personalized learning, Journal of School Health **41:** Feb., 1971.

Gagne, R. M.: Some new views on learning and instruction, Phi Delta Kappan **7:** May, 1970.

Galdston, I., editor: The epidemiology of health, New York, 1953, Health Education Council, New York Academy of Medicine.

Grandsen, A. N.: How children learn, New York, 1957, McGraw-Hill Book Co.

Grout, R. E.: Health teaching in schools; for teachers in elementary and secondary schools, ed. 5, Philadelphia, 1968, W. B. Saunders Co.

Hanna, L. A., Potter, G. L., and Hagaman, N.: Unit teaching in the elementary school, New York, 1955, Holt, Rinehart & Winston.

Harris, C. W., editor: Encyclopedia of education research, ed. 3, New York, 1960, Macmillan, Inc.

Hochbaum, G.: Research in behavioral sciences, presented at the Regional Institute on the Science of Health Education at the University of California at Los Angeles, June 12-14, 1961.

Hochbaum, G.: Learning and behavior; alcohol education for what? Alcohol Education Conference Proceedings, March, 1966, U.S. Department of Health, Education, and Welfare.

Hochbaum, G.: Effecting health behavior, presented at the annual meeting of the New York State Public Health Association, Buffalo, May 23, 1967.

Hochbaum, G.: How we can teach adolescents about smoking, drinking, and drug abuse? Journal of Health, Physical Education, and Recreation **39:** Oct., 1968.

Hochbaum, G.: Changing health behavior in youth, School Health Review, Sept., 1969.

Hochbaum, G.: Health behavior, Belmont, Calif., 1970, Wadsworth Publishing Co., Inc.

Hochbaum, G.: Human behavior and nutrition education, Nutrition News **40:** Feb., 1977.

Jordan, A. M.: Educational psychology, ed. 4, New York, 1956, Holt, Rinehart & Winston.

Katz, J.: Responsible decision making, Health Education **6:** March/April, 1975.

Kegeles, S. S.: Why people seek dental care; a review of present knowledge, Journal of School Health **51:** Sept., 1961.

McKennell, A.: Implication for health education of social influences on smoking. American Journal of Public Health **59:** Nov., 1969.

Mossman, M.: How we can motivate in health education, Journal of Health, Physical Education, and Recreation **24:** Sept., 1953.

Ripple, R. E., editor: Learning and human abilities; education psychology, New York, 1964, Harper & Row, Publishers, Inc.

Rosenstock, I. M.: Motivation bases for health education practices, presented at the fifty-first annual meeting of the Wisconsin Anti-Tuberculosis Association in Milwaukee, Wis., April 24, 1959.

Rosenstock, I. M.: Psychological forces, motivation, and nutrition education, American Journal of Public Health **59:** Nov., 1969.

School Health Education Study: Health education; a conceptual approach to curriculum design, 1967, St. Paul, Minn., 3M Education Press.

Strang, R.: The six steps of learning healthful living, Journal of Health, Physical Education, and Recreation **27:** Feb., 1956.

Tyler, R. W.: Health education implications from behavioral sciences, Journal of Health, Physical Education, and Recreation **31:** May-June, 1960.

11 Methods and techniques in health teaching

Health cannot be given to people, it demands their participation.
RENÉ SAUD

Now that the role of the learner in health education has been considered, let us look at the role of the teacher in the behavior modification process with specific reference to the learning process.

The teacher is the most important single factor in the health education program. The responsibility for organizing, guiding, and directing the learning toward health objectives rests with the teacher. This is accomplished through a familiarity with a wide assortment of teaching activities and experiences. The selection of those methods and techniques that will most efficiently and effectively aid learning and lead to health-educated pupils is necessary. The variety of procedures used by teachers to achieve the practices, attitudes, and knowledge goals of healthful living are called methods or methods of teaching.

WHAT IS METHOD?

"Method" is a broad term in teaching referring to the organized and systematized ways used by teachers to achieve purposes or objectives. They are often said to be the "how to" of teaching. "Techniques" is a concrete word describing more specific ways to attain goals. They may be called activities, experiences, or teaching/learning activities. In health education, these procedures help to interpret and translate scientific information to pupils.

The mere selection of appropriate activities or experiences by the teacher does not assure effective learning. These related factors must also receive consideration:

1. The maintenance of good pupil relationships provides an atmosphere conducive to learning. Understanding of children's physical, emotional, social, and intellectual characteristics, treating pupils fairly and firmly, and using democratic procedures contribute to an appropriate social climate in the classroom.

2. Teachers must recognize and provide for differences in abilities, aptitudes, and achievements in pupils. Some students may need more help in learning how to floss and brush teeth. Others may require special guidance to complete survey and research projects.

3. Methods may be teacher or pupil centered. Teacher-centered methods are those dominated by the teacher and are usually more formal in approach. They may include recitations, question and answer sessions, and lectures. Pupil-centered methods refers to the nondirective processes that allow for greater student participation. They may include demonstrations, excursions, constructive activities, and peer group involvement. Greater emphasis must be given to those activities involving pupils if health attitudes and behavior changes are to occur.

WHAT ARE THE TYPES OF METHODS?

Methods are difficult to categorize because the variations and combinations used by teachers are so numerous. In addition, their close relationships to instructional materials add to the complexity of grouping. Nevertheless, the types listed are classifications

245

that have been found effective and useful in health instruction programs in elementary schools.

1. Problem solving
   a. Brainstorming
   b. Values clarification
2. Construction activities
3. Creative activities
4. Demonstrations
5. Discussions
   a. Questions and answers
      (1) Question box
      (2) Quizzes—examinations
      (3) Self-tests
   b. Experience charts and records
   c. Buzz groups
   d. Problem solving—answers to questions
6. Dramatizations
   a. Dramatic play
   b. Role playing or sociodrama
   c. Plays
   d. Puppet shows
   e. Stories and storytelling
7. Educational games and simulations
8. Excursions
9. Experiments
10. Individual and group reports
11. Illustrated presentations
12. Resource people—guest speakers
13. Show and tell time
14. Surveys
15. Others—films, filmstrips, tape recordings, videotapes, slides, and additional instructional aids

Problem solving

Problem solving is perhaps the most important and practical method available for teacher use in the development of pupil health behaviors—in helping students make decisions. It is a general process whereby children learn to solve personal and community health problems through the use of the scientific approach. Pupils learn how to investigate, to reason, and to think reflectively so that they can differentiate facts from fiction and truth from superstition. It includes the use of a variety of activities, such as discussion, sociodrama, experimentation, dramatic play, and storytelling.

Several illustrations of health problems that may be solved are: How can we protect ourselves from disease? Who are some of the people who help us to stay healthy? What foods do we need for growth? Should we drink alcoholic beverages? Should we smoke? How can we prevent accidents?

The sequential steps that teachers can use to guide pupils in solving health problems are:
1. Recognition of the problem
2. Definition of the problem
3. Selection of methods of procedure
4. Collection of pertinent data
5. Selection, interpretation, and organization of data
6. Preparation of conclusions or alternatives
7. Application of conclusions or alternatives to the solution, problem, or plan of action
8. Possible evaluation of solution or solutions

Brainstorming, a type of problem solving. Brainstorming is a group attempt to solve a well-defined problem by offering any solution that comes to mind, no matter how extreme. It attempts to generate ideas quickly and in large quantity by the free association of ideas.

These procedures should be followed:
1. Encourage a free flow of ideas no matter how far out. Permit freewheeling.
2. Do not permit critical judgments, negative comments, or evaluations.
3. Restate the problem and start sorting out and refining ideas.
4. Evaluate the ideas objectively and narrow them to one or more solutions.
5. Summarize, and assign responsibilities.

These problems are illustrations of ones suitable for brainstorming: How can we encourage pupils to refrain from smoking cigarettes? How can we improve safety at school? How can we convince pupils to refrain from the misuse of drugs?

This procedure has value because it allows for freedom of expression, an exchange of ideas, and creative thinking. It has limitations in that the teacher may find it difficult to maintain class control, and it may not be productive if the class is too large. It also demands clarification of ideas, well-planned organization, and follow-up for effective results.

Value clarification, a type of problem solving. Value clarification involves a series of strategies or methods for helping students learn about values. It does not attempt to teach values per se. Illustrations of strategies can be found in Chapter 11. The seven criteria* used in the process are found in Chapter 9.

Value clarification will help students to critically review their own as well as society's values. It will aid pupils in identifying the concept of self and in searching for meaning in life.

Construction activities

Construction activities involve pupil-teacher planning as well as pupil participation in the preparation of a variety of items (using paper, wood, cardboard, glue, crayons, and other materials). Illustrations of specific items that may be made include a fire alarm box, a traffic light standard with stop and go signals, papier-mâché models of fruits and vegetables, plaster-of-paris models of teeth, the heart, and other organs of the body, and construction of paper models of the Basic 4 foods. These items have use in dramatic play, sociodramas, exhibits, bulletin board displays, and other techniques of teaching.

Creative activities

The free expression of children's thoughts, ideas, and feelings through such media as stories, poems and verses, dramatic plays, murals, and other creative activities may be useful and productive in the health instruction program. (See Chapter 11 for illustrations.)

Demonstrations

Demonstrations are procedures that help to make abstract verbal descriptions and symbols more concrete and meaningful in health education. They may include involvement of the sense of sight and touch as well as the auditory sense. They are helpful ways to improve the teaching process and may be performed by teachers or pupils.

Five important reasons for the use of demonstrations in teaching are the following:
1. They stimulate interest and thereby motivate learning.
2. They help to clarify learnings.
3. They help improve and speed up the learning process.
4. They may be used to initiate a unit.
5. They provide a visual image helpful in retention of things learned.

Some demonstrations usable in health education are (1) the importance of oxygen in fires; (2) the proper way to brush teeth; (3) the safest way to ride a bicycle on sidewalks, streets, and highways; and (4) the proper use of fire extinguishers.

Discussions

The discussion as a method of teaching is probably the most familiar and commonly used procedure in health instruction. All activities and methods include or should include some type of discussion. These methods generally permit children to ask questions, make recitations, perform surveys, and participate in numerous other ways in the teaching process. They provide opportunities for the exchange of information between pupils and teachers. Group discussion is especially valuable since it is conducive to helping children to gain understanding and respect for each other's feelings and viewpoints.

Discussions need teacher guidance, and several of the following helpful points should aid in directing the conversation along constructive channels:
1. Encourage and stimulate pupil questions since they provide information about needs, interests, and concerns. Pupils should be helped to think through their own experiences and relate them to the discussion.
2. Try to get all children in the class to participate or be involved.
3. Do not hurry discussion.
4. Listen carefully to all contributions and relate them to the topic. Compliment and

---

*Raths, L. E., Harmin, M., and Simon, S. B.: Values and teaching; working with values in the classroom, Columbus, Ohio, 1966, Charles E. Merrill Books, Inc.

encourage children who make significant remarks. It may be necessary to have students amplify their statements.

5. When groups are reluctant to engage in discussions, mention of a personal experience or anecdote may help to get children to participate.

Discussions may take place in a variety of ways, and the suggestions that follow merely serve to illustrate the numerous variations that may be used in the health instruction program.

Questions and answers. Questions may serve to introduce a health area, they may be part of the teaching process used during the presentation of a unit or lesson, and they may serve as a review or summary of a class discussion.

The best results are obtained when careful thought, planning, and organization are given to building sets of questions. As a general rule, question and answer periods and sessions should be planned in detail and in advance as carefully as other teaching procedures.

QUESTION BOX. Occasionally, children are reluctant to ask questions in class because they fear embarrassment or for other reasons. This situation can be solved by having a receptacle of some kind available where pupils may anonymously place questions of interest or concern. This procedure may be especially appropriate when the topic of sex education or social hygiene is being considered in class.

QUIZZES. Quizzes can be oral, written, or performance in nature. They have value when used for drill, review, or grading purposes. They serve to motivate learning and are important in the instruction program. They have evaluation limitations since they tend to measure only the cognitive learning (understandings) acquired by pupils.

SELF-TESTS. Self-tests refer to a series of teacher-prepared, easily answered questions that help to stimulate discussion about a particular health topic. The number and difficulty of questions can vary, depending on the purpose of the test and the grade level in which it is used.

These tests are not given for grading pur-

poses. They have value because they can be duplicated and distributed at the start of the class and immediately get all pupils participating and thinking about the lesson. They may also be used to initiate a unit as well as to help determine additional class activities.

The following is an illustration of a partial self-test:

What do you know about tuberculosis?

Please circle the correct answer to the statements that are listed below. If you do not know the answer, circle the letter "D."

1. Tuberculosis is caused by a germ.   T   F   D
2. Tuberculosis is a contagious, or communicable, disease.   T   F   D
3. A person with a persistent cough may have tuberculosis.   T   F   D
4. Tuberculosis can be cured.   T   F   D
5. You can have tuberculosis without feeling sick.   T   F   D
6. The tuberculin test is used to find people with tuberculosis.   T   F   D

Experience charts and records. Experience charts and records are lists of phrases or brief stories that are dictated by children to the teacher who records their suggestions, or ideas, or thoughts on the blackboard or on large sheets of paper. This procedure has been used in the primary grades to introduce reading, but it also serves as a good technique when teaching health education. It is usable at other grade levels as a way to list or record questions that need to be answered about a particular health topic. It may be considered part of the problem-solving technique in teaching.

An illustration of a partial experience chart used in the first grade shows the following:

Milk

Milk is good for us.
Milk helps us grow.
Milk helps us play.
Milk makes us strong.
Drink milk each day.

Buzz groups. The buzz group method is one in which the class is divided into small groups of from five to eight pupils to discuss a specific problem or series of problems for a limited time, probably of 3 to 5 minutes' duration. Each subgroup selects a chairman to keep the discussion on the topic and to give everyone an opportunity to speak. A recorder is chosen who not only will jot down key points but will also be prepared to present these verbally to the entire class on request. The teacher's role during the buzzing is to move from group to group to be certain that the topic is being discussed, that students know what is expected of them, and to clarify questions relating to the problem under discussion. At the conclusion of the buzz groups, the teacher permits the spokespersons to report their answers, and a pupil summarizes the main points on the blackboard. Further discussion is encouraged by the class members during the summary period.

This technique has a number of important advantages for use in the health instruction program:

1. It provides a way to have several committees in class study different aspects of a given topic.
2. It allows greater pupil participation in the discussion.
3. It provides an atmosphere conducive to discussion.
4. It may serve as a diagnostic procedure to find out what pupils know about a particular topic.
5. It may lead to further pupil activities or experiences.

Buzz groups may be used (1) to discuss a particular problem or question; (2) to determine what action to take regarding a particular problem or question; and (3) to determine questions to ask a resource person who may be coming to class the following day.

Illustrations of several problems suitable for this method are the following: Should we drink alcoholic beverages? Is exercise good for us? Should we smoke cigarettes?

This procedure has limitations especially if pupils have no background information about the discussion topic; it may result in a rehash of ignorance. Also, it takes careful planning for the best results, for the prevention of a few students dominating the conversation, and for the confining of the comments to the topic. Selection of a subject about which students have controversial opinions increases the chances of success for this method.

Problem solving. Problem solving is a teaching technique whereby children are presented with specific health questions or situations and they attempt to provide solutions through class discussions. An illustration of this activity can best describe it. A teacher may present the following situations for pupil reactions:

1. What would you do if you were injured at school?
2. What would you do if you were injured a long way from home?
3. What would you do if a friend tried to persuade you to smoke a cigarette?

A modification of this procedure would be to present a problem in written form, such as the following:

> You were playing in the school yard at lunchtime and cut your leg on a sharp object. The wound was bleeding quite a bit, and you were in pain. Place a check in the box beside the statement below that would best describe what you would do. Be prepared to tell why you would take this action.
>
> 1. Take out my handkerchief and wrap it around the cut. ☐
> 2. Wash the cut with water. ☐
> 3. Press my hand on the cut to try to stop the bleeding. ☐
> 4. Report to the nurse or to my teacher. ☐
> 5. Wait until I arrived at home before doing anything. ☐
> 6. Not do anything. ☐
> 7. Go home. ☐

Critical review of quotations found in the literature and analysis of newspaper articles, lyrics from popular songs, scenes from movies, and value strategies are additional problem-solving possibilities.

Dramatizations

Dramatizations are ways for children to express their feelings and urges through make-believe, imitation, and imagination. It is believed that children are more likely to remember facts when they are portrayed or when they participate in portraying them. These procedures are interesting to children and apparently contribute to the development of health attitudes and values since pupils tend to identify themselves with characters in the situations.

Dramatic play. Dramatic play is an informal, spontaneous, natural way for children to act out what they have been reading, discussing, or seeing in health.

Children who have visited a fire station or read about one may construct an imaginary station in the classroom and play fire fighter. A visit to a grocery store may result in such a store being established in school. The presence of the school doctor may encourage children to establish a corner in the room as a physician's office.

Role playing or sociodrama. Role playing or sociodrama is a more formalized procedure than dramatic play. It is spontaneous and unrehearsed and focuses on a health problem of interest or concern. It provides a considerable amount of emotionalism and realism that apparently communicates to individuals.

The steps to follow in conducting a sociodrama generally include the following:

1. Selection of a problem of interest and importance to children
2. Explanation of the technique in simple terms
3. Provision of enough of the story to set the scene
4. Selection of children to participate
5. Definition of the problem and role of each pupil
6. Definition of the audience role
7. Cues to begin or opening remarks needed by first actors to get started
8. Stopping sociodrama at the point where action drops or when discussion should be started; may be after a 2- or 3-minute presentation
9. Conducting discussion afterward, asking such questions as: "What was being presented?" "What was good about the way the situation was handled?" "What might have been changed in the situation?"

Illustrations or dramatizations suitable in health education include (1) walking across the street; (2) riding a bicycle on the street;

(3) helping a person who is lost; (4) how a person behaves when teased by someone; and (5) how to say no.

Plays. Plays are more formal in nature because they have a prepared script and involve memorization of dialogue. They may or may not be pupil-written. They can serve as culminating activities with presentations made to parent groups or to school assemblies.

Puppet shows. When children are involved in making the puppets and planning the stories, the result on health behaviors can be very beneficial. These experiences are enjoyed by young children both as spectators and as participants. They have great attitudinal effects on pupils. Puppets may also be used in dramatic play or with spontaneous dialogue.

Many areas including dental health, nutrition, and safety provide suitable materials for these shows.

*Stories and storytelling.** Children enjoy stories and storytelling to the extent that various health topics can serve as themes. They can be used to initiate a unit in health, or they may be part of the on-going activities. They help stimulate questions and answers.

Some illustrations of how this procedure may be used are (1) read stories about fear, courage, honesty, truthfulness, and other phases of mental health; (2) read stories about fire and traffic safety; (3) prepare a puppet or a construction paper character having some such name as Bozo the dog, Chippy chipmunk, or Ronny raccoon and create a story in which this animal discusses mental health or nutrition; (4) prepare a flip chart with a series of humorous or otherwise interesting drawings that relate to how to take care of your eyes, ears, or feet; and (5) show pictures of toothbrushes, wash cloths, combs, and other such items and encourage pupil discussions relative to the importance of these items to health.

---

*See Chapter 12 for specific story references.

*Educational games and simulations.** These activities are ways to stimulate interest in health education by increasing student attention and making learning an active process. The techniques may be used by individuals or groups of individuals. They are found in many forms and include crossword puzzles, anagrams, quiz shows, bingo, nonverbal and verbal communication, tic-tac-toe, and baseball. They have received increased attention in recent years, and numerous commercial materials are available. Teachers must learn to be selective in those games to be used in the classroom. They should contribute to the achievement of the established health education goals.

Excursions and field trips. Excursions are designed to enrich classroom teaching procedures by making health more meaningful. Field trips may be limited to the school plant and the school neighborhood, or they may be distant journeys requiring bus transportation.

Some places to visit that may be part of the health instruction program are the school lunchroom, the school grounds, a grocery store, the corner crosswalk, the first-aid station, a dairy, a hospital, a dentist's office, and the health department.

Experiments

Experiments are procedures that use the scientific method to test suggested truths or to illustrate known truths. They are ways to solve problems and may also be classified as demonstrations. They differ from demonstrations because the techniques employed are more exacting and precise and controls are used to ensure valid results. The specific sequential steps may include the following:
1. Define problem to be solved or the hypothesis to be tested.

2. Select methods of procedure to be used.
3. Identify and assemble necessary materials needed.
4. Conduct experiment.
5. Collect and record data.
6. Select, organize, and interpret data.
7. Prepare conclusions.

Experiments stimulate interest and attention in learning. They provide realism to abstract concepts and make learning more meaningful.

Following are illustrations of experiments that have been helpful in the health instruction program:

1. The effect of good and poor diets on growth and development may be shown by the white rat feeding experiment. This demonstration may be done with kindergarten or first-grade children to encourage the drinking of milk and to discourage the consumption of excess sweets. Details of the exact procedures are available from the National Dairy Council.*

2. The importance of washing hands with soap may be demonstrated through the use of a series of sterile agar plates (petri dishes from science department). Children place fingers in one dish before washing with soap and water and in a second dish after washing. The dishes are then incubated or kept in a warm place for 24 hours or longer, and the extent of germ growth can be compared in the two dishes.

Individual and group reports. Individual and group reports are methods whereby oral or written reports, or both, are made about assigned or special interest health topics by individual pupils or groups of pupils. They involve critical reading and analyses, research, independent study, interviews, investigations as well as excursions or field trips. Questions and answers become necessary since they may precede, be part of, or follow the reports. They may include panel and forum presentations and independent study.

---

*Specific activities are found in Chapter 12. These references provide teacher information. Packer, K. L.: Peer training through game utilization, Journal of School Health **45:** Feb., 1975. Sleet, D. A.: The use of games and simulations in health instruction, California School Health **13:** Jan., 1975.

---

*National Dairy Council, 111 N. Canal St., Chicago, Ill. 60606.

Illustrated presentations. Illustrated presentations are activities whereby teachers present phases of health using audiovisual materials such as charts, models, pictures, and specimens. Children should be encouraged to participate in discussions and provided opportunities to ask questions.

An example of this procedure would be the use of food models on a flannelboard to illustrate the Basic 4 food groups or appropriate breakfasts, lunches, and dinners.

The use of chalk, both colored and white, could be used effectively to make cartoons, sketches, and schematic drawings of germs, body parts, foods, maps, illustrated slogans (germs hate soap), charts, and a variety of other valuable and useful visual presentations.

Resource people

The use of community resource people who are experts in their chosen fields often enriches the health instruction program. Such individuals may include physicians, dentists, health officers, police officers, fire fighters, and nurses.

The following points should be discussed with speakers who are invited to schools:
1. The choice of topic appropriate to that being covered in class
2. The grade level of the class
3. The nature of the vocabulary to use
4. The use of audiovisual aids whenever possible
5. The use of demonstrations, experiments, and illustrations whenever possible
6. Permission for children to ask questions

If speakers have difficulty complying with these points, or if it is impossible to review them in advance, it may be advisable to have a question and answer session. This will necessitate some advance pupil discussion or preparation of questions.

Peer group action. This is a method whereby students prepare materials for use or are able to discuss one or more health topics with their peers in formal and informal educational settings. By way of illustration, these procedures may include the preparation of audiovisual materials for presentation, the conduct of rap sessions, participation and leadership in a variety of discussions, and writing and producing newspaper articles and special bulletin materials for distribution.

This approach has had a measurable degree of success with students having drug problems. Former drug users have been able to reach drug users more effectively in selected situations. Junior high pupils have been able to improve communications with their peers or young people in sixth grade. However, the concept is conceivably useful in the areas of venereal disease, family health, and mental health if knowledgeable and interested students are involved. This pupil participation idea is worthy of consideration in the upper grades and possibly also in the intermediate grades.

The survey provides excellent opportunities to integrate health with language, art, and arithmetic. The survey forms will need to be prepared by pupils, and oral and written reports plus research may also be necessary. In addition, arithmetic tabulations and computations must be completed.

Some areas in health that lend themselves to surveys are: (1) the types and amounts of snack-time foods consumed by pupils; (2) the amount of candy and soda consumed daily, or weekly, by children; (3) the kinds of foods eaten for breakfast, lunch, and dinner by children; (4) the extent to which students smoke cigarettes or use drugs; and (5) the safety hazards in the school or home.

Show and tell time. Show and tell time is an appropriate time to discuss health matters as well as other topics. This activity is especially useful in the primary grades for children to tell about visits to dentists or physicians, accidents at home, or fires that happened in the community. Some children with parents who are physicians, dentists, fire fighters, police officers, or health officers may have special health items that they will bring to school and share with their classmates, such as stethoscopes, teeth, models, charts, books, and pamphlets.

Surveys. Surveys are procedures whereby students use checklists, interviews, questionnaires, and opinionnaires to collect information about the nature and extent of pupil or community health problems or practices. They may be considered as part of the problem-solving process.

Others

There are many variations of the methods of teaching described in this chapter that can be used in health education. Teacher ingenuity and creativity are necessary to develop the variety of other possible techniques. Communication media including television, radio, tape recordings, films, and filmstrips, videotapes, and slides as well as models, charts, exhibits, displays, bulletin boards, posters, flannelboards, and other audiovisual aids may be combined with the procedures just presented to provide numerous additional activities and experiences.

WHAT METHODS SHOULD TEACHERS USE?

There is no one best method or combination of methods to be used in the health instruction program. If any procedure is to be singled out as a basis from which to start selecting, perhaps the problem-solving approach must be given first consideration. This is a meaningful and scientific way to teach health education, it involves other activities, and it is behavior centered as well as pupil centered.

The process of developing health-educated individuals is complex and difficult. The techniques teachers employ should be those, however, that help pupils to understand the concepts needed to acquire the practices, attitudes, and knowledge for healthful living. It is important therefore that teachers be familiar with the nature, values, and limitations of many methods so that they may choose the ones that will aid pupils to achieve these objectives.

Teachers should review the following questions and use them as criteria when selecting procedures for the health instruction program:

1. Will the objectives be achieved?
2. Will they have educational value?
3. Will pupils participate actively?
4. Will interest be attracted and maintained?
5. Will information be communicated to pupils?
6. Will the teacher feel comfortable in using the procedures?
7. Will the methods be appropriate for the abilities and aptitudes of pupils?
8. Will the methods be suitable for the grade level?
9. Will they be adaptable to the supplies, equipment, and facilities that are readily available?

Kindergarten–primary grades

The health education program at kindergarten–primary grades should be centered around the daily activities that occur in school, the home, and the community, such as safety, disease control, nutrition, rest and sleep, the doctor, the police officer, the fire fighter, and the nurse.

Health can be integrated very easily into other areas of the curriculum, such as language arts, social studies, and science; however, there will always be need for direct teaching.

The methods selected for these grades should be those that include doing, experiencing, and observing. The techniques that will achieve the best results will probably include reading, stories, games, problem solving, excursions, discussions, show and tell periods, creative activities, construction activities, questions and answers, experience charts and records, and dramatizations.

Intermediate grades

Children in intermediate grades have acquired a new level of curiosity and enthusiasm. They begin asking more questions and want to know the "whys" of health. They are seeking more exact answers to their questions.

The growth changes occurring in pupils provide the need for learning about the structure and functions of the human organism. Girls particularly need information about menstrual hygiene.

The beginning of group activities and the

wider use of community resources and problem-solving procedures become possible and should be considered for use by teachers in their health instruction programs.

Health continues to be integrated to some extent with other subjects, but more direct teaching begins to be necessary.

The methods that teachers may use in their programs include discussions, problem solving, educational games, surveys, excursions, illustrated lectures, role playing, experiments, demonstrations, resource people, and individual and group reports.

Upper grades

Children in the upper grades are adventuresome, want to experiment, and desire more activity than ever before in their lives. Therefore, the health experiences must go far beyond the confines of the textbook. Pupils can be involved in cooperative planning and sharing of experiences.

The early adolescent period indicates the need for additional content areas to be included in the health instruction program. Tobacco, alcohol, and the use of drugs begin to have added meaning for these children, although these areas should receive consideration in the lower grades. In addition, exercise takes on importance, with dental and nutritional problems and venereal disease having special significance.

Some of the methods that may be included in the health instruction program are surveys, panels, debates, excursions, peer group action, exhibits, tape recordings, independent and group work, demonstrations, experiments, buzz groups, and problem solving.

ARE INCIDENTS METHODS?

Incidents by themselves are not methods. However, they are teachable moments that stimulate learning by setting the stage for meaningful health education. They can serve to initiate units or lessons. They may be considered as health problems that lend themselves to solutions through the use of the problem-solving process as well as other procedures. They lend themselves to both formal and informal educational approaches. Therefore, they may be considered to be a part of method.

Teachers must be constantly alert for the numerous occasions that happen in schools, in homes, and in communities that are usable in health instruction programs. The newspapers, magazines, and television are also sources in addition to student and adult reports. Teachers who consistently capitalize on these motivating events will undoubtedly be more successful in getting children to acquire the appropriate health behaviors.

The teacher must recognize that there are values as well as limitations in the use of incidents in health teaching. When they are improperly used, they may result in serious emotional disturbances among children. A teacher who discusses the cleanliness habits or the decayed teeth of a particular pupil in class not only may embarrass the child but also may make the child unnecessarily conspicuous before the other classmates. From a psychologic viewpoint, therefore, this action may be very harmful to the child. The teacher must use discretion in choosing incidents as well as the appropriate occasion for capitalizing on such situations. Incidents in health teaching may be used in several ways:

1. To discuss individual health problems with pupils in private or with parents.

2. To discuss health and safety problems that have been observed in school or elsewhere without reference to any special pupil or groups of pupils.

3. To discuss special events or occasions involving health and safety that will take place in the school or in the community.

4. To discuss a particular pupil health problem when the child is not in the room. This is probably the rare occasion but may be necessary for the protection of the child. For example, if a child has had an epileptic seizure in class, it will be necessary for the teacher to seek the support of the child's classmates to help this pupil when necessary. This attack could occur on the playground or on the way home when the teacher or other adult was not nearby. Therefore, a brief explanation of the nature of seizures

and first-aid procedures is important. This action may help to prevent the pupil from being injured and being rejected by the other classmates.

The following incidents that occur in the school setting illustrate opportunities available for health instruction:

1. Students smoking in school.
2. Many children absent because of the "flu."
3. Pupils come to school with colds.
4. Children prepare refreshments for a party at school.
5. A student tells how a friend's hand was burned while playing with matches.
6. The school conducts a fire drill.
7. A child reports a visit to the dentist.
8. Pupils make fun of children wearing eyeglasses or hearing aids.
9. The food served for lunch at school.
10. Children have their vision and/or hearing screened at school.
11. A student asks about dental health or nutrition in TV commercials.
12. A child is bitten by a dog on the playground.
13. A student has an epileptic seizure in class.
14. An accident occurs to a student on the way to or at school.
15. Students eating candy and sweets in excess.

A third-grade teacher who took advantage of a report in the newspaper of a bicycle accident that occurred to a school child and resulted in a broken arm will serve to illustrate how to use an incident in the instruction program. The morning after the accident the teacher asked the class how it happened. Discussion brought out such matters as careless riders, unsafe conditions, and unsafe equipment. The conversation led the pupils to list the actions that often lead to accidents: bicycle riding, car driving, walking, living in school, and living at home. The teacher than asked the question: "If these may lead to accidents, how can we act safely?" The pupils began to mention safety rules but finally decided they needed more information to be able to answer this question

satisfactorily. At this point the teacher suggested that continued planning should go on the next day.

When the discussion resumed the following day, the children decided to participate in a variety of experiences to learn more about safety. These are some of the activities they selected:

1. Read stories in safety books and pamphlets.
2. Create bulletin board displays of safety posters.
3. Create a checklist of "Ways to make my home safe."
4. Invite a police officer to visit the class to discuss safety.
5. Conduct a culminating activity that dramatizes a typical day of children who do not practice safety and a typical day of children who do.

Special community and school events are also important occasions to motivate for health education in schools. The "Monthly Health Specials Calendar" approach that follows offers useful suggestions.

MONTHLY HEALTH SPECIALS*

September
Find safest way to school
Walk *left* on rural highways
Bus safety
Bike safety
Classroom safety
Doctor, nurse, and dental hygienist are your friends
Emphasize good nutrition
Wash hands before eating
Know phone numbers: home, police, and fire department
National Child Safety Week

October
Fire Prevention Week—discuss fire drills. Emphasize home clean-up for fire safety
Halloween safety

---

*Adapted from Schneeweis, S. M., and Jones, R.: Time linked health problems; the monthly health specials calendar approach for use in grades K-6, Journal of School Health **38:** Oct., 1968. (Reprinted by permission of editor, Journal of School Health, with minor revisions.)

November
Winter hazards

December
Christmas tree: use safe lights, turn off if no one
in the room; inspect lights carefully
Vacation safety
Smoking and alcohol education

January
Snow and ice are still with us
Stress good sportsmanship and courtesy and their
relationship between popularity and good mental health

February
Dental Health Week
First aid

March
High water and dangerous slippery banks: *stay
away*
Vacation safety again
Bike safety
Save Your Vision Week

April
Cancer drive: relate this to dangers of smoking,
polluted air, and emphasize early examinations
of adults
Good-Vision Week
Bike Safety Campaign
*Beware of strangers; never get in a car with an
unknown person*

May
Child Health Week
Mental Health Week
Stress swimming and other water safety
Mention farm animals and their danger
First aid

June
Sunburn is a real burn! Poison ivy is a danger
Water safety
Camping safety

Other seasonal events also offer opportunities for health education: (1) the appropriate time to discuss safety to and from school,
bicycle safety, and playground safety may be
when children return to school in September; (2) fall and winter may be significant times to discuss respiratory diseases and
other communicable diseases; and (3) spring
may be the time when camping, picnic, and
water safety become especially important.

IS THE USE OF THE HEALTH TEXTBOOK A METHOD?

The health textbook is a very important
teaching aid that should serve as a reference
or resource to provide information necessary
to solve health problems. It should be used
in conjunction with pupil activities and experiences and therefore may be considered
to be a part of or related to method. It may
be used in the preparation for discussions,
panels, individual and group work as well
as in other ways. It can help to provide continuity and direction to learning experiences.

A textbook, however, should not be used
as a passive reading lesson. Children will not
acquire the necessary health behaviors if
their experiences are limited to a 10- or 15-
minute daily reading assignment in a health
text. This procedure is contrary to the principles of learning discussed in Chapter 10.
Teachers must be more imaginative and creative and use a variety of the methods and
activities described in this chapter if the goals
of health education are to be achieved.

WHAT ARE THE RELATIONSHIPS BETWEEN METHOD AND MATERIAL AIDS?

Material or teaching aids such as models of
the teeth, health films, and filmstrips, flannelboards, exhibits, or displays of the contents of first-aid kits are valuable supplementary items that enrich learning experiences. They are aids to learning that make
abstract health concepts become specific,
concrete, and meaningful in the lives of students; they serve to attract and maintain attention; they help to stimulate interest in the
teaching process; they assist in encouraging
greater student participation in the learning process. Teachers should be familiar with
the variety of such items that are available
and use many of them in their teaching.
Chapter 12 provides a comprehensive coverage of the nature of these aids.

Instructional aids should not be considered
teaching methods in themselves. However,
they are important and necessary supplementary and complementary aspects of the

procedures used in learning. They are part of the "how to" methods of teaching.

At times it is difficult to distinguish between methods and teaching aids. An example or two serves best to illustrate this point. A film by itself is a teaching aid. When children are expected to look for specific information as they view the film and, after its showing, discuss what they saw, then it becomes part of the teaching process. Therefore, discussion may be the method used in the learning, with the film being a part of this procedure. A flannelboard and food models are teaching aids. When these items are used in a discussion to demonstrate the food items needed for an adequate breakfast, they become a method.

The use of a variety of teaching aids can greatly contribute to the emphasis on pupil-centered methods of teaching. They will assist in providing more pupil participation in the learning process.

WHAT TEACHING TECHNIQUES ARE USABLE IN HEALTH INSTRUCTION?*

The wide variety of specific teaching techniques that are presented next will aid the teacher in the achievement of the objectives in health education. They include more than 1,200 ideas for use in the instructional program. They are organized alphabetically into fifteen subject areas, and the appropriate grade level group for each activity is identified.

When the procedures for health teaching

are selected, it will be helpful to keep in mind these essentials:

1. The purposes of health education go beyond an emphasis on information alone. They also consider the development of health attitudes and practices.
2. The principles of learning described in Chapter 10 are important.
3. The specific technique or combination of techniques to be used should help to achieve a desired goal or goals.
4. Activities should be continually evaluated to determine the extent of learning taking place.

Despite the many and varied types of activities presented, the procedures that follow do not provide a comprehensive coverage of all health teaching experiences, nor do they include the use of films and filmstrips. Rather they serve a fourfold purpose:

1. To provide specific, tested techniques that will give spark and vitality to the health instruction program. The numerous experiences listed have been used by many teachers in their classrooms.
2. To provide a broad selection of activities for those with limited or extensive teaching experience.
3. To provide suggestions of teaching techniques that will stimulate the creative and imaginative teacher to modify, change, or devise completely new procedures.
4. To provide methods that may be used to initiate units or as culminating activities.

It should be noted that the following teaching procedures have been organized in a functional and practical manner for easy reference by the teacher. The letters or numbers found on the right of the page in the activities or experiences that follow refer to the *suggested* grades or grade level in which they may be used: P, primary; I, intermediate; U, upper.

---

*An excellent culminating activity that involves much student, parent, and community participation is the conduct of a *health fair*. The reference at the end of this chapter prepared by the American School Health Association is one worthy of review.

ALCOHOL

Grades

Bulletin board	1 Illustrated display of accidents and other losses attributed to alcohol.	U
	2 Illustrated display of the content of alcohol found in the various kinds of beverages.	U
Buzz group	3 Conduct a buzz session on the questions "Should I drink alcoholic beverages?" "Why do people drink alcoholic beverages?"	6, 7, 8
Chart	4 Prepare a chart or poster that shows the effect of alcohol on the body; the level of alcohol in the blood after beverages consumed.	6, 7, 8
Demonstration	5 Place a small (3-inch) goldfish in a solution of ½ ounce of alcohol in ¾ pint of water (the amount in a 12-ounce bottle of beer). In almost 20 minutes the fish will be "under the influence" (floating to the surface). When the effect of the alcohol can be seen, remove the fish and place in fresh water to be revived.	I, U
Discussion	6 The physiologic, psychologic, and sociologic effects of alcohol on the human body.	6, 7, 8
	7 The nutritional elements found in a glass of milk, an ounce of whiskey, and a bottle of beer.	6, 7, 8
	8 The nature of the alcohol content in beer, wine, and whiskey.	6, 7, 8
	9 Collect ads from newspapers and magazines on alcoholic beverages and analyze them in class.	U
	10 Safe and unsafe use of alcohol.	U
	11 Predisposing factors to alcoholism.	U
	12 Effects on families of individuals with alcohol problems.	U
Dramatization	13 High school drama class depicts scenes of pressures put on sixth-, seventh-, and eighth-grade students to drink alcoholic beverages. Follow with discussion of junior high school pupils' suggestions for handling such situations.	6, 7, 8
Exhibit	14 Display whiskey, wine, and beer glasses and discuss the amount of alcohol contained in each beverage and in each glass.	6, 7, 8
	15 Display a variety of magazines, pamphlets, and other materials for students to read, do research, and prepare oral and written reports on alcohol.	U
	16 Pupils display labels taken from medicine bottles and other containers and prepare a list of the amount of alcohol found in these substances.	U
Graph	17 Compare the amount of money spent on beverage alcohol and the amount spent on education, cancer, tuberculosis, and other health projects.	U
Guest speaker	18 Invite a member of Alcoholics Anonymous to discuss the services rendered by this organization to help alcoholics.	U
	19 Invite a physician to discuss the physiologic effects of alcohol on the human body.	U

ALCOHOL—cont'd   Grades

			Grades

Individual and group reports
20 Pupil committees write letters to organizations having materials on alcohol and request copies for use in class.   6, 7, 8

21 Pupils prepare oral and written reports on recent magazine articles about alcohol.   6, 7, 8

22 Pupils prepare oral and written reports on the effect of alcohol on a person in sports, driving an automobile, flying, typing, and using industrial skills.   U

23 Pupils prepare individual and group reports on such topics as the preserving quality of alcohol, alcohol as a fuel, alcohol in medicine, and alcohol as a disinfectant.   U

Interview
24 Interview a member of the sheriff's office or police department to find out the effect of alcohol on the crime rate and the accident rate in the community.   U

25 A pupil committee interviews a physician and the health officer on the benefits and adverse features of the use of alcohol.   U

Panel
26 Have a panel discussion on the topic "Why people drink alcoholic beverages."   U

Problem solving
27 Pupils do research and prepare oral and written reports about a series of problems such as: "Why do people drink?" "Should teenagers drink alcoholic beverages?" "What effect does alcohol have on the body?" "What effect does alcohol have on the mind?" "Is alcohol a food?" "What are the uses of alcohol?" These may also serve as introductory questions to stimulate student discussion to determine ways to find solutions.   U

Reports
28 Pupils prepare reports in regard to Alateen and Alanon programs; relationships of alcoholism and nutritional problems; state laws; community resources to treat alcoholism; alcohol and use in religious ceremonies.   U

Resource persons
29 Invite member of Alcoholics Anonymous to class.   U

30 Have police officer talk about alcohol intoxication tests.   U

Role playing
31 Saying no when offered an alcoholic beverage.   U

32 Pressures of peer groups to consume alcoholic beverages.   U

Scrapbook
33 Pupils make scrapbooks to include pictures, magazines articles, newspaper articles, stories, and other items about the use and effect of alcohol.   U

Self-test
34 Pupils complete a self-test and conduct a discussion afterward.   U

What do you know about alcohol?

Circle the correct answer to the right. If you do not know the answer, circle the letter "D."

1. Alcohol is a narcotic drug.	T	F	D
2. Scientists consider alcohol to be a good food.	T	F	D
3. Alcohol has good uses outside the body.	T	F	D
4. A person can get drunk on beer.	T	F	D
5. A person can do things better after a few drinks.	T	F	D

ALCOHOL—cont'd

Grades

6. A drink of whiskey helps to overcome a cold.   T F D
7. Alcohol slows down digestion.   T F D
8. Football coaches permit their players to drink small amounts of alcohol.   T F D
9. More accidents are caused by drivers with "just a few" drinks than by drunk drivers.   T F D
10. The use of alcohol is related to the crime rate.   T F D
11. Drinking is related to the causes of divorce.   T F D
12. If people want to drink, it is their own business.   T F D
13. Drinking is a good way to solve a difficult problem.   T F D
14. Most people begin to drink because they like the taste.   T F D
15. It is easy to tell who may become an alcoholic.   T F D
16. Alcohol is a stimulant.   T F D
17. Alcohol is a disinfectant.   T F D

Survey   35 Conduct a survey among pupils to find out the kinds and amounts of alcoholic beverages they have tasted or now drink.   U

Tape recording   36 Have students interview an exalcoholic about attitudes toward use of alcoholic beverages.   U

COMMUNITY HEALTH

Bulletin board   1 Display illustrated drawing or pictures of the functions of various community health agencies.   I, U

2 Show the life cycle of the mosquito or the fly.   I, U

Chart   3 Make illustrated charts and posters about community health helpers.   P

4 List ways that children can help to promote good health in the community.   P, I

5 Make a chart listing the professional, official, and voluntary health agencies in the community.   I, U

Checklist   6 Prepare a checklist for use in rating the school health environment and the community health environment.   U

Construction   7 Make a bear's head out of papier-mâché and a large ice cream carton have the mouth open for paper deposits—"Litter Bear."   P, I

Demonstration   8 The correct use of the drinking fountain.   P, I

9 How water may be purified by filtration as illustrated in Fig. 11-1.   I, U

10 Have pupils examine some swamp water under a microscope and a second sample of this same water after it has been treated with chlorine.   U

11 Show how a small amount of oil on water forms a thin layer that causes mosquito larvae to die because they cannot penetrate the film to breathe. Obtain swamp or other stagnant water containing mosquito larvae for this demonstration.   U

Diorama   12 Prepare a diorama showing the locations of the agencies and the helpers involved in community health.   P

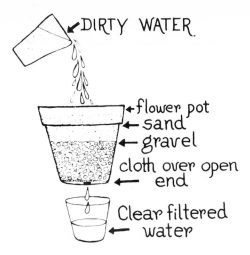

Fig. 11-1

	COMMUNITY HEALTH—cont'd	Grades
Discussion	13 Discuss and illustrate the pictures and stick men drawings the various kinds of community helpers who take care of our health, such as the milkman, the fire fighter, the police officer, the doctor, the nurse, and the dentist.	P
	14 Collect pictures of ponds, lakes, rivers, and reservoirs and ask the class whether they think it is safe to drink water out of or to swim in these places.	P, I
	15 The proper use and maintenance of drinking fountains and lavatories.	P, I
	16 The maintenance of a healthful school environment including cleanliness, lighting, heating, and ventilation.	P, I
	17 The danger of petting strange animals and the procedures to follow if bitten by one.	P, I
	18 The importance of sanitation including the disposal of lunch papers and refuse in the school and classroom.	P, I, U
	19 The community rules and regulations concerning garbage and rubbish disposal.	I, U
	20 The relationship of water supply to the sewage disposal systems in schools, homes, and rural areas.	I, U
	21 The importance of restaurant sanitation.	I, U
	22 The responsibilities of individuals to keep public places clean, such as picnic grounds, parks, campgrounds, and public rest rooms.	I, U
	23 The effects of water pollution and how local health laws protect against pollution.	I, U
	24 The need for periodic health examinations.	I, U
	25 The use of chemical sprays and dusts in agriculture and the possible dangers involved.	I, U
	26 Ways used by the city to remove and dispose of garbage and trash.	I, U
	27 The sanitary procedures necessary for swimming pools.	I, U

COMMUNITY HEALTH—cont'd Grades

Dramatization	28 Prepare and present a play to the Parent-Teachers' Association on the work of the health department.	I, U
	29 Prepare and present a play to a school assembly that will dramatize community health problems with possible solutions.	I, U
Drawing	30 Make drawings showing the sanitary procedures used in the school cafeteria.	I
Excursion	31 Take an excursion to the lavatories in the school and discuss use and maintenance.	P
	32 Visit a grocery store or food market to observe how perishable foods are stored and how cleanliness is practiced.	P
	33 Take a trip to a dairy to observe the sanitary procedures used in the handling of milk.	I, U
	34 Visit a water purification plant, a sewage disposal plant, or a health department.	I, U
	35 Visit food markets, restaurants, and other establishments to observe sanitary ways of handling and dispensing food.	I, U
	36 Visit a local hospital.	I, U
Exhibit	37 Display larvae, eggs, pupae, and adult mosquitoes and flies to observe development.	I, U
	38 Display pamphlets, books, and other reading material relating to community health.	I, U
Experiment	39 To demonstrate the need for refrigeration in preserving foods, obtain two glasses of milk and cover them. Put one in the refrigerator and leave the other outside at room temperature. Compare the milk in each glass for several days, noting the differences in appearance, texture, and taste.	I, U
Guest speaker	40 Invite the custodian to discuss ways that he or she uses to protect the health of pupils in school.	I, U
	41 Invite a member of the mosquito abatement office to discuss the control of mosquitoes and flies in the community.	I, U
	42 Invite members of the health department staff such as sanitarians, laboratory technologists, statisticians, and health officers to discuss community health.	I, U
	43 Invite a sanitarian from the local health department to discuss health laws regarding public eating places, public rest rooms, and the sale of food in the community.	I, U
	44 Have a guest speaker from the community health council or committee describe the organization and its functions.	U
	45 Have a panel of speakers discuss possible health careers, such as nurses, doctors, dentists, and dietitians.	U
Individual and group reports	46 Write an individual or group letter to the city water department requesting literature on how water is filtered and purified.	I, U
	47 Pupils write a group letter to the health department asking about its role in the health of the community.	I, U
	48 Write a group letter to the local health officer requesting materials that tell how he or she helps to protect the health of the community.	I, U

COMMUNITY HEALTH—cont'd   Grades

49 Pupils prepare a list and conduct a study of the common in-   I, U
sects and animals that carry disease and create sanitation
problems.

50 A pupil committee writes to the mosquito abatement office for   I, U
information concerning the control of mosquitoes and flies.

51 Report on the procedures used to make water safe for drink-   I, U
ing in the community.

52 Investigate the nature of air pollution and the role of the health   I, U
department in this problem.

53 Pupils write to the World Health Organization, the U.S. Pub-   U
lic Health Service, and the state department of public health
for information about their services and activities.

54 Consult the local health officer and report on the morbidity   U
and mortality statistics of the community.

55 Pupils report on the health heroes in history and their con-   U
tributions to community health.

56 Investigate ways that the community is protected against dis-   U
ease from people who come from foreign countries by ship and
plane.

57 Report on the services rendered to the community by such   U
agencies as the heart and tuberculosis organizations.

58 Pupils write reports on the methods of sewage disposal in the   U
community and the problems related to these procedures.

59 Write reports on ways to purify water and compare them with   U
the procedures used in the community.

Interview   60 Pupils interview parents on the major community health   I, U
problems.

61 Interview health officials and obtain information about food   I, U
poisoning.

62 A committee of pupils visits the cafeteria manager to discuss   I, U
ways used to sanitize dishes, dispose of garbage, and store
food.

63 A committee of pupils interviews someone from the county or   U
city health department for information about housing laws.

Mural   64 Draw a mural showing the location and functions of the various   P, I
community health helpers.

Panel   65 Have a panel discussion of the major community health prob-   U
lems and present viewpoints of the nurse, physician, health
officer, and others.

Posters   66 Make illustrated posters and charts about keeping clean public   I, U
places, such as parks, public rest rooms, and campgrounds.
Include slogans: "Did you use the garbage can?" "Did you
leave the campground clean?"

67 Pupils prepare drawings and posters after a trip to the dairy to   I, U
observe the procedures used in the sanitary handling of milk.

Scrapbooks   68 Prepare scrapbooks containing pictures and newspaper and   I, U
magazine articles of community health helpers.

69 Make illustrated booklets of the work of the health department   I
or a local hospital or both.

COMMUNITY HEALTH—cont'd

Grades

Show and tell	**70** Have a child tell of a recent visit to a hospital.	P
Sociodrama	**71** Children dramatize an unclean classroom or improper sanitation in the cafeteria or a restaurant.	I
Story	**72** Write a cooperative story about "Jeremiah Germ" who delights in bad health habits that help him get around the community.	P
Survey	**73** A pupil committee surveys the school environmental conditions, such as light, heat, and flies, that influence health.	I, U
	74 Have a committee survey the community to determine the "clean-up" needs and plan a campaign.	U

CONSUMER HEALTH*

Attitude opinionnaire

1 Prepare a series of statements as illustrated below: U

Check the appropriate box for each statement below (SA = strongly agree; A = agree; N = neutral; D = disagree; SD = strongly disagree).

	SA	A	N	D	SD
1. A physician is the best person to see when ill.	☐	☐	☐	☐	☐
2. Nurses provide reliable health information.	☐	☐	☐	☐	☐
3. People should treat themselves when ill.	☐	☐	☐	☐	☐
4. Acupuncture helps people with certain illnesses.	☐	☐	☐	☐	☐
5. Special foods and diets help people with arthritis.	☐	☐	☐	☐	☐
6. Books and pamphlets are good places to find out about health.	☐	☐	☐	☐	☐

Bulletin board

2 Display health products advertised in newspapers and magazines for student review and analysis.   I, U

3 Display magazine and newspaper articles related to consumer health students bring to class.   I, U

4 List local consumer health agencies and organizations and the services they render. Include addresses and telephone numbers.   I, U

Discussion

5 Pupils bring a variety of labels from health products to class for discussion.   I, U

6 Pupils bring advertisements of health products to class for critical analysis.   6, 7, 8

7 Television and radio advertisements of health products.   6, 7, 8

8 The Pure Food, Drug, and Cosmetic Law.   U

9 Health food fads and fallacies.   U

10 Superstitions and quacks in health.   U

11 Role of the physician, nurse, dentist and other health practitioners.   P, I, U

12 Use of products in the medicine cabinet at home.   P, I

*Teacher information is available in Cornacchia, H. J.: Consumer health, St. Louis, 1976, The C. V. Mosby Co.

CONSUMER HEALTH—cont'd   Grades

	13 Alternative healing philosophies—acupuncture, faith healing, chiropractice, and others.	U
	14 Self-diagnosis and self-medication.	I, U
	15 The intelligent health consumer.	P, I, U
	16 Reliable sources of health information.	P, I, U
	17 Community agencies and organizations to protect the health consumer.	U
	18 Food fads—vitamins, wheat germ, yogurt, and others.	I, U
	19 Use of aspirin and aspirinlike compounds.	P, I, U
Excursion	20 Visit a Food and Drug Administration laboratory.	6, 7, 8
Exhibit	21 Display a variety of items that are available in the various health food stores and discuss.	6, 7, 8
	22 Display labels of a variety of over-the-counter drugs available in drugstores.	6, 7, 8
	23 Have a place in the classroom where pamphlets and publications relating to consumer health are available for pupil use.	6, 7, 8
	24 Have the Food and Drug Administration, the Arthritis Foundation or other organizations display gadgets and items sold by quacks in the community.	U
Guest speaker	25 Invite the school nurse or a physician to discuss answers to such questions as "How can I choose a competent physician?" "Should I choose my own medication at the drugstore?" "What are the various kinds of specialists who can help me when I am sick and what do they do?"	I, U
	26 Invite a speaker from the Food and Drug Administration to relate how that organization protects the health of the consumer.	6, 7, 8
	27 Invite speakers from such organizations as the federal Food and Drug Administration, the Better Business Bureau, the state Food and Drug Administration, the Post Office Department, the Federal Trades Commission, or the American Medical Association to discuss how they protect the health of the consumer.	6, 7, 8
Individual and group reports	28 Children prepare lists of the health products, or the products that affect health, advertised on radio and television as well as in newspapers and magazines.	I, U
	29 Pupils collect lists of superstitions, sayings, or customs related to health and health practices.	6, 7, 8
	30 Pupils prepare reports on the meaning of the terms "quack" and "nostrum."	I, U
	31 Write to the Food and Drug Administration, the Better Business Bureau, the American Medical Association, and other organizations for information and materials about consumer health.	U
	32 Pupils write reports on the different kinds of health specialists found in the community.	U
	33 Pupils prepare individual and group reports on consumer health found in current magazine articles.	U
	34 Compile a list of community sources from which reliable and accurate health information can be obtained.	U

CONSUMER HEALTH—cont'd   Grades

		Grades
	35 Students prepare a list of services rendered by community health agencies and organizations protecting the consumer.	I, U
	36 Students prepare reports analyzing health publications available for sale.	U
Interview	37 A committee of pupils interviews a member of the Food and Drug Administration, the Better Business Bureau, the Post Office, and other agencies that play a role in consumer health.	U
	38 A pupil committee interviews a representative from the advertising department of a local newspaper to learn whether newspapers have criteria for accepting advertising for health products and services.	U
Panel	39 Have a panel discussion of the question "What are the dangers of self-medication?" Present viewpoints of parent, nurse, and physician.	6, 7, 8
	40 Have a panel discussion on the question "How should I choose a physician?" Present viewpoints of parent, nurse, and physician.	6, 7, 8
Self-test	41 Prepare a self-test on superstitions, quackery, or health fads.	U

Nutrition facts or fiction?

Place a check mark in the box under the appropriate answer.

	FACT	FICTION	DON'T KNOW
1. Dry cereals are necessary for body energy.	☐	☐	☐
2. Raw eggs are more nutritious than cooked.	☐	☐	☐
3. Eating an egg a day is harmful.	☐	☐	☐
4. Fish and celery are brain foods.	☐	☐	☐
5. Frozen orange juice has less nutritive value than fresh.	☐	☐	☐
6. Vegetable juices have magic health-giving qualities.	☐	☐	☐
7. All fruits and vegetables should be eaten raw.	☐	☐	☐
8. It is dangerous to leave food in a can that has been opened.	☐	☐	☐
9. Water is fattening.	☐	☐	☐
10. Drinking ice water causes heart trouble.	☐	☐	☐
11. Wine makes blood.	☐	☐	☐
12. If one vitamin pill a day is good, two or three are better.	☐	☐	☐
13. Meat is fattening.	☐	☐	☐
14. Toast has fewer calories than bread.	☐	☐	☐

		Grades
Survey	42 Students ask parents and friends about the kinds and extent of use of over-the-counter drug products purchased in drugstores.	U
	43 Students ask parents and friends about the kinds and extent of use of foods purchased in health food stores.	U

DENTAL HEALTH

Grades

Bulletin board

1 Display a collection of magazine pictures about dental health.   P, I

2 Display illustrated captions on dental health such as the following: P, I

> Here is little Billy
> Doesn't he look silly?
> He was pulled out by Carol
> When he fell in a barrel.
> I would have been just fine
> If I had kept my place in line
> To the faucet I did run
> Broke this tooth and that's no fun.
> Here's a tooth so very loose
> As you can see it's not much use.
> 'Cause Tommy refused to look ahead
> And ran into someone else's head.

3 Prepare posters or displays on dental health as illustrated in Figs. 11-2 to 11-5.   P, I, U

4 Students help the teacher in the preparation of a health chart of practices that contribute to dental health as follows: P, I

PRACTICES	PRODUCTS NEEDED	SERVICES NEEDED
Brush teeth	Brush	See dentist twice
Floss teeth	Toothpaste	yearly or when
	Dental floss	problem develops

Brush-in

5 Provide toothbrushes and toothpaste to be used in practicing toothbrushing procedures. Use disclosing tablets to determine effectiveness.   P, I

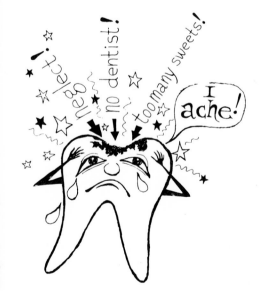

Fig. 11-2

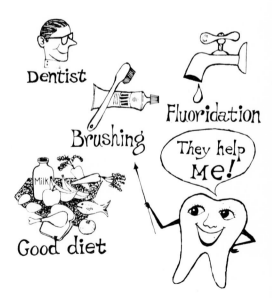

Fig. 11-3

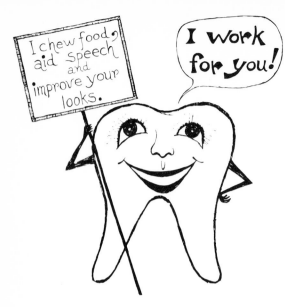

Fig. 11-4

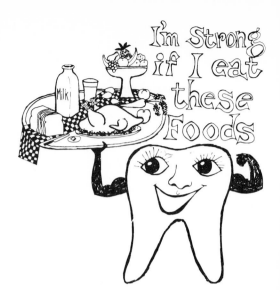

Fig. 11-5

DENTAL HEALTH—cont'd

Grades

Checklist

6 Children prepare a daily brushing chart to be taken home and hung in the bathroom to record when their teeth have been brushed.

P, I

7 Have students complete and discuss "How do I rate?"

I, U

How do I rate?	YES	NO
1. I have had a thorough examination of my teeth in the last 6 months.	☐	☐
2. I have my teeth x-rayed regularly.	☐	☐
3. All dental treatment recommended by my dentist has been completed.	☐	☐
4. I brush my teeth or rinse my mouth with water immediately after eating.	☐	☐
5. I understand the importance of having missing teeth replaced.	☐	☐
6. I do not eat sweets between meals.	☐	☐
7. I have my teeth cleaned by a dentist or dental hygienist regularly.	☐	☐
8. I know that sugar in candy and soft drinks can lead to tooth decay.	☐	☐
9. My teeth have been treated with a fluoride solution at the recommended ages.	☐	☐

Construction

8 Children make large construction paper toothbrushes. Each day the child reports the removal of plaque from brushing, the child may hang the brush on the wall-long toothbrush holder.

P

Debate

9 Have a debate or panel discussion on fluoridation of the water supply.

U

DENTAL HEALTH—cont'd

Grades

Demonstration

10 Teacher demonstrates the proper way to brush teeth, and students practice the technique using the flexed fingers of one hand on the cheeks and lips. Distribute toothbrushes and small tubes of toothpaste for all children to take home and use.   P, I

11 Make tooth powder in class. Students mix the following ingredients in the proportions indicated: 1 teaspoon salt, 2 to 3 teaspoons baking soda, and a drop or two of oil of peppermint, wintergreen, or cinnamon. Pupils take home some of the mixture to use when brushing teeth.   P, I

12 Have pupils show the acidity or alkalinity of the mouth using nitrazine paper. Give pupils strips of paper, instructing them to soak sterile cotton swabs with saliva and apply to the paper. The degree of acidity or alkalinity can be determined by comparing the resulting color of the paper strips with the color chart provided by the manufacturer. A pH of 7 indicates a neutral mouth, less than 7 indicates an acid mouth, and greater than 7 shows an alkaline mouth.*   P, I, U

13 Demonstrate the proper way to brush the teeth using a large toothbrush and a large set of teeth. Children participate in a toothbrush drill using tongue blades instead of toothbrushes. Pupils also practice rinsing their mouths and swallowing—"swishing and swallowing." Pupils may also be given disclosing tablets to take home and use.†   P, I

14 Show spoonful amounts of sugar found in candy, soft drinks, and other foods by placing equivalent quantities in test tubes or other containers. Each container should be labeled and placed on exhibit.   I, U

Discussion

15 The value of certain foods, such as apples, celery, carrots, and oranges, as tooth cleaners.   P

16 Display and discuss magazine pictures brought by children showing good and bad foods for teeth using "the happy and sad tooth" chart.   P

17 The loss of primary teeth (deciduous) as a normal process unless there is tooth decay or an accident.   P

18 The importance of teeth in speaking after having children pronounce such words as thirsty, thank you, thistle, and sister Susie sitting on a thistle.   P

19 Show and discuss pictures of people smiling. Illustrate how some of these people would look with missing teeth by blackening a few teeth.   P

20 The reasons why the dentist is a friend.   P

21 Have the class discuss how teeth grow by examining a model of the teeth and jaw.   I, U

22 The types and functions of teeth, using models: incisor—cuts, cuspid—tears, bicuspid—crushes, molar—grinds.   P, I

23 The qualities and care of a good toothbrush. Draw on blackboard or bring models of toothbrushes to school.   P, I, U

---

*Rich, R.: Tests for acidity of the mouth in relation to susceptibility to dental caries, Journal of School Health **33:** Feb., 1963.

†Your dentist or local dental society can provide information about securing a supply of these tablets.

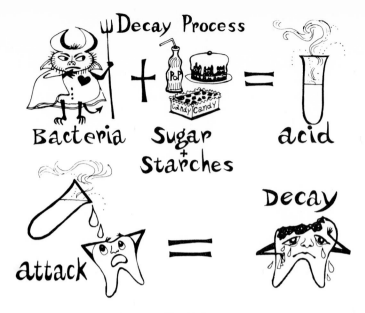

Fig. 11-6

	DENTAL HEALTH—cont'd	**Grades**
	24 During discussion of teeth have pupils label mimeographed diagrams.	I, U
	25 The value of the use of tooth pastes or tooth powders.	I, U
	26 Fluoridation	U
	27 Discuss the decay process, using the illustration in Fig. 11-6.	P, I, U
Dramatization	28 Children set up a dentist's chair and dramatize cleaning teeth and visiting a dentist. A discussion should precede this activity on how to clean teeth and why visits to the dentist are necessary.	P
	29 To show that acid will weaken substances containing calcium (such as tooth enamel), place a whole egg in a bowl of vinegar (acetic acid) for about 24 hours. The eggshell should become soft as the vinegar decalcifies the shell.	P, I, U
	30 Dramatize a visit to the dentist's office.	P
	31 Have class write a play on dental health and present it to the Parent-Teachers' Association or at a school assembly.	P, I, U
Drawing	32 Children draw, color, and possibly animate different teeth as well as different parts of teeth.	P, I
Excursion	33 Visit the community water plant and observe how water is fluoridated.	U
Exhibit	34 Display pencils, unshelled nuts, buttons, and other hard objects and discuss the dangers to teeth when these items are bitten or chewed.	P, I
	35 Display an explorer and mouth mirror and other implements used by the dentist to examine the teeth and discuss these implements.	P, I

DENTAL HEALTH—cont'd

		Grades
	36 Build a toothbrush holder and supply each child with a new toothbrush (possibly obtain from the Parent-Teachers' Association) for noon brushing. Be certain that each brush is properly labeled with each child's name on it.	P, I
	37 Display several types of toothbrushes.	I, U
	38 Display booklets, pamphlets, teeth, models, and other items relating to dental health.	I
	39 Display x-ray films and discuss their use in dental care.	I, U
	40 Obtain extracted teeth from a dentist and display to illustrate decayed teeth.	I, U
	41 Display models of orthodontia showing before and after results.	U
	42 Exhibit mouth protectors used in sports such as football and boxing.	U
	43 Show the relative amounts of sugar in different foods, such as candy bars and soft drinks.	U
Experience chart	44 Prepare an experience chart or record listing significant points about dental health, such as:	P

Teeth are our helpers.
Teeth must be cleaned.
Teeth help us to chew.

	45 Prepare a chart listing the foods that are good for teeth.	P
Experiment	46 Observe the progress of decay in two apples by breaking the skin of one and leaving the other intact. Place both apples in a place where they can be seen for a few days and relate what happens in the dental decay process.	P, I
	47 Have each child eat a cracker and with the tongue feel the coating of food on the teeth. Then have each student eat a piece of carrot, celery, or apple and note how much cleaner the teeth feel.	P, I
	48 Demonstrate the relative value of brushing the teeth, swishing with water and swallowing, and chewing such raw fruits and vegetables as apples, carrots, and celery right after eating a snack. Have six children each eat a chocolate cookie. One should then brush using water and no dentifrice, a second should swish with water and swallow, a third should eat an apple, a fourth should eat a piece of raw celery, a fifth should carrot, and a sixth should do nothing. All pupils should receive a paper cup that is ¾ full of water and be instructed to rinse their mouths (using water in small amounts) and empty into a second cup. The amount of chocolate food debris in each cup will serve as a measure of the cleansing effectiveness of the different methods used.	I, U
Flannelboard	49 To show the presence of bacteria in the mouth, sterilize some gelatin (sweetened with sugar) in a pressure cooker for 15 minutes (or heat in oven at 100° to 120° F. for 1 hour). Prepare two shallow dishes of the gelatin. Carefully scrape between the teeth and near the gum line to remove food debris (may use a toothpick). Place these scrapings in one dish. Cover both dishes, label, and place in a warm place. After several days	I, U

DENTAL HEALTH—cont'd

Grades

fungus growth should appear in the dish exposed to the mouth bacteria, but little or none will be seen in the uncontaminated dish.

50 Comprise a story of how a rabbit or other animal took care of its teeth and illustrate the procedures using a flannelboard.　　　P

51 Prepare models to compare the parts of a tooth with a hard-cooked egg or an apple.　　　P, I

　　Enamel—skin of apple or egg shell
　　Dentin—white of apple or egg white
　　Pulp—core of apple or egg yolk

52 Discuss appropriate foods for dental health by preparing models for use on the flannelboard and include poor food (candy and soft drinks) models, but do not put sandpaper on the backs of these items. When an attempt is made to place them on the board, they will fall off, indicating their poor quality.　　　P, I, U

53 Show the parts of the tooth and how decay proceeds by using colored flannel cutouts with black for decay, gray for a filling, pink for the pulp, yellow for the dentin, white for enamel, and red for infection and abscess. Use name tags (enamel, dentin, crown, and others) made of paper with sandpaper backing to identify the flannel parts.　　　P, I, U

54 Illustrate the decay process (Fig. 11-6).　　　P, I, U

55 Illustrate the progressive stages of dental caries.　　　P, I, U

Field trip　　56 Students visit a dentist's office.　　　P, I

Flip chart　　57 Make a flip chart that shows the importance of retaining all of one's teeth. Show pictures of appetizing foods, such as steak, apples, oranges, and celery. Also illustrate types of baby food that would have to be eaten if children did not have teeth.　　　I, U

Floss-in　　58 Demonstrate proper way to use dental floss and have students practice this skill in class. Relate to brush-in and use of disclosing tablets to determine effectiveness.　　　P, I, U

Guest speaker　　59 Invite a dentist or dental hygienist to class to discuss dental care.　　　P, I, U

Individual and group reports

60 Children write brief summary paragraph in answer to the question "What must we do to take care of our teeth?"　　　P, I, U

61 Children prepare lists of good dental snack-time foods.　　　P, I, U

62 A pupil committee sends a composite letter to the American Dental Association requesting materials on dental health.　　　I, U

63 Pupils write reports on the values of x-ray films in dental health.　　　I, U

64 Pupils investigate the use of fluorides in preventing tooth decay.　　　U

65 Pupils write a group letter to the water commission requesting information about the natural supply of fluorides in the water supply.　　　U

66 Students identify foods consumed in 1 day and determine the amount of sugar in each item and total the daily intake. Provide plans for reduction of amount eaten.　　　I, U

DENTAL HEALTH—cont'd

			Grades

Kit
  67 Prepare a plaque control kit containing a toothbrush, flossing material, and disclosing tablets for use at school or at home.
   P, I, U

Models
  68 Children construct plaster-of-paris models of their own teeth.
   P, I

Mural
  69 Make a mural in which each child draws a self-portrait and writes a slogan under the picture describing good dental health practices.
   I

Poems
  70 Create original poems.
   P

> We brush the teeth as they grow
> Down from the top and
> Up from below.
> Your teeth look swell
> When you brush them well.
> But your teeth decay
> When you keep the brush away.

Puppets
  71 Children participate in puppet shows emphasizing a visit to the dentist, brushing the teeth properly, or eating the proper foods for dental health.
   P

Scrapbooks
  72 Children prepare scrapbooks of picture cutouts showing good and bad teeth as well as proper and improper foods for dental health; also drawings of toothbrushes, dental floss, and toothpaste.
   P, I

Show and tell
  73 Children share a visit to the dentist or the experience of losing a tooth.
   P

Songs
  74 Create simple toothbrushing or dental health songs.
   P

> TUNE: *A Hunting We Will Go*
> A brushing we will go,
> A brushing we will go,
> We'll brush our teeth so white and clean,
> A brushing we will go.

> TUNE: *Mulberry Bush*
> This is the way we brush our teeth,
> Brush our teeth, brush our teeth,
> This is the way we brush our teeth
> Right after eating food.

Stories
  75 Have children make up a short story about the care of the teeth.
   P

Survey
  76 Survey the class to determine how many pupils have visited the dentist within the past year.
   I, U

  77 Have children keep records of the amount of candy, soft drinks, and other such items consumed and estimate the total amounts of sugar being eaten.
   I, U

Tasting party
  78 Have a bunny rabbit party in which celery, green peppers, and carrot sticks are served and discuss their importance in helping to clean the teeth.
   P, I, U

  79 Plan a dental health program for parents and serve nutritious snacktime foods.
   P, I, U

DISEASE CONTROL AND PREVENTION

Grades

Bulletin board

1 Display a list of good health rules and practices that will protect children from disease. — P

2 Display illustrations of animals and insects that carry disease. — P, I

3 Display pictures or drawings showing how to cover the face when coughing or sneezing. — P, I

4 Prepare posters to illustrate ways to protect others from communicable diseases, such as: — P, I

> Catch that sneeze (use of handkerchief or tissue)
> Cut the apple to share it (rather than taking a bite)
> Use your own comb or towel or washcloth

5 Display the signs, symptoms, control, and treatment of a particular disease. Different diseases can be featured. Community health organizations often have materials to help with the bulletin board. — U

6 Prepare pictures of such items as soap, washcloth, toothbrush, comb, and towel. Place caption below reading "We need these to keep clean." — P

7 Display the hands of all the children in class by tracing them on paper and making cutouts. Place the caption below to read "We wash our hands." — P

Chart

8 Prepare a chart that lists the ways germs are transmitted from one person to another: talking, sneezing, coughing, dirty hands and objects, carelessness in handling foods, utensils, and dishes. — P, I

9 Make a "Good health habits" chart to include statements with illustrations of the following: — P

> My hair is combed.
> My face is clean.
> I wash my hands and nails frequently.
> My clothes are neat and clean.
> My shoes are clean.

Choral speaking

10 Children participate in choral speaking. — P

> **My hanky**
> See my hanky white as snow,
> I use it when my nose I blow,
> It's not to play with,
> Oh, my, no!!

Construction

11 Prepare a disease prevention railroad train for bulletin board display using construction paper. The various freight cars should be hauling a comb, toothbrush, handkerchief, washcloth, soap, and other items needed. Each car can be labeled "Comb car," "Toothbrush car," and other appropriate names. The total train might be called "The disease prevention train" or the "Getting ready for school train." — P, I

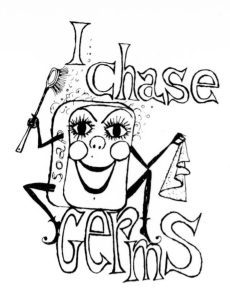

Fig. 11-7

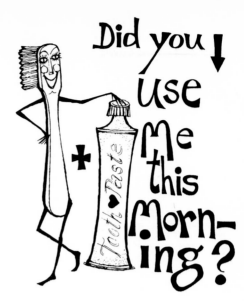

Fig. 11-8

	DISEASE CONTROL AND PREVENTION—cont'd	**Grades**
Demonstration	12 The proper way to blow the nose.	P, I
	13 The way to cover coughs and sneezes.	P, I
	14 The proper way to wash hands.	P, I
	15 The proper use of handkerchief or tissue.	P, I
	16 How to use a paper bag as a sanitary way to discard disposable tissues and other contaminated objects.	P, I, U
	17 Darken the classroom and flash the light from a movie projector on the wall so that the dust particles in the air may be seen. This will show how germs may be spread by the dust to which they attach.	I, U
	18 Have a member of the health department demonstrate tuberculin testing.	I, U
	19 The use of the clinical thermometer in class and its importance in illness.	I, U
	20 Demonstrate how germs may be transferred by putting fluorescent dye on some coins or other appropriate objects with several pupils handling the items. Have one or two of these pupils wash their hands with soap and water. Using "black light" (ultraviolet) in a darkened room, observe the hands of the children who handled the objects as well as those who washed their hands. If the dye remains on the hands, it will be clearly visible by glowing in the "black light" and thus showing how germs may be spread. The washed hands may or may not fluoresce, depending on the thoroughness of the washing. Ultraviolet light may be damaging if shone directly into the eyes. The nurse may have a Wood's light for use in this demonstration.	I, U

DISEASE CONTROL AND PREVENTION—cont'd

		Grades
	21 Show pictures of a boy washing hands, a girl washing hands, and hands being washed with soap. Discuss how and when to wash hands. Demonstrate the proper way and follow by having all children practice the proper way to wash hands.	P
	22 Demonstrate the proper way to wash the hands and face.	P
	23 Make soap in the classroom.	P, I
	24 Show the proper way to clean and file fingernails.	P, I
	25 Have children use a magnifying glass to examine the creases and folds of the skin and the dirt on one hand. After washing the hand have pupils again examine the skin.	I
	26 Examine samples of different kinds of clothing material with magnifying glass. Discuss seasonal appropriateness of each.	I
	27 Demonstrate "hidden dirt" on the skin of a child who appears to be clean but has perspired by washing an area of the skin with rubbing alcohol using a piece of cotton. Show the cotton to the class after the demonstration.	I, U
	28 Display two beakers containing warm water in one and cold water in the other with each having a tablespoon of oil and a tablespoon of liquid soap. Stir both beakers and compare the results. Warm water disperses the oil globules more effectively and hence is better for washing.	I, U
	29 Using charts and models, study the structure of the skin and relate this to cleanliness and disease control.	I, U
Discussion	30 Disease control in terms of sleep and rest requirements.	P
	31 Briefly discuss some of the common childhood diseases, their symptoms, prevention, and control.	P
	32 The need for immunizations.	P
	33 Why children should stay at home when not feeling well.	P, I
	34 How to protect ourselves and others from contracting contagious diseases.	P, I
	35 The importance of washing hands before lunch and after the toilet. Have children practice these habits at the appropriate times.	P, I
	36 Cleanliness in handling and consuming food; washing of fruits and vegetables before eating and refusing to share bites of food or to eat food that has been dropped on the floor.	P, I
	37 The causes of disease.	P, I
	38 Colds and other contagious diseases in terms of prevention.	P, I
	39 Beneficial and harmful germs. Beneficial germs give cheese its flavor, make bread rise, and turn apple juice to cider. Harmful germs cause disease and illness.	P, I
	40 The importance and significance of poliomyelitis immunization.	P, I, U
	41 The use of disinfectant in the control of disease.	I, U
	42 The methods that help to destroy bacteria; soap and water, pasteurization, sterilization, light and air.	I, U
	43 Tuberculin test and its meaning.	I, U
	44 Food poisoning and how it may be prevented.	I, U
	45 The heart and heart disease using a model of the heart and a chart of the circulatory system.	U
	46 Weather and seasonal changes that require different kinds of clothing.	P, I

	DISEASE CONTROL AND PREVENTION—cont'd	Grades

47 Pictures of appropriate shoes and clothing for work and play as well as for different kinds of weather.   **P, I**

48 The correct disposal of tissues.   **P, I**

49 Such questions as "Why should I keep clean?" "What should I do before I eat?"   **P, I**

50 Need, frequency, and methods of bathing.   **P, I**

Dramatization

51 Dramatize a visit to the doctor to be immunized or to obtain treatment for a contagious disease.   **P**

52 Getting ready for school using towels, soap, nail file, mirror, nail brush, comb and brush, cloth to wipe shoes, toothbrush, and clean handkerchief.   **P**

Excursion

53 Visit the school health office and meet the school nurse.   **P**

Exhibit

54 Display pamphlets and materials on communicable diseases for student use.   **I, U**

55 Display samples of clothing for use in different kinds of weather. Have children discuss and select appropriate apparel for the weather indicated by the teacher or by pupils.   **P**

Experience chart

56 Prepare an experience chart about good health rules and practices in preventing and controlling communicable diseases.   **P**

Experiments

57 To show the existence of germs on the hands, wash with soap and water and place salt on them. Try to rub off the salt until none is visible. By touching the tongue to the hands it can be shown that salt still remains. Wash hands again with soap and water and touch tongue to hands to show that the salt has been removed.   **P, I**

58 To discover the conditions that may affect the growth of germs, have pupils wet two pieces of cloth and place one in a dark, warm place and the other in sunlight and air for one week. The results will show that warmth, moisture, and darkness help molds and bacteria to grow whereas sunshine prevents this process.   **P, I**

59 To discover that hands are germ carriers, have pupils with dirty hands touch a piece of bread and place it in a labeled jar. Have children with freshly scrubbed and dried hands touch another piece of bread and place it in a second labeled jar. After a week or more, the piece of bread that was touched with the dirty hands will have much more mold than that touched with clean hands.   **P, I**

60 To discover how germs are spread, push a needle into the moldy part of an orange. Pierce a second orange with the contaminated needle. Clean and sterilize the needle by boiling and pierce a third orange. Label all oranges and observe the changes that occur daily for a week or more. Mold will grow on the contaminated orange.   **I, U**

61 To discover the presence of germs, wash, dry, and sterilize (heat directly on an electric plate at medium temperatures for 1 hour on each side) two petri dishes (may use metal lids and glass squares). Prepare a sterile solution by dissolving ½ ounce of plain gelatin in 1¾ cups of water and boil for 1 hour. Pour this substance into the petri dishes. Cough into one petri dish   **I, U**

DISEASE CONTROL AND PREVENTION—cont'd   Grades

and cover. Merely cover the second dish. Place these dishes in a warm dark place and observe them daily for 1 week. Colonies of bacteria will develop in the contaminated dish.

62 To discover that sunlight kills bacteria, inoculate two petri   I, U
dishes (prepared as previously described) from a dish where bacteria are growing. Place one dish in the open sunlight and the other in a warm dark place. After one dish has been in the sunlight for several hours, place it in the dark, warm, place with the other dish. Examine the two dishes each day for several days.

63 Using a magnifying glass, study the molds that have grown on   I, U
stale bread, fruit, or other material. Bring a microscope to class for each child to view this mold.

64 To show the growth of germs, boil some small, peeled potatoes   I, U
until still firm and place one in each of four sterile pint jars with lids. Maintain one jar as a control, but contaminate the potatoes in the other three jars by (a) rubbing with dirty hands, (b) rubbing with hands after washing with soap and water, and (c) rubbing with tissue after blowing nose. Put lids on all jars, label, and place in a warm but visible location. Observe daily the growth of bacteria and compare with the control potato.

65 Touch different articles in the classroom with swabs and touch   I, U
these to petri dishes containing agar. Incubate the dishes so that the germs will grow. Ask a laboratory technologist from the health department to identify some of the germs.

66 To teach the importance of cleanliness, put some dust on a   I, U
sterile agar petri dish (may use gelatin if agar not available), cover and place in a warm, dark place. Use a sterile petri dish as a control, cover, and place with the first dish. Observe results daily for about one week and compare the growth of germs.

67 To show how flies spread disease, have one crawl across a   I, U
sterile agar petri dish (may use thin layer of gelatin if agar not available), cover and place in a warm, dark place. Use a sterile petri dish as a control; cover, and place with the first dish. Observe results daily for about 1 week and compare the growth of germs.

Finger plays   68 Children participate in finger plays.   P

Here is my little washcloth,	Here is Johnny, ready for bed,
Here is my bar of soap.	Down on the pillow he lays his head.
This is the way I wash my face,	He pulls up the covers over him tight,
Until it's clean, I hope.	This is the way he sleeps all night.
This is the way I brush my teeth,	Morning comes, the sun is bright,
Until they are so white.	Back with a kick the covers fly.
I drink my milk and eat my cereal	He jumps up and gets dressed
So when at school I feel just right.	And goes to school to play with the rest.

Flannelboard   69 Use paper dolls on a flannelboard to illustrate the appropriate   P, I
clothing for school and different kinds of weather.

Guest speakers   70 Invite the health officer or nurse to dicusss communicable   P, I, U
diseases.

DISEASE CONTROL AND PREVENTION—cont'd

		Grades

71 Invite guest speakers from the heart, cancer, and tuberculosis associations to discuss the nature of chronic diseases.   U

72 Invite a nurse, dermatologist, or other physician to discuss skin problems or care of the skin.   U

Individual and group reports

73 Children write a brief summary paragraph or two in answer to the question "Why is it necessary to wash our hands and when should this be done?"   P, I

74 Children write a brief report on "Why I should stay home when I am ill."   I, U

75 Pupils read about such health heroes as Leeuwenhoek, Koch, and Pasteur and write about their contributions to the control of disease.   I, U

76 Pupils read and write reports about communicable diseases transmitted by insects or animals to man including methods of control.   I, U

77 Pupils write to the health department, requesting materials about the control of diseaeses.   I, U

78 Pupils prepare written reports for publication in the school newspaper on tuberculosis, poliomyelitis, colds, and other communicable diseases.   I, U

79 Form pupil committees to report on diseases such as tetanus and smallpox.   I, U

80 Pupils read and write about harmful bacteria in drinking water, milk, or food.   I, U

81 Pupils write reports on television or radio programs they have seen or heard on the control of disease.   I, U

Interview

82 A pupil committee interviews health department officials about the prevention and control of disease in the community.   I, U

Mobile

83 Make a mobile showing a toothbrush, comb, washcloth, nail file, and other items needed for cleanliness and disease control.   P

Pantomime

84 Discuss the various procedures a child should follow when getting ready for school. Have children pantomime these procedures and let the class guess the activities being dramatized.   P

Poem

85 Children or teacher or all create poems.   P, I, U

If you cough,
Or if you sneeze,
Cover your mouth
With a tissue, please.

Cover your mouth when you sneeze,
'Cause if you don't
Someone might get the disease.

The man with the flying sneeze

Germs fly thorough the air with the greatest of ease,
Whenever you cough or whenever you sneeze.
So don't be a goose,
A clean handkerchief use,
Anytime with a flying sneeze.
     Ah - - Chooooooooo - - - - - -

DISEASE CONTROL AND PREVENTION—cont'd

Good food we should eat,
And get plenty of sleep.
When water is deep,
Away from it keep.
Be on the alert
And don't be a jerk
Anytime with a flying sneeze.

Dirt

Dirt is fine:
   For gardens and roads,
   For worms and toads,
   For puppy to dig—
   And maybe for pig—
   For cats
   For rats
   For night-flying bats,
   For lambs
   and clams
   and even for dams,
   For slugs and snails,
but
     Under my nails,
   Not mine!
DORIS HAMMER

			Grades
Posters	86	Children make posters about the control and prevention of communicable diseases.	P, I, U
Problem solving	87	Jimmy and his parents are going on a camping trip for a week where there are no modern facilities such as tap water, electricity, or other conveniences. Help Jimmy answer the following questions: How can we keep clean? How can we obtain safe drinking water? What should we do if we get a cut knee? What other things must be done to protect ourselves from disease?	I, U
Puppets	88	Make two puppets and call them "Healthy Harry" and "Sick Sam." Dramatize children coming to school who feel sick.	P
Quiz	89	Show students a series of pictures and have them orally tell or write the answers to these questions:	P, I

PICTURES	QUESTIONS
Washing hands	1. When do we do this?
Brushing teeth	2. When do we do this?
Going to bed	3. How much sleep do we need?
Coughing or sneezing	4. What must we do?
Wearing raincoat	5. Why do we need this?

Research	90	Children read and write reports on how disease germs are spread and controlled.	I
	91	Committees prepare oral and written reports on the following diseases: heart, cancer, diabetes, asthma, allergies, and arthritis.	U

	DISEASE CONTROL AND PREVENTION—cont'd	**Grades**
Riddle	92 Make up riddles such as "I'm thinking of something we should do after we play and before we eat. What is it?"	P, I
Scrapbooks	93 Prepare scrapbooks of magazine and newspaper articles and pictures relating to communicable diseases.	I
	94 Pupils collect magazine articles, pictures, and other information on chronic diseases and prepare scrapbooks.	U
Self-test	95 Prepare a self-test on the prevention and control of disease.	I, U
Show and tell	96 Children report experiences about illnesses at home.	P
Sociodrama	97 The school health examination.	P, I
	98 Conduct a sociodrama on the immunization procedure.	P, I
	99 The procedures for the proper handling of foods.	P, I
	100 The role of the nurse and the doctor in the prevention of disease.	P, I
Stories and songs	101 Prepare creative stories and songs about the doctor, nurse, and health habits.	P
Survey	102 Survey the nature of illness and the extent of immunizations of the children in class.	I, U
Television box	103 Construct a television box and prepare a series of panels on various aspects of cleanliness. Children or teacher could make the panels, which might include soap, comb, washcloth, children washing, and others. Have a television show when everything is ready.	P

DRUGS*

Advertisements	1 Students bring drug "ads" to class for analysis.	U
Brainstorming	2 Have students identify ways they can contribute to the control of drugs in the school and the community.	U
Bulletin board	3 Display magazine and newspaper articles brought to class by pupils.	U
	4 Display illustrations of popular drugs used and abused.	I, U
	5 Display pamphlets and other reading materials and permit students to select items they wish to read or report on.	U
	6 Display of ways how to say no.	I, U
Buzz groups	7 Discussion questions: Should students use drugs? Should marijuana be legalized? Why do students use drugs? Does "everybody's using drugs" mean everyone should do so?	U

---

*For additional techniques, see Cornacchia, H. J., Smith, D. E., and Bentel, D. J.: Drugs in the classroom; a conceptual model for school programs, ed. 2, St. Louis, 1978, The C. V. Mosby Co.

DRUGS—cont'd

Grades

Comparative analysis

8 Have students seriously think about something they like to do above all else—art, music, read, football—and ask them to jot down in several brief, concise phrases their feelings of what this activity does to and for themselves. Teachers list all the phrases on the chalkboard without reference to the activity. Give students a copy of a list of phrases extracted from drug abusers about their feelings of what drugs do for them. Compare this list with the chalkboard list, which might include:

U

> It makes you aware.
> My mind is broadened.
> It does something to my perception.
> I notice differences more.
> It increases my potential.
> The world is more interesting.
> It gives you a sense of awe of nature.
> It's an intense total experience.
> You appreciate your senses better.
> It puts me in a world by myself.
> I don't understand why people find boredom in living.
> I am totally involved in the environment.

Ask students to identify the similarities and differences in the two lists and give the reasons why. This procedure should encourage a discussion of alternatives to drugs rather easily and profitably.

Discussion

9 The kinds of medicines that are used by members of the family such as cough medicine (codeine), sleeping pills, aspirin, and others. Also talk about the effects of these drugs on the body: sleep induction, sedation, relief of pain. — I, U

10 Read current newspaper articles about drugs and have pupils prepare questions that they wish to have answered. List these questions on the blackboard and have pupils determine how to find answers. — U

11 The importance of taking drugs under parents' and doctors' supervision. — P, I

12 The effect of coffee, tea, and cocoa on the body. — P, I

13 Why people use drugs. — U

14 The physiologic effects of drugs such as marijuana, heroin, morphine, barbiturates, amphetamines, volatile chemicals, hallucinogens and others on the body. — I, U

15 Sociologic factors, including laws of drug use and abuse. — U

16 Drug usage by students in schools. — U

17 Poisonous substances in the home. — P, I

18 Emergency procedures when poisonous substances are ingested. — P, I, U

19 How young people are introduced to drugs. — I, U

20 The federal and state regulations concerning the sale and use of drugs. — U

Dramatization

21 A student is urged by friends to ingest an unknown substance. — I, U

Exhibit

22 Display a variety of containers that contain drugs obtainable at drug stores. — U

DRUGS—cont'd   Grades

	23 Display a variety of pamphlets, magazine articles, and other materials for pupil use in writing and preparing reports.	U
Field trip	24 Students attend a court session involving illegal drugs.	U
	25 Students visit and talk with drug abusers.	U
	26 Entire class visits a teenage rehabilitative resource center.	U
Guest speaker	27 Invite a member of the sheriff's office, the local police department, or the state narcotics office to discuss narcotic drugs.	U
	28 Invite a physician or pharmacist to come to class to discuss the effects of drugs on the human body.	U
	29 Invite a drug abuser to class.	U
Individual and group reports	30 Vocabulary lists and definitions of such drugs as narcotics, heroin, morphine, marijuana, barbiturates, amphetamines, hallucinogens, volatile substances.	U
	31 Use of drugs by individuals and their effects on the body.	I, U
	32 Oral and written reports on the uses of drugs in medicine.	U
	33 Origins of drugs.	U
	34 Federal, state, and local laws about the sale and use of drugs.	U
Music	35 Have students relate rock music, or music in general, to the drug scene.	U
Newspaper articles	36 Students collect articles about drugs for discussion in class.	I, U
Interview	37 A committee of pupils interviews a physician to obtain information about the values, dangers, and abuses of the use of drugs.	U
Panel	38 Have a panel discussion describing the effects of such drugs as aspirin, sleeping pills, and tranquilizers on the human organism.	U
Peer group	39 Upper grade students prepare presentation for sixth grade pupils or seventh-eighth graders.	U
Posters	40 Students plan a drug education program for schools, using a variety of posters.	U
Pretest	41 Give a pretest to determine the extent of pupils' knowledge about drugs.	U
Problem solving	42 Place the following terms on the blackboard (or assign pupils to locate their meaning): bennies (benzedrine pills), coke (cocaine), cook a pill (heat opium for smoking), fix (injection), get high (smoke marijuana), hemp (marijuana), horse (heroin), junk (narcotics), mainliner (addict), pusher (peddler), and weed (marijuana cigarette). Ask pupils to identify these words. Continue the discussion by defining the terms and providing additional information about drugs. Pupils may raise further questions that need exploration.	U
	43 Procedures to be followed to ensure the proper use of medicines.	P, I
	44 If you discovered your brother, sister, or friend using drugs, what would you do? What should you do?	U

DRUGS—cont'd   Grades

45 What might be the consequences if you are attending a party or in a car where drugs are being used?   U

Puppets   **46** Prepare stick or other types of puppets and dramatize use of medicine in the home.   P

Questions and answers   **47** Pupils prepare anonymous questions that they would like answered about drugs.   U

Rap session   **48** Provide opportunities for students to meet voluntarily in small groups or on a one-to-one basis with a school person who communicates easily with students and is knowledgeable about the drug scene.   U

Reports   **49** Have students prepare reports on: my philosophy of life; what I value; peer pressure and drug use; drug laws and minors.   U

Records   **50** Play records of rock bands related to drugs. Prepare verses to songs and discuss contents.   U

Role playing   **51** Students dramatize trying to influence others to use illicit drugs, and class analyzes the situation presented.   U

52 Students dramatize a parent giving medicine to a sick child.   P

53 Students dramatize someone refusing an offer to smoke a marijuana cigarette.   I, U

Scrapbook   **54** Pupils make scrapbooks containing drawings, newspaper and magazine articles, and written reports on drugs.   U

Sociodrama   **55** Conduct a sociodrama of a peddler who approaches a group of pupils at a soda fountain and tries to sell them marijuana cigarettes.   U

Student information center   **56** Establish a location in school manned by students where pupils seeking information may go for help.   U

Survey   **57** Students attempt to discover the extent of the use of drugs in school.   U

Tape recording   **58** Interview drug users and abusers, physicians, and others.   U

Television   **59** Students view a current program about drugs and prepare report for class.   U

CARE OF THE EARS

Bulletin board   **1** Display drawings or pictures that show how the ears help us to hear.   P, I

2 Prepare a bulletin board showing the head of a clown and place a large pupil-drawn ear on the clown. Put a caption at the top of the display "We use our ears to:" and then put various other statements around the clown, such as "use the telephone," "hear bells," "hear danger signals," and "enjoy music."   P, I, U

Cartoons   **3** Draw cartoons illustrating rules about the care of and hazards to the ears.   P, I

CARE OF THE EARS—cont'd   Grades

Demonstration

4 The proper way to wash the ears. P

5 The proper way to blow the nose. Have children practice the procedure following the demonstration. P, I

6 Show a drum and relate it to the functions of the eardrum and sound vibrations. P, I

7 Demonstrate lip reading to show how handicapped a deaf person might be. Discuss the importance of protecting one's hearing. P, I

8 How a drum head may be punctured from a severe blow and relate the possibility of this occurring to the eardrum from a loud noise or blow. P, I, U

9 Sound vibrations using a tuning fork. Drop a rock in water to show how vibrations travel in all directions. I, U

10 Test hearing using the whisper and watch test. I, U

Discussion

11 How infections, accidents, and foreign objects may affect hearing. P, I

12 How the ear helps us to hear. P, I

13 The need for reporting pains or other symptoms of ear problems. P, I

14 The dangers of putting objects in the ear. P, I

15 How we hear. Use rhythm instruments to produce sounds and relate these to hearing. P, I

16 How to protect ears from loud noises such as yelling in someone's ear, and the television or radio turned on too loud. P, I, U

17 The structure and function of the ear, using charts and models to illustrate. I, U

18 The prevention of ear injuries when swimming, blowing the nose, cleaning the ears, playing, and blows to the ears. I, U

19 How colds and other diseases may result in deafness. I, U

20 How to help the person with poor hearing; hearing aids, talking into the good ear, making distinct words for the lip reader, and removing wax from the ears. I, U

21 Motion sickness. I, U

Dramatization

22 Dramatize hearing testing or a doctor's examination of the ears. P

23 Have children dramatize the following procedures: proper way to blow nose, wash ears, whispered conversation, loud voice, and normal conversation. P, I

24 Dramatize a situation in which a person is wearing a hearing aid and is overly conscious of it. Bring out the relationships of hearing problems to emotional stability and the importance of understanding on the part of friends. U

Exhibit

25 Display an otoscope (instrument to look into ears) and discuss how the doctor uses this instrument. P, I

26 Permit children to examine an ear model. P, I

27 Display several types of hearing aids. I, U

Experience chart

28 Prepare an experience chart on the care of the ears. P

CARE OF THE EARS—cont'd   Grades

Game	29 Play "listening" game. Have each child blindfolded or with closed eyes and ask individual players to identify different sounds: bell, bottle half full of water being shaken, horn, clock, crumpling of paper, and others.	P
	30 Play the game "ask-it-basket." Divide the class into two teams and place in a basket questions prepared on the care of the ear. Team captains draw one question at a time and ask the opposing team for answers.	I, U
	31 Have pupils prepare a list of common terms relating to the ear and use these words to construct a crossword puzzle.	I, U
Guest speaker	32 Invite the audiometrist to demonstrate hearing testing and discuss care of the ears.	P, I, U
	33 Invite the teacher for the hard-of-hearing to discuss hearing.	I, U
Individual and group reports	34 Pupils prepare written reports on care of the ears.	I, U
	35 Pupils prepare oral and written reports about people who have succeeded in life despite hearing difficulties.	U
Posters	36 Prepare a series of posters showing how the ear may be injured.	I, U
	37 Prepare drawing of the ear and label the major parts.	I, U
Pretest	38 Give a pretest to determine the extent of pupil understanding of the structure, function, and care of the ears.	I, U
Story	39 Children and teacher cooperatively write stories about the care of the ears.	P
Tape recording	40 Record voices on the tape recorder and permit children to hear their own voices.	P, I, U

EXERCISE AND BODY MECHANICS

Bulletin board	1 Display drawings or pictures of proper sitting, standing, and walking posture	P, I, U
	2 Display charts of the muscles and bones (skeleton) with captions or illustrations showing their relation to exercise, movement, and body mechanics.	P, I, U
	3 Display a series of pictures or drawings of beneficial activities and exercises.	I, U
Debate or panel	4 Have a debate or panel discussion on the "Soft American." Bring in viewpoints of physicians, parents, and others.	U
Demonstration	5 Children observe own posture in a full-length mirror.	P, I, U
	6 The correct way to pick up objects.	P, I, U
	7 Correct sitting, standing, and walking posture. Conduct drills in which pupils practice these procedures.	P, I, U
	8 Correct body alignment using a plumb line.	I, U
	9 Have pupils walk attempting to carry a book on their heads after they have assumed the correct posture.	I, U

EXERCISE AND BODY MECHANICS—c

10 To show the effect of exercise on pulse rate, ha
own pulses' while sitting or at rest. Permit them
aisles and jump up and down about ten times
own pulse rates. Ranges of pulse rates before
cise can be noted on board with individual
relationships to exercise discussed.

11 Conduct posture parade monthly in which th
the boy or girl demonstrating the best walkir
dren should determine in advance how they p
selection.

12 To show the effect of exercise on breathing and oxygₑₙ
have children count the number of breaths they normally take
per minute using a watch with a sweep second hand. Have
pupils stand in the aisles, jump up and down about ten times,
and again count the number of breaths needed after exercise.

Diorama	13 Prepare a diorama of suitable physical education activities and exercises using pipe cleaners for figures.	I, U
Discussion	14 The importance and need for exercise in the maintenance and development of physical fitness.	P, I, U
	15 The relationship of muscles and bones to good body mechanics.	P, I, U
	16 The factors that influence posture such as food, sleep, exercise, and mental attitudes.	I, U
	17 The relationships of exercise and eating to good posture.	I, U
	18 The types of exercise and sports activities that are beneficial.	I, U
	19 The importance of muscular strength in preventing fatigue and in performing daily activities.	I, U
Game	20 Have pupils play "Indians" by walking on a straight line with heads held high. The leader (the "chief") has children vary their arm positions while walking; out to side, overhead, or bent at elbow in front of chest.	P, I
	21 Play "puppet" and "pull" self straight up as though using an imaginary string at the top of the head.	P, I
	22 Children stand against a wall and try to make their heads, shoulders, hips, and heels touch the wall. Follow this action by having pupils walk away from the wall retaining this position.	P, I, U
Guest speaker	23 Invite the physical education teacher or supervisor to discuss and demonstrate good body mechanics.	P, I, U
	24 Invite the physical education teacher or supervisor to visit the classroom to discuss "keeping in condition" and its importance in daily living.	I, U
Individual and group reports	25 Pupils write or give oral reports on such topics as "How I exercise each day," "The sport I like best."	I, U
	26 Pupils prepare written or oral reports on the values of exercise.	I, U
	27 Children prepare written reports about their favorite sports and list the parts of the body that are exercised most in these activities.	I, U

EXERCISE AND BODY MECHANICS—cont'd   Grades

28 Pupils make a posture model (use heavy cardboard) for use in the discussion of body mechanics.   I, U

29 Make a mural of the variety of kinds of beneficial pupil activities and exercises.   I, U

Music   30 Walk to music, exhibiting good posture.   P, I

Poems, songs, and plays   31 Children create poems, songs, and plays about exercise and its values.   P

Posters   32 Make posters showing the importance of exercise in daily living.   P, I

Scrapbook   33 Make a series of drawings and collect magazine pictures and stories demonstrating proper body mechanics.   P, I

Shadowgram   34 Children make shadowgrams of each other. Using a piece of craft paper as large as a child, with two students holding the paper, have a third pupil stand between the paper and a source of light. A fourth boy or girl outlines the shadow of the third child using a piece of charcoal or crayon. Discuss these drawings individually in terms of good body mechanics.   I, U

Stories   35 Children write illustrated stories of how exercise helps us.   P, I

Survey   36 Survey the amount of exercise pupils receive by completing the following:

How much exercise do I get?

Fill in the amount of time in hours or in fractions of hours.

	S	M	T	W	Th	F	S
Riding bicycle or walking to and from school							
Playing at recesses							
Playing before school, in the morning, and at noon							
Exercising during the physical education class							
Active playing after school and before bedtime							
TOTALS							

    Grades

37 Survey the kinds of activities in which pupils participate.   U

Television box   38 Make a television or motion picture box and have children prepare a series of pictures showing the importance of exercise and body mechanics.   P

CARE OF THE EYES

Bulletin board	1 Display pictures and drawings about care of the eyes.	P, I
Chart	2 Prepare a chart containing important terms to know about the eye.	I, U
	3 Have pupils complete the names of the parts of the eye on a mimeographed diagram.	I, U
Demonstration	4 The correct way to carry objects such as sticks, knives, and tools.	P, I
	5 The procedure for removing foreign objects from the eye.	P, I, U
	6 The proper lighting needed for reading and working.	P, I, U
	7 Have a child read or look at a book or picture in direct sunlight or under a bright light. Discuss such questions as "Why is it difficult to read?" "Do your eyes hurt?" "Must you squint or frown to see?"	P, I, U
	8 Blindfold a child, turn him around several times, and have him try to walk to different places in the room. Discuss blindness.	P, I, U
	9 The importance of sight by having children cover their eyes and explain their reactions to a variety of situations.	P, I, U
	10 Teacher or nurse demonstrates the vision screening procedure.	P, I, U
	11 Demonstrate the blinking response using one pupil in class. With the corner of a soft paper, touch the lashes near the inner corner of one eye. Have children note the blinking reaction. Discuss the closure of the eyelid when sand lands on the eyeball, which is accompanied by a flow of tears to try to flush away the particle.	P, I, U
	12 Completely darken the room for a few minutes and then lighten it. Discuss what happens to sight when you first enter a darkened movie theater and also when later you first come into the bright sunlight.	P, I, U
	13 Demonstrate or draw a comparison between the function of the eye and a camera.	I, U
	14 Display various types of paper showing those with low and high gloss and discuss their importance in vision.	I, U
	15 Use a light meter to show the amount of light in the classroom.	I, U
	16 Have pupils hold their thumb at arm's length and look at it. Have pupil close their right eye and line up their thumb with the corner of the room. Without moving the arm, have them close their left eye and look with the right eye. Pupils should see a different view with each eye, demonstrating that binocular vision helps to adjust to space relationships.	I, U
	17 Have pupils close one eye and hold a pencil from 12 to 14 inches from the other eye. Have pupils look at the pencil and then at a distant object and report how the pencil appeared in each instance. Pencil looks blurred when the eye is focused a distant object or the reverse is true. This indicates the need for occasional resting of the eyes because muscles are involved in eye focusing changes.	I, U

CARE OF THE EYES—cont'd

Grades

18 Have pupils look at a neighbor's eye in a darkened room. Lighten the room quickly and have pupils note contractions of the pupils of the eye. The eye must adjust to various amounts of light; therefore a well-lighted room involves fewer eye adjustments and is less fatiguing. — I, U

19 Where the optic nerve enters the eyeball, there is a blind spot that can very easily be demonstrated. Have pupils draw a black dot (¼ inch in diameter) on a white sheet of paper, and about 1½ inches to the right draw a black cross (¼ inch). Have the pupils close their left eye and stare steadily at the black dot with their right eye while the paper rests on the table. Have pupils pick up the sheet of paper and move it slowly toward the eye while staring at the dot. They will find a point where the image of the cross to the right will disappear. The blind spot for the left eye can be found by closing the right one and staring at the cross. When the sheet is brought close to the eye, the black spot will disappear. — I, U

20 With curtains or blinds drawn, hold a lighted 40-watt electric lamp exactly 2 feet above an open book. This is approximately the amount of illumination needed for comfortable reading. Show that light rapidly diminishes as the lamp is moved further away. At a distance of about 3 feet a 100-watt bulb is needed to provide the same illumination that a 40-watt bulb gives at 2 feet. — P, I, U

Discussion

21 The possible danger to the eyes of throwing things including sand, rocks, and dirt. — P, I

22 The importance of vision to animals, showing pictures to illustrate. — P, I

23 An accident on the playground that resulted in an injury to a child's eye. — P, I

24 The importance of wearing glasses when necessary. — P, I, U

25 Show pictures of artists, surgeons, pilots, and others and discuss the importance of vision in their work. — P, I, U

26 Care of the eyes and television. — P, I, U

27 Have children roll a sheet of paper to make a cylinder and look through it with one eye. Discuss tunnel vision. — P, I, U

28 The importance of symptoms of vision difficulties such as inability to see the blackboard, words look fuzzy, or vision is blurred. Emphasize importance of notifying parent or teacher when these signs appear. — P, I, U

29 The hazards to vision of looking directly at the sun. — P, I, U

30 The ways eyes are protected in various sports. — P, I, U

31 The structure and function of the eye, using charts and models. — I, U

32 The importance of periodic eye examinations. — I, U

Dramatization

33 Dramatize the school nurse doing the vision screening test on a child. — P, I

34 Dramatize the correct sitting distance and lighting for various television. — P, I

35 Dramatize good reading habits and a visit to an eye doctor. — P, I

CARE OF THE EYES—cont'd

			Grades
Exhibit	36	Display a model of the eye and permit children to take it apart and put it together.	P, I
	37	Display samples of Braille material and discuss how a blind person uses it to learn to read.	P, I, U
	38	Display various materials used in the vision screening program and discuss.	P, I, U
	39	Display pamphlets, magazines, and other reading materials on vision and make available for reading and research.	I, U
	40	Display different styles of glasses including sunglasses and goggles used to protect the eye in various activities.	I, U
Experience chart or record	41	Make an experience chart or record about the care of the eyes.	P
Game	42	Play the game "Pin the tail on the donkey" and discuss the importance of vision.	P, I
Guest speaker	43	Invite the school nurse to discuss vision screening.	P, I, U
	44	Invite an eye doctor to discuss care of the eyes.	I, U
Individual and group reports	45	Pupils prepare oral or written reports about signs and symptoms of vision problems as well as common eye difficulties.	I, U
	46	Pupils prepare oral or written reports on eye infections; conjunctivitis, styes, and others.	I, U
	47	Pupils prepare oral or written reports on the various kinds of eye specialists in the community.	I, U
	48	Pupils write reports on the various ways eyes are protected in sports.	U
Mural	49	Make a mural on care of the eyes or hazards to the eye.	P, I
Panel	50	Have a panel discussion of the various ways eyes are protected in sports. Get opinions on football, basketball, baseball, and others from appropriate sources.	U
Poems, stories, and plays	51	Create poems, stories, and plays about care of the eyes.	P
Posters	52	Make a series of pictures or drawings about proper lighting for reading as well as care of the eyes.	P, I
Self-test	53	Give self-test on the structure and function of the eye.	I, U

Self-test illustration

eyeball	pupil	retina
iris	lens	optic nerve

Fill in the blanks using the words above.

_____ Small, dark, round hole in center of eye.
_____ Carries pictures from retina to brain.
_____ Moves up, down, and sideways.
_____ Light passes through lens, falls on lining at back of eyeball.
_____ Front part of eyeball, blue, brown or gray (in color) in circle.
_____ Behind the pupil and inside the eye.

<table>
<tr><td></td><td></td><td align="right">Grades</td></tr>
</table>

	CARE OF THE EYES—cont'd	Grades
Show and tell	54 Children relate a visit to an eye doctor or tell how wearing glasses helps those who need them.	P
Sociodrama	55 Role-play parents and children watching a television program, a visit to an eye doctor, having to wear glasses, and others. Discuss the significance to vision.	P, I
Survey	56 A pupil committee determines the amount of light in the classroom, halls, and other areas of the school using a light meter.	I, U

FAMILY HEALTH

Bulletin board	1 Collect pictures of boys and girls of approximately the ages of students in class for a display illustrating differences in size and body build among children of the same age.	I
	2 Show pictures of ways families spend their time in recreation and during holidays.	I
	3 Collect pictures on family life and magazine and newspaper articles about birth and display them.	I, U
	4 Show pictures of happy families and have students describe what makes the families happy.	P
Charts	5 Construct a chart showing varying ages when boys and girls mature.	I
Discussion	6 What can I do to help my family be happy?	P
	7 Ways in which the community helps the family.	P
	8 Differences in growth rates between boys and girls.	I
	9 Inherited characteristics, such as eye and hair color, and curly or straight hair.	I, U
	10 Meaning of "growing up."	I
	11 Anonymous questions prepared by students.	I, U
	12 Living things come from living things.	P
	13 Family rules and family problems.	I, U
	14 Home responsibilities.	I, U
	15 What family members can do to show love, especially at certain times.	P, I
	16 Family customs, traditions, race, religions, and patterns.	I, U
	17 Care of pets.	P
	18 Nature and function of the endocrine glands.	I, U
	19 Secondary sex characteristics of boys and girls as they relate to body shape, size, and growth.	I, U
	20 Moral and ethical values and their relation to sexual activities.	U
	21 Different ways of reproduction, asexual and sexual.	I, U
	22 Human reproduction.	I, U
	23 Good sources of information on sex, reproduction, and family living.	I, U
	24 Attraction of sexes and venereal disease.	U
	25 Ways to resolve family conflicts.	P, I
	26 Animal and plant reproduction.	P
	27 Compare the development of human babies before birth with animal babies.	P

FAMILY HEALTH—cont'd   **Grades**

	28 Family changes due to death, divorce, or separation.	P, I
	29 Responsibilities at home, at school, and elsewhere.	P
	30 Freedom and responsibility.	I
	31 Terms, such as mating, stud, heat, foal.	I, U
	32 Puberty and maturity.	I, U
	33 Love—marriage, children, family.	U
	34 Sex drive, birth process, masturbation, wet dreams, behavior on dates, marriage.	U
	35 People, organizations, and agencies that help people with family problems.	U
	36 Behavior on dates.	U
	37 Steady dating.	U
	38 Determination of personal values.	I, U
Demonstrations	39 Have male and female guinea pigs or hamsters in the classroom. Pregnancy of the female will offer an opportunity to discuss the creation of new life.	P
	40 Hatch chicks from eggs.	P
	41 Observe the growth of seeds in relation to new life.	P
	42 Observe the growth of frog eggs.	P
Display	43 Make available pamphlets and magazine and newspaper articles about sex, reproduction, and values, for student optional reading.	I, U
Drawings	44 Illustrate ways in which families have good times together.	P
	45 Children draw their own family groups and list various family patterns.	P
	46 Illustrate pupil's own family or animal families.	P
	47 Depict mother's, father's, or own work.	P
Exhibit and health fair	48 Students prepare bulletin board displays, posters, charts, and other visual materials for display and exhibit these materials at school. Pupils should be available to discuss their projects, to provide information requested, and to distribute pamphlets.	I, U
Field trip	49 Tour the school building and include a visit to boys' and girls' bathrooms. This should lead to a discussion of anatomic differences of boys and girls and correct names of body parts.	P
	50 Visit a farm and observe the animals.	P
	51 Visit a local museum, hospital, or clinic to view exhibits of before birth and birth of a baby.	P, I, U
Films	52 Observe films on birth and growth of animals.	P
	53 See and discuss films on human growth, menstruation, and reproduction.	I, U
Guest speakers	54 Invite a physician or nurse to discuss reproduction, childbirth, and other matters.	I, U
	55 Invite ministers, priests, and other religious representatives to discuss moral and ethical values.	I, U
Graph	56 Prepare a graph that shows the heights and weights of class members; compare with national norms.	I

FAMILY HEALTH—cont'd

		Grades
Mural	57 Develop a mural showing animals and human beings caring for babies.	P
Pretest	58 Develop a test relating to puberty, mate selection, reproduction, sex drive, and other matters.	U
Problem solving	59 Develop relevant situations with alternative solutions concerning dating, behavior on dates, selection of marriage partners, sexual relations. Use these as a basis for class discussion.	U
	60 Have children try to provide answers to these questions: How do you grow? What helps you grow? Why do you grow?	I
Individual and group reports	61 Rh factor, sex drive, marriage, dating, and others.	U
	62 Different ethnic, religious, and cultural backgrounds of people.	I, U
	63 What things do I do that make my family happy or unhappy?	P, I
Puppets	64 Prepare a skit to show how parents help us.	P
Question box	65 Provide a box in an appropriate location for students' anonymous questions.	I, U
Role playing	66 Provide skits relating to family roles of mothers and fathers, getting along with brothers and sisters, helping to care for a new baby.	P
	67 Develop skits depicting manners and etiquette.	P
Scrapbook	68 Include illustrated materials "All about me," all the items in terms of family, friends, and things that cause different emotional responses.	I
Story	69 Prepare an open-ended story about the family, its activities, responsibilities of children. Allow pupils to fill in some of the words.	P
	70 Teacher starts with "I love my father and mother because . . ."	P
	71 Read appropriate stories about families and family relations.	P, I
Transparencies	72 View and discuss materials available from 3M Company.	P, I, U

CARE OF THE FEET

Bulletin board	1 Prepare a bulletin board display using magazine pictures and drawings of appropriate types of shoes for play, school, parties, and other occasions.	P, I, U
Chart	2 Prepare a chart listing the important rules to consider when purchasing shoes.	P, I, U
	3 Prepare a chart listing the important rules to consider in caring for the feet.	P, I, U
Demonstration	4 The proper way to walk with the feet parallel and have children practice this method.	P, I, U
	5 The proper way to wash and dry the feet.	P, I, U

CARE OF THE FEET—cont'd

		Grades
	6 To demonstrate the proper way to walk, have a pupil make footprints on paper and make cutouts of these prints. Draw a straight line on the floor with chalk and have the pupil tape the footprints to the floor so that the inside of each print is parallel to the line and the toes point straight ahead. Now permit the child to walk the chalk line stepping in the footprints.	I, U
	7 Have pupils trace the outline of their shoes on a piece of paper. Have them remove the shoes and trace the outline of the foot on top of the shoe outline. Compare the two drawings and determine whether the shoe is the proper size.	I, U
	8 The importance of the feet to posture. Illustrate how walking with pronated or inverted feet may cause undue back and leg pressures with possible result that posture will be affected.	I, U
	9 High and low foot arches by having pupils walk on pieces of paper with wet feet.	I, U
Discussion	10 The importance of changing shoes and socks when wet.	P, I, U
	11 The proper way to cut toenails.	P, I, U
	12 The importance of drying the feet properly.	P, I, U
	13 The proper care of the feet.	P, I, U
	14 The importance of shoes and socks or stockings that fit well and provide the best protection for the feet.	P, I, U
	15 The signs and symptoms of foot problems and whom to see when they appear.	P, I, U
	16 How posture is affected by shoes that do not fit properly or are in poor condition.	P, I, U
	17 How to prevent athlete's foot and what to do about it when you have the condition.	I, U
	18 The importance of the bones and arches of the feet to posture and walking using a chart, drawing, or model.	I, U
Dramatization	19 Dramatize buying a new pair of shoes.	P, I, U
Exhibit	20 Display a variety of shoes for different kinds of activities.	P, I
	21 Display an instrument used in a shoe store to measure feet for new shoes. Have pupils determine their correct sizes and compare these with the shoes they are wearing.	I, U
	22 Display various types of materials found in socks, such as wool, nylon, and cotton, and discuss their significance in foot care.	I, U
Experience chart or record	23 Prepare an experience chart or record to show the proper ways to care for the feet.	P
Guest speaker	24 Invite a shoe salesman to discuss the way to select a properly fitting shoe.	I, U
	25 Invite a chiropodist to discuss the care of the feet.	U
Poems and plays	26 Children write poems, jingles, and plays about the proper care of the feet.	P
Posters	27 Make drawings or posters illustrating the importance of properly fitting shoes and socks.	P, I

	CARE OF THE FEET—cont'd	**Grades**
Scrapbook	28 Prepare a scrapbook of magazine pictures and drawings of different styles of shoes for various activities and also stories about the care of the feet.	P, I
Story	29 Have children create a story about the kinds of shoes to wear for various types of weather.	P

GROWTH AND DEVELOPMENT

Bulletin board	1 Teacher prepares a series of large drawings that show the progressive stages of the development of a chick embryo into a full-grown chick. Appropriate colors may be necessary to make these illustrations more attractive.	P, I
	2 Children collect pictures showing differences in growth patterns of adults for a bulletin board display: midgets and giants as well as tall and short persons. Discuss these differences as they relate to the pupils themselves.	P, I, U
	3 Pupils bring to class pictures of well-known, important people and prepare a bulletin board display of these individuals. Discuss the differences in body build.	I, U
	4 Teacher prepares a display showing the relationship of cells, tissues, organs, and systems to the organism as shown in Fig. 11-9.	I, U
Buzz group	5 Have a buzz group discussion about the meaning of the term "growing up."	I, U
Demonstration	6 Put several articles in a bag and observe whether children can identify the articles by merely touching them and not seeing them. This introduces the fact that the nerves send messages to the brain.	I

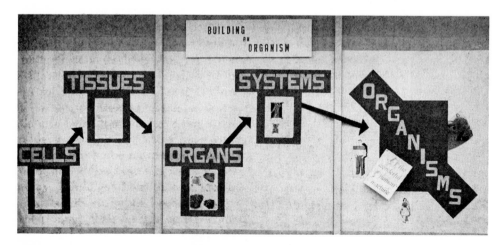

Fig. 11-9. Growth and development bulletin board. (Courtesy Jefferson Union Elementary School District, Daly, Calif.)

GROWTH AND DEV

7 Bring an earthworm to class and
and its only means of locomotio.
Mention that without a skeletal sys.
probably move around like an earthv
concept that each part of the skeleton is
lar function and that muscles are neces.

8 Demonstrate what happens when a person.
suring the size of the chest before and after
breath.

9 Bring a stethoscope to class to demonstrate ho
uses this instrument.

10 Line up pupils in class and have them note the diff
height. Discuss the fact that children do not have u
growth rate due to many factors: heredity, nutrition, .

11 Dissect a hog's or cow's heart and identify its parts.   .., U

Discussion	12 Provide an illustrated discussion of the nervous and digestive systems using suitable charts and models.	I, U
	13 Provide an illustrated discussion of the respiratory system using suitable charts and models.	I, U
	14 Provide an illustrated discussion of the heart and the circulatory system using suitable charts and models.	I, U
	15 Provide an illustrated discussion of the muscles of the body, using suitable charts and models. Demonstrate how muscles fasten to bones.	I, U
	16 Discuss the nature and function of the skeletal system, using suitable charts and models.	I, U
	17 Discuss the endocrine glands and their role in growth and development.	I, U
	18 Discuss and compare the human body with a machine (automobile). Mention the intake of fuel and the conversion to energy.	I, U
	19 Disassemble a model of the human torso and ask pupils to identify the separated parts. Pupils might also try to reassemble the torso at the conclusion of this discussion.	I, U
	20 Provide pupils with diagrams of the nervous, digestive, respiratory, skeletal, and circulatory systems and have them label the parts.	I, U
	21 Growth as an individual matter and show the differential patterns.	I, U
	22 The story of heredity.	I, U
	23 Ask such questions as: How do you know you have a heart? How big is your heart? What is pulse? Can you feel it? How many times does your heart beat, and how many times do you breathe in one minute?	I
Display	24 Bones from a variety of animals including human beings and have students try to identify them.	I, U
Dramatization	25 Dramatize a small boy trying to pick a fight with a large boy. Discuss the implications in terms of growth and development.	I, U

26 Child
298
Methods and materials in health
Drawings
Exhibit

		Grades
	...ren draw, color, and label various systems and organs of the human body.	I, U
	27 Display pamphlets and other publications on growth and development in the classroom for review by interested children.	P, I, U
	28 Display animal bones obtained from a meat market. Show some cross sections and longitudinal sections of bones.	I, U
Experiment	29 Demonstrate how baby chicks, ducks, or other animals grow when given the proper food. The white rat experiment may also be used to illustrate the growth process.	P, I
	30 Provide a flannelboard and a box containing cutouts of the bones of the human body. Permit children to try to build the human skeleton on the flannelboard.	I, U
Films	31 Show and discuss such films as "Human Growth," "Story of Menstruation."	I, U
Game	32 Play the game "Who am I?" A child describes the function of a particular organ of the body and pupils try to identify the organ. Another version of this game is to have children mention bones of the body and then have other pupils name bones to which they attach.	I, U
Graph	33 Construct a giraffe out of plywood and place measurements on its neck. Have children periodically measure themselves and record these findings on a graph that they have prepared.	P
	34 Have each child prepare a height and weight graph. Children take their measurements once a month and plot their findings. Separate graphs using height and age or weight and age may also be advisable to make and use.	I, U
Guest speaker	35 Invite the school nurse to meet with the girls to discuss menstruation.	I, U
	36 Invite the school nurse to come to class to discuss the process of human reproduction.	I, U
	37 Invite a physician or other qualified person to class to discuss sexual growth with the boys.	U
Individual and group reports	38 Pupils compile a list of causes for individual differences in growth.	I, U
	39 Pupils find the means of the words "heredity" and "environment."	I, U
	40 Pupils prepare lists of the characteristics they have inherited and acquired.	I, U
Model	41 Children make clay models of different organs of the body after they have seen pictures or drawings of these parts.	I, U
	42 Children make a stethoscope using the material shown in Fig. 11-10. Have pupils hold funnel firmly over the heart and listen to heart sounds. Discussion of structure, function, and related diseases could follow.	I
	43 Display real organs or plastic models of the heart and other body organs.	I, U

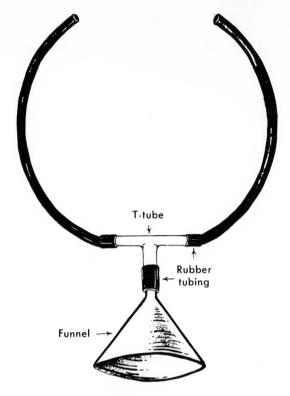

Fig. 11-10. Stethoscope model.

	GROWTH AND DEVELOPMENT—cont'd	**Grades**
Problem solving	44 Encourage pupils to raise questions about growth and development and list these on the blackboard. Have pupils determine ways to find answers to the listed problems.	I, U
	45 Present these or similar questions to pupils for discussion: What does "growing up" mean? How do individuals grow? Do boys and girls grow at the same rate? Why doesn't everyone grow at the same rate? How does one know when growth is taking place? What factors are involved in growth?	I, U
Question box	46 Provide a question box for pupils' anonymous questions about menstruation, reproduction, and other aspects of growth and development.	I, U
Self-test	47 Prepare a self-test on the various aspects of growth and development, systems of the body, endocrine glands, heredity.	I, U

MENTAL HEALTH*

Bulletin board	1 Collect and display pictures and drawings of happy children and families as well as of people showing kindness.	P, I
	2 Display work by each child as often as possible to encourage responsibility in doing his or her best work.	P, I

*See Chapter 12 for games.

MENTAL HEALTH—cont'd   Grades

		Grades
	3 Display a list of class helpers for a week, eventually giving everyone in class a chance to be a leader.	P, I
	4 Prepare a bulletin board of examples found in newspapers and magazines that show good deeds, good sportsmanship, and other qualities.	P, I, U
	5 Display an illustrated list on the hobbies of the children in class.	P, I, U
	6 Prepare a bulletin board with a variety of illustrated mental health phrases such as "Meet friends halfway," "Be cheerful," and "Control your anger."	I, U
	7 Display pictures of a variety of emotions with the caption: "Emotions we live with."	P, I
	8 Pupils collect for display magazine and newspaper articles that describe mental health problems of concern to pupils.	U
	9 Prepare the display illustrated in Fig. 11-11. The teacher can prepare questions in first panel and pupils can bring pictures for second panel and also help to obtain definition and lists for third panel.	I, U
Brainstorming	10 Students prepare lists of problems they consider important and develop plans to resolve them.	I, U
Buzz group	11 Conduct a buzz group discussion on the character traits a pupil likes or dislikes in a person.	U
	12 Have a buzz group discussion of how boys and girls may become better acquainted.	U
	13 Discuss such questions as: what is reality? Does "everybody's doing it" mean everyone should do it?	U
Checklist	14 Pupils complete checklists and teacher either holds individual conferences with pupils or anonymously discusses some of the problems in class. Some sample statements on this list might include:	I, U

> I do not get along well with my parents.
> I am frequently embarrassed when with others.
> I usually do not know how to act in company.
> I usually feel inferior to my classmates.
> I lack self-confidence.

		Grades
Consequences	15 Students periodically prepare written statements for discussion to the questions that follow regarding any or all of the actions identified or others deemed appropriate: *Questions*—Do you consider the consequences before taking action? Should you? How frequently? Why? What are the possible consequences of your actions? *Actions*—smoking; using marijuana; using heroin; selecting dates; getting angry or emotional with friends or others; refusing the help of parents, teachers, and others when problems arise; sex activities; eating foods that may be harmful to health; racial and ethnic prejudice	I, U
Demonstration	16 Choose a child to be "big brother" or "big sister" to a new pupil during the first week in school.	P

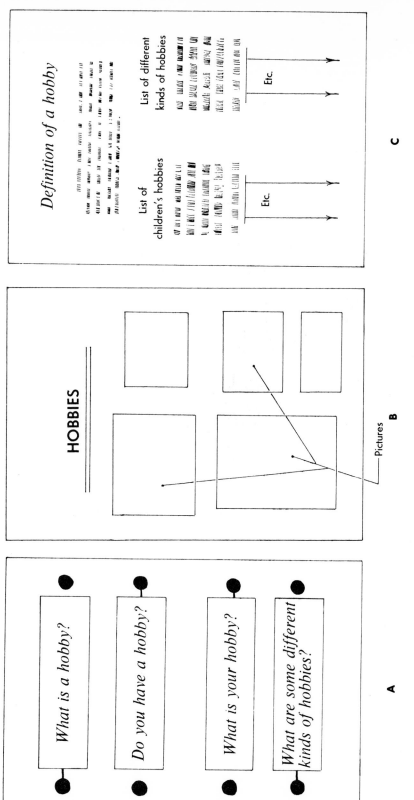

Fig. 11-11. Mental health bulletin board. **A,** Left panel. **B,** Middle panel. **C,** Right panel.

MENTAL HEALTH—cont'd

		Grades
	17 Demonstrate ways for children to "let off steam" through such activities as play, music, hobbies, creative work, dramatization, and talking about things.	P, I, U
	18 Teacher provides opportunities for all children to have chances in leadership roles.	P, I, U
	19 Teachers provide a warm, friendly atmosphere in the classroom with many centers of interest.	P, I, U
Discussion	20 Children have opportunities to experiment with planning, to carry out plans, and to evaluate results of a variety of experiences.	P
	21 Talk about how to make friends.	P
	22 Ways to be helpful at home, happy times with the family, and ways to be unselfish about listening to the radio and television.	P
	23 The use of the words "please" and "thank you."	P
	24 The necessity for proper rules and manners in the cafeteria.	P, I
	25 Children's feelings and the need for control over such actions as crying easily, temper tantrums, and fighting.	P, I
	26 Behaviors in class and in school in terms of getting along with one another and related problems.	P, I
	27 What it means to be a leader and a follower.	P, I
	28 When playing games in physical education, discuss the need to rotate positions to give opportunities for all.	P, I
	29 Discuss what to do when one feels sad, what to do to help others who are unhappy, and ways to behave when something unfortunate happens.	P, I
	30 The need to forgive children who have made mistakes.	P, I
	31 The need for the development of self-responsibility by keeping desk clean, hanging clothes in closet, taking care of pets.	P, I
	32 The quality of friendship.	P, I
	33 How people differ in their abilities to do things.	P, I, U
	34 Have class elect officers, with children establishing rules on voting and rules of behavior.	I
	35 Ways to cope with and solve problems* when they arise. What specific procedures should a pupil follow when faced with a situation for which he can find no answer.	I, U
	36 What it means to put oneself in another person's shoes.	I, U
	37 How people can be considerate of the feelings of others and how to handle hurt feelings.	I, U
	38 Honesty and truthfulness.	I, U
	39 Develop standards for acceptable behavior in the classroom, on the playground, to and from school, on the bus, in the library, on study trips, and at home.	I, U
	40 Children who are embarrassed by physical defects and what others can do to help these individuals.	I, U
	41 Inadvisability of keeping emotional tensions, worry, and fear bottled up inside. Discuss the need for friends to talk to, hobbies as outlets, being able to face up to problems, and other solutions.	I, U

Inside/Out is a series of 30 films that are 15 minutes each in length and are designed for 8- to 10-year-old children. *Self-Incorporated* is a series of 15 films that are 15 minutes each in length and are prepared for 11- to 13-year-old children. These series are available from National Instructional Television Center, Box A, Bloomington, Ind. 47401.

MENTAL HEALTH—cont'd   Grades

42	Have pupils prepare a list of qualities they like in a person as well as those qualities they do not like and post these on the bulletin board or put them in the school newspaper.	I, U
43	The following personality traits: kindness, helpfulness, reliability, tactfulness, cheerfulness, good sportsmanship, good manners, intelligence, sense of humor, loyalty, and honesty.	I, U
44	Evaluate ways boys and girls have of gaining acceptance through such means as conforming to clothing fads, using current slang, forming clubs, and participating in school-sponsored social activities, plays, and other projects.	U
45	Discuss the question "At what age should one start dating?"	U
46	Habits and ways of behaving that will give parents confidence in allowing boys and girls increasing freedom to make decisions and to participate in activities outside the home.	U
47	Reactions to other individuals who do not act, look, or believe as you do.	U
48	The values of people.	U

Dramatization

49	Dramatize the following: thoughtfulness, courtesy, self-reliance, sharing, playing and working together, helping at school, following directions, respecting each other's property, lost and found, self-control, rudeness, good manners, and criticism.	P, I
50	Dramatize emotional behavior exhibited such as anger, fear, jealousy, sorrow, hate, love, and temper.	P, I
51	Dramatize such incidents as the following:	P, I, U

> Things that make me happy.
> Things that make others happy.
> Things that make me sad.
> Problems on playground or in classrooms.
> Things I like to do.
> How to make new friends.
> Other kids can always do thing I can't do.
> It's not my fault others won't play with me.

52	Dramatize introductions to and conversations with other people in public places, bus, school, dance, party, theater, and street.	U
53	Dramatize how it feels to be different from others in terms of race, nationality, beliefs, and customs.	U

Drawings

54	Have children make drawings illustrating: things I love; how I feel when hurt, scared, and angry; when I've wanted something I couldn't get.	P, I
55	Draw a picture illustrating a way to be helpful to someone.	P, I
56	Draw pictures of objects or animals that make us afraid.	P

Emotion box

57	Prepare an emotion box and have students periodically complete form in which their names, dates, types of emotion experienced, and the reason for same is identified. Teacher occasionally reviews and uses the material as a basis for class discussion and problem solving without indicating students by name.	I

MENTAL HEALTH—cont'd

Grades

Exhibit	58 Display pictures brought to class by children of places they would like to visit or where they would like to live. Discuss the reasons these places have been selected.	I, U
Finger paint	59 Provide children opportunities to finger paint to help release tensions and to explore creative abilities.	P
Flannelboard	60 Use the flannelboard to illustrate situations of fair play and good sportsmanship and to create stories about fear, anger, hate, friendship, and others.	P, I
Good-deed box	61 Prepare a good-deed box and have children deposit in writing good things that they have seen classmates do during the day. At the end of the day the teacher reads these to the class without mentioning names.	P, I
Guest speaker	62 Invite a psychologist or psychiatrist to discuss the meaning of the term "personality."	U
Individual and group reports	63 Children write brief stories or reports on "How to be a better leader or follower."	P, I
	64 Children write a brief summary paragraph or two in answer to the question "Why should we learn to get along with others?"	P, I
	65 Pupils complete an individual written assignment on the topic "When my feelings were hurt."	I, U
	66 Prepare oral or written pupil reports on good manners and courtesy.	I, U
	67 Write a brief paragraph about good citizenship and draw pictures to illustrate.	I, U
	68 Prepare reports on jealousy, prejudice, anger, and others for the school newspaper.	I, U
	69 Boys make up lists of the qualities they like and dislike in other boys and have the girls do the same. Discuss the common characteristics found in both lists and their meanings to the pupils.	I, U
	70 Pupils prepare written reports about what they do well and what they would like to improve in themselves.	I, U
	71 Pupils write about and discuss the following: what makes me angry, happy, sad, or afraid; what I wonder about; three persons I love; three wishes; what I would like to change at home or at school; what I like about people; what I like about my friends.	I, U
	72 Pupils write reports about the racial, religious, and other prejudices they have noticed that people have against individuals.	I, U
Mobile	73 Using colored construction paper, children trace and cut out their hands and feet as well as other parts of the body they consider important. Various lengths of string are attached to each cutout and attached to a coat hanger or short pieces of dowling and hung around the classroom.	P, I

MENTAL HEALTH—cont'd   Grades

Murals   **74** Make murals, charts, and booklets that emphasize sharing in   P, I
terms of carrying dishes to the table, going to the store, taking
care of pets, making the bed, hanging up clothes, putting away
food, running errands, and putting things away.

Music   **75** Use of various types of music to help calm and relax children   P, I
to help create a beneficial classroom atmosphere.

76 Discuss the meaning of lyrics found in a variety of popular   U
songs.

Poems   **77** Prepare original poems.   P

> So little hands, be careful please
> Of everything you do
> For if you are sent to bed
> I'll have to go there too.

78 Read poems.   P, I, U

Joy*

> Joy is like a magic cup,
> I lift it to the sky,
> And all the more I offer up,
> The fuller joy have I.

A smile*

> A smile is like a little wedge
> That often keeps us from the edge
> Of getting sad, or feeling blue—
> I love to see a smile, don't you?

Words*

> I love the sound of kindly words—
> I try to make them sing,
> And I hope I never send one out
> To be a hurtful thing.

Politeness*

> Hearts, like doors, will open with ease
> To very, very little keys,
> And don't forget that two of these
> Are "Thank you, Sir," and "If you please."

A level head*

> It takes a level head to win,
> A level hand, a level eye,
> But sometimes, even when you try
> Your level best, thing go awry.
> You drop the ball, you miss your aim,
> You slip a cog and queer the game.
> Then comes the test. Don't make excuse;
> Don't crumple; stand up in your shoes.
> Remember, in a certain sense,
> It takes a level head to lose.

---

*Los Angeles City School Districts, California: Speech in the elementary school, pub. No. 479, 1949, Office of the Superintendent of Schools, p. 190, 262, 263.

MENTAL HEALTH—cont'd   Grades

| Problem solving | 79 | Describe a human relations episode to the class, such as lying, stealing, rudeness, or poor sportsmanship, and have children write or orally discuss how they would solve the problem. | I, U |

| Puppets | 80 | Make stick, paper bag, or hand puppets and prepare stories or plays around such themes as fear, anger, and jealousy. | P, I |
| | 81 | Construct a shadow box or puppet stage with children working together. | P, I |

Questionnaire 82 Students complete short answers to the following: I, U

Happiness is —————————————————————.
Sadness is —————————————————————.
I am fearful of —————————————————————.
I am angry when —————————————————————.

Question box 83 Have a question box in class and encourage children to put in questions concerning worries, fears, and other areas of trouble that they would like discussed.   I, U

Reports 84 Students write about: "Me as I see myself"; "Me as I would like to be"; "When I wanted something I could not have, what did I do?" "What should I have done?"   I, U

Role playing* 85 Teacher acts out such emotions as anger, fear, and hate. Students are requested to close their eyes before the teacher performs and on signal to open them as the demonstration occurs. Pupils try to identify the emotion and discuss beneficial and hazardous uses.   P

86 Students act out such situations as how to make friends; getting along with others; facing dangers; solving problems.   I, U

Scrapbook 87 Children prepare a scrapbook or notebook with illustrated writings on "What to do when I get angry," "How to play fairly."   P, I

88 Prepare a scrapbook of pictures and magazine and newspaper articles that illustrate good sportsmanship.   I

Self-test 89 Have pupils complete the following: I, U

Friendliness test

	YES	NO
Do you smile easily?	☐	☐
Are you a good listener?	☐	☐
Are you courteous?	☐	☐
Are you a good sport?	☐	☐
Do you refuse to tell tales?	☐	☐
Do you have a hobby?	☐	☐
Can you laugh at a joke on yourself?	☐	☐
Are you usually in a good humor?	☐	☐
Can your friends depend on you?	☐	☐
Do you try to talk about what interests other people?	☐	☐

*Also refer to Hawley, R.: Value exploration through role playing, Amherst, Mass., 1974, Educational Research Press.

MENTAL HEALTH—cont'd   Grades

			Grades
Show and tell	**90**	Provide time for jokes, funny stories, and riddles.	P
	91	Provide opportunities for all children to show and tell something as frequently as possible.	P
Sociogram	**92**	Prepare a sociogram to find out if children in the classroom have friends. Have each child list the three children he or she would like to sit near.	P, I
Stories*	**93**	Read, make up, and discuss stories showing thoughtfulness of individuals to other individuals, about fears, cooperation, sharing, fair play, courtesy, sportsmanship, honesty, truthfulness, courage, friendliness, and other personality traits.	P
	94	Tell and read stories about helping at home, sharing of toys, caring for baby, and family living.	P
	95	Read and discuss stories of famous people who have overcome handicaps and failures such as Edison, Helen Keller, Pasteur.	I, U
	96	Have students write an ending to an unfinished story. Have several read aloud and follow with discussion.	P, I
	97	Read and discuss such stories as:	P

"Boo, Who Used to Be Afraid of the Dark," Leaf Munro
"Noise in the Night," Anne Alexander
"A Friend Is Someone You Like," J. W. Anglund
"Having a Friend," Betty Miles
"Behave Yourself," B. A. M. Briggs

	98	Read stories† about death and dying.	P, I, U
Survey	**99**	Conduct a survey regarding the qualities or traits that the pupils like in their friends. Have a committee tabulate the results and prepare a chart for display titled "Our best friends."	I, U
	100	Conduct a survey of interests, tabulate, and prepare a series of discussion questions on the findings. Some sample questions that could be included are the following:	I, U

I wish I had better grades.
I wish I didn't get headaches when I read.
I wish I didn't get into trouble at school.
I wish I could change some of my teachers.
I wish my folks didn't quarrel at mealtime.
I wish my parents got along better.
I wish my parents really loved me.
I wish I could take my friends home.
I wish my father could spend more time with me.
I wish I weren't afraid of things.

Tape recordings	**101**	Record conversations of a group of children and then have pupils listen to the tone of voices. Point out the emotions expressed and consider ways to modify them.	P, I

---

*See Chapter 12.
†See the death education references in Chapter 12.

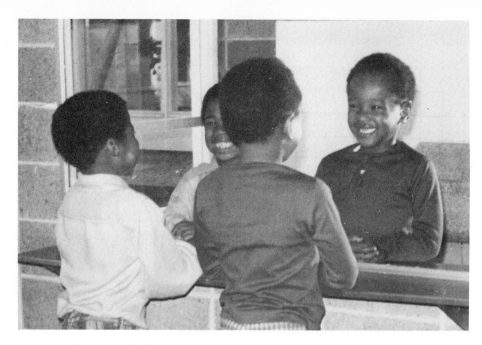

Fig. 11-12. Self-concept identification. (Courtesy Miss Betty Jane Mobley, teacher, Tacoma Public Schools, Tacoma, Wash.)

<table>
<tr><td></td><td></td><td align="center">**MENTAL HEALTH—cont'd**</td><td align="right">**Grades**</td></tr>
</table>

Television box	102	Make a television box with a series of drawings illustrating captions such as the following:	P

> This little girl is too lazy to make her bed.
> Are you a good sport?
> Are you helpful at home, at school?
> Do you lose your temper and fight?
> Do you cry easily?
> Are you kind to others?

VALUE CLARIFICATION PROCEDURES*

Clarifying of values	103	Have students write their opinions regarding such questions as: Are people treated fairly in this school or community? Is money the most important thing in life? What do you really believe in? Do you want war or peace, violence or rational action? Do people treat others justly, honestly, and equally? What do you want to be? Discuss the above questions and raise others in an attempt to help in the clarification of values.	U
Consequences	104	Have students prepare reports or discuss these behaviors: self-medication and self-diagnosis; smoking; use of marijuana or heroin; sexual intercourse; destroying or damaging someone else's property; stealing a book or money; having no friends; being a failure; telling people untruths; conflicts with	I, U

*Adapted from Simon, S. B.: Promoting the search for values, School Health Review **2:** Feb., 1971; also, Raths, E. L., Harmin, M. and Simon, S. B.: Values and teaching; working with values in the classroom, Columbus, Ohio, 1966, Charles E. Merrill Books, Inc.

MENTAL HEALTH—cont'd   Grades

parents; being rude to friends and others; venereal disease; exceeding the speed limit while driving an automobile. They should respond to these questions: Do you consider the consequences before you act? Should you? Why?

DUSO*   105 Developing Understanding of Self and Others involves a   P
                    variety of activities, including a story, role playing or pup-
                    pets, posters, and discussion picture. It focuses on such de-
                    velopmental tasks as self-identify, self-acceptance, feelings of
                    adequacy, responsibility, and value judgments.

Incomplete   106 Have students complete such questions as those that follow   I, U
questions   and discuss answers using the value clarification technique:

                    I believe the three most important things in life are _____.
                    If I could change the school program, I would _____.
                    If I could be any person in the world, I would be _____.
                    If I had three wishes, they would be _____.
                    If I could change myself, I would _____.

Me   107 Students select words, pictures, symbols, and the like from   P, I
                    magazines and newspapers that represent who they are and
                    prepare a collage of these items on large pieces of construc-
                    tion paper.

Language of   108 Pupils write five words that describe themselves on a sheet of   I, U
self   paper. They turn over this paper and write five words they
                    wish would describe themselves. Discussion may take place
                    in class.

Self-confidence 109 Students check rating to the right of the following for discus-   I, U
chart   sion:

	NO				YES
	1	2	3	4	5
Am easily upset emotionally.	☐	☐	☐	☐	☐
Dislike meeting people	☐	☐	☐	☐	☐
Find criticism hard to take.	☐	☐	☐	☐	☐
Have trouble solving problems.	☐	☐	☐	☐	☐
Feel inferior most of the time.	☐	☐	☐	☐	☐
Will not try anything if it means failure.	☐	☐	☐	☐	☐

Self-rating per- 110 Students cooperatively prepare a self-rating scale that con-   I, U
sonality scale   tains such criteria as: makes friends easily; talkative; moody
                     or happy-go-lucky; accepts responsibilities; good sport; is
                     considerate. An individual self-analysis is followed by class
                     discussion.

Things I like   111 Students identify the five things they like to do in order of im- I, U
to do   portance on a sheet of paper. They indicate using a dollar
                    ($) sign if they cost money to do, indicate the date last per-
                    formed, and place an X beside those they enjoy doing with
                    others. These may be discussed in class.

---

*Dinkmeyer, D.: Developing understanding of self and others, Circle Pines, Minn., 1970, American Guidance Service, Inc.

MENTAL HEALTH—cont'd

Grades

Unfinished sentences	112 Provide students with a variety of unfinished sentences to be completed such as: "If I were older . . ." "I wish . . ." "I would like to be . . ." "My favorite fun is . . ." "I make mistakes when . . ." Children can be encouraged to respond to answers by choice in class.	I, U
Value analysis	113 Ask students a series of questions and following responses ask why to: What aspect of health do you value most? If you had to give up one of your senses, which one would it be? If you had six months to live, what would you do? What do you like or dislike about yourself?	U
Value challenges	114 The teacher periodically raises value issues with students by introducing provocative, controversial statements found in newspapers, magazines, books, and elsewhere about values. Quotations, pictures with or without captions, scenes from plays or movies, lyrics from songs, and advertising slogans may also be used. These should be duplicated or shown to students for reading and viewing and followed by a series of questions such as: what is your reaction to the statement, item, photo, or scene? Would you be proud of this action? Was it right or wrong? Why? Does it make you want to change your life? How would you have helped? How would you have handled it?	I, U
Value questionnaire	115 Prepare a series of questions for student responses and discussion such as: What do you most like to do with your free time? What adult qualities do you admire? Where will you be and what will you be doing in 10 years? What injustices exist in the community? How do you feel about money and and material possessions? Would you marry outside your race or religion?	U
Value report card	116 Students turn in weekly anonymous 4 by 6 inch value cards on which they describe things they care about deeply, or value highly. One card is turned in each time containing one value. Some cards are read and discussed in class periodically.	U
Value time diary	117 Students maintain a time diary for 1 week; a daily chart divided into 30-minute time blocks. Actual uses of time are identified. This information should be considered personal and not for viewing by anyone. An attempt should be made to help student locate those things they most like to do, to discover wasted time, to identify inconsistencies, and to focus on the difference between what one says and what one does. After students tabulate and clarify activities, students make individual efforts to determine what they really value.	I, U

Who am I?   **118** Students write about themselves and discuss those questions   I, U
they wish, such as: What are my emotions like? How can
they be controlled? What do I look like? How can I tell?
Which is the most important: money, security, education?
Can I change what I look like? Which is the most important:
money, security, education? Why? What do I want to be?
How can I get there? What makes me sad, glad, angry, hate-
ful, worry?

NUTRITION

Bulletin board   **1** Prepare a display of new foods tried by children. Include the   P
food item, a picture or drawing of the food, and the name of
the student who had eaten the food.

2 From cereal boxes and milk and other cartons construct a food   P
train with an engine and four cars containing the Basic 4 foods.
Place food models made from construction paper, clay, papier-
mâché, or cutouts from magazines in the cars.

3 Prepare a bulletin board display depicting a rocket ship and in   P, I
the pilot's seat insert animated fruits or vegetables. Illustrated
caption might read:

Mr. Carrot: "Fly high with me and grow big and strong."
Mr. Milk: "I fly high and fast because I give lots of pep and energy."

The captions and food items can be changed periodically.

4 Prepare bulletin board displays, showcase exhibits, dioramas,   P, I, U
and others using real foods, food models, attractive pictures,
children-made cutouts, and papier-mâché models showing:

A well-balanced breakfast, lunch, or dinner
Wholesome "snack" foods
Milk products, such as whole milk, skim milk, dried milk, cottage
    cheese, cream, butter, and indicate their importance
Foods containing vitamins, minerals, proteins, carbohydrates, and fats
Food sanitation including the preparation, serving, cleanup, washing
    of utensils, and the storage of food
Meals or foods to be served in the school lunchroom
Recent newspaper and magazine articles
The amount of sugar contained in various kinds of candy and soft
    drinks
A model of the Basic 4 boy and girl having the foods they need pinned
    to them
World food problems

5 Construct a "Mr. Breakfast" (Fig. 11-13) out of construction   P, I, U
or drawing paper as follows:
Hat—bowl of cereal
Head—an orange
Body—bottle of milk
Hands—fruits, eggs, bacon, and bread
Arms—may substitute bananas
Legs—may substitute bacon strips

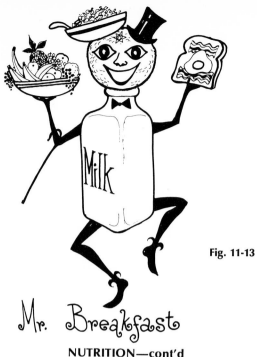

Fig. 11-13

Mr. Breakfast

NUTRITION—cont'd

Grades

6 Assign a group of students the responsibility of locating pictures and newspaper and magazine articles related to nutrition. Students should provide statements or comments below each item.

I, U

Chart

7 Prepare a cooperative chart, or charts, on the kinds of foods (carbohydrates, fats, proteins, minerals, and vitamins) with food pictures to illustrate.

P, I

8 Cut pictures of foods from magazines and make a Basic 4 classification chart for the classroom.

P, I

9 Prepare a chart of the food nutrients as follows:

U

NUTRIENT	WHAT IT DOES	FOODS IN WHICH FOUND
Proteins		
Vitamins		
Carbohydrates		
Fats		
Minerals		

NUTRITION—cont'd   Grades

Demonstration	10 Make butter from cream and serve on bread to children in class. Permit each child a chance to shake the jar containing the cream.

P

11 Make giant paintings of favorite fruits or vegetables on paper bags. Cut holes for the head and arms and have children wear these bags while they tell pupils in other classes what they like about these fruits and vegetables.

P

12 With the help of parents or teachers, prepare and serve a nutritious breakfast.

P, I

13 With Parent-Teachers' Association members, plan, prepare, and serve a meal that contains foods from a foreign country.

I, U

14 Children participate in the planning and preparation of nutritious foods for class or school parties. Avoid the usual cakes, candies, and soft drinks, substituting such items as fruit, fruit juices, popcorn, and nuts.

I, U

15 Pupil committee tries to improve the attractiveness of the cafeteria through the use of posters, table settings, and flowers.

I, U

16 Demonstrate ways to test foods for content.

I, U

Starch—Soften, crush, and dissolve foods in water. Place in a test tube with some water and add a drop of iodine (1% solution). If solution turns blue, starch is present.

Fat—Place foods on pieces of paper. Remove foods and place papers on radiator to heat. Fatty foods will leave grease spots.

Protein—Burn foods in direct flame of Bunsen burner. Protein foods (raw, lean meat; cheese; dried beans) will emit odor of burning feathers. May need to burn a feather first so that pupils recognize odor.

Minerals—Burn various foods on a small asbestos or metal plate. High mineral content foods (dried milk, beans, peas, and egg yolk) will leave a gray ash containing one or more minerals such as calcium. Nonmineral foods such as sugar will leave only a small residue of black carbon.

Water—Expose fruits, leafy vegetables, and other foods containing high water content to air and they become shriveled after a while. They may be weighed before and after dehydration to determine the amount of water lost.

Discussion

17 Establish the EE and FF clubs. Have children read the cafeteria lunch menu each day and compare this with the balanced food chart found on the bulletin board. Upon their return from lunch, pupils report themselves as EE (eat everything) or FF (fussy feeder) members. Discuss why they acted as they did.

I

18 Discuss and help plan a school lunch menu.

I, U

19 Discuss a well-balanced lunch in class and select menus to show foods containing the necessary vitamins and minerals needed for growth. Pupils discuss items purchased in cafeteria and best ways to spend money to obtain proper foods.

I, U

20 Obesity, weight reducing, and vitamin pills.

U

21 The kinds and purposes of foods necessary for growth as well as the deficiency diseases.

U

22 Participate as a member of a school health advisory committee to help solve school nutrition problems.

U

NUTRITION—cont'd

Grades

Dramatization   **23** Dramatize visits to the dairy, grocery store, and food markets by constructing a store having shelves filled with empty food cans, boxes, and other such items. Also play house and dramatize foods eaten for breakfast, lunch, and dinner.   P

24 Children prepare and participate in plays, radio, and television broadcasts presenting various aspects of nutrition.   P, I, U

Drawings   **25** Have children draw pictures of foods, using a worksheet like the one below.   P

MILK	ORANGE JUICE	BUTTER
BREAD	CELERY	MEAT
EGGS	APPLE	CARROTS

Excursions   **26** Visit the dairy, grocery store, and local food markets to observe the availability and storage of different foods.   P

27 Visit the school lunch room to observe foods being prepared for the noon meal.   P, I

28 Observe the sanitary methods used in the preparation, serving, and storage of foods in a restaurant or in the school cafeteria.   I, U

29 Visit milk or food processing plants.   I, U

Exhibit   **30** Prepare a display or exhibit of well-balanced breakfasts, lunches, and dinners using real foods or food models.   P, I, U

31 Construct a man or woman from a variety of dairy product cartons.   I, U
Head—cottage cheese carton
Buttons—other cheese cartons
Body—ice cream carton
Legs—milk cartons
Arms—cubed butter wrappers or cartons

32 Have a "Food Fair" during which children display various kinds of foods, adequate lunches, dinners, and breakfasts, and appropriate snack-time foods. Pupils may construct murals, bulletin board displays, write-ups for the newspaper, and invitations to parents.   I, U

33 Set up a nutrition corner displaying pamphlets, books, magazines, and other materials for pupil reference and use during the nutrition unit.   I, U

NUTRITION—cont'd   Grades

Experiment 34 Place grass seed in a sponge, add some water, and watch the   P, I
                sprouts grow. This activity shows the need of food for growth.

            35 Participate in the white rat experiment to learn the impor-   P, I
                tance of food for life and growth.

            36 Soak a corn seed in water overnight, remove the bran coat,   I, U
                and then discuss the significance of this outer coat to the white
                part underneath.

            37 Use two sibling rats, conduct a feeding experiment in which   I, U
                one of the rats receives milk to drink and the other receives
                coffee in addition to food. The rat drinking the milk will grow
                and look much better than the coffee-fed rat.

            38 Soak a small uncooked bone in vinegar for three days. The   I, U
                mineral matter will dissolve and the bone will lose its strength
                and firmness so that it can be easily bent. This experiment
                demonstrates the presence of minerals (especially calcium and
                phosphorus) in bones. It points out the importance of minerals
                in the diet.

Finger play 39 Prepare finger play, such as: P

TUNE: *Mulberry Bush*
This is the way we drink our milk,
Drink our milk, drink our milk,
This is the way we drink our milk,
Every night and morning.

This is the way it makes us grow,
Makes us grow, makes us grow.
This is the way it makes us grow,
Every single day.

Flannelboard 40 Read the following poem and have children (as many as pos-   P
                  sible) place the appropriate foods mentioned on the board.

End

Three little pigs and their dinners

There were three little pigs so happy and gay,
As each started to go his way one day.
Said the first little pig, in his house of straw,
"Now I can eat all the candy I want, hurrah."
So he filled his tummy with candy and cake,
'Till it began to ache and ache.
"Oh I wish I had listened to Mommy," he said,
As he rolled over and over in his bed.

The second little pig in his house of twigs,
Said, "Now I have no Mommy to make me eat figs."
So he had doughnuts, popsicles, and root beer.
Soon he yelled loud, "Oh dear! Oh dear!
My tooth is aching, my tummy's in pain.
I'll never do that, no never again."

The third little pig, remembering what his Mommy said,
Had meat, fresh vegetables, milk, and bread.
He ate oranges and apples, singing their praise,
As he felt peppy and strong all of his days.
"I'm always healthy, happy, and strong
I get my sleep and nothing goes wrong."
MARY STULTZ

NUTRITION—cont'd Grades

41 Place the following food pictures on a flannelboard and have children prepare three different breakfasts: oranges, whole wheat bread, butter, cocoa, eggs, bacon, milk, and cereal. — P, I

42 Have food models available and permit children to show the foods they ate for breakfast, lunch, dinner, and snack-time, and also the foods they should eat for breakfast, lunch, dinner, and snack-time. — P, I

43 Use food models to illustrate the Basic 4 foods as well as a balanced breakfast, lunch, and dinner. — I, U

44 Pictures from magazines are brought to class and children cut out good food items. Pupils paste these foods on cardboard plates, shellac them, and use them to play "Going to the cafeteria" and "What to eat." — P

Individual and group reports

45 Pupils prepare lists of foods they like and dislike and make comparisons with the Basic 4 food groups. — I, U

46 Read and write words and sentences about nutrition. — P

47 Children write a brief summary paragraph or two in answer to the question "What are the proper kinds of foods to eat, and why must we eat them?" — P, I

48 Serve as a class committee member to meet with the school lunch manager to learn how nutritious lunches are prepared and report findings in oral or written reports to the entire class. — I, U

49 Pupils write letters of request to various companies for available nutrition materials for use in class. — I, U

50 Prepare magazine articles regarding school lunch menus, weight reduction, and other important phases of nutrition for publication in the school newspaper. — U

51 Analyze weight-reducing procedures advertised in newspapers and magazines. — U

52 Analyze several newspaper or magazine advertisements about foods and food products. — U

53 Pupils prepare lists of food fallacies and do research to discover why these are considered to be such. — U

54 Students prepare notebooks of food pictures cut out of newspapers and magazines and grouped according to the Basic 4 food groups. — P

55 Students identify one favorite food and determine the nutrients, caloric value, and contributions to health. — I, U

Mobile

56 Make a food mobile illustrating individual foods found in the Basic 4. — P, I

57 Teacher prepares a large block (at least 12 inches square) and places pictures of the Basic 4 food groups on each side. The block is hung as a mobile during the time that nutrition is being discussed. Manila cardboard can also be used to construct the block because it can be folded and stored more easily. — P, I

NUTRITION—cont'd   Grades

Model   58 With colored construction paper, teacher and children make a   P
5-foot "Mr. Breakfast." The following day the teacher mimeo-
graphs the model on a smaller scale, the children color it, put
their names at the bottom, and take it home to their parents.

59 Prepare food models from clay, sawdust mixtures, cardboard,   P, I
newspaper clippings, and other materials to be used for exhibit
purposes or in the discussion on nutrition.

60 Prepare papier-mâché fruits and vegetables using real foods   P, I
as forms. These items can be used in dramatic play and in the
discussion of nutrition.

Panel   61 Participate in a panel discussion of the problem "Diet and its   U
relationship to weight control."

Poem   62 Create original poems about nutrition, such as the following: P

There was an old woman
Who lived in a shoe.
She had so many children
But she knew what to do.
She fed them milk, fruit,
And vegetable greens.
So they were the best children
You have ever seen.

Iggildy, piggildy, wiggildy, doo!
I'm Mr. Carrot, How do you do!
I'm lean and crisp.
I come in a bunch.
Eat me and see that I'm so good to munch.
I'm good for teeth.
I make them chew.
I make them exercise.
That's what I do.
I'm good for eyes to see things, too!

Oodle, doodle, humpty dumpty!
I'm white and smooth and never lumpy.
Drinking me keeps you in trim.
Drink me well 'cause I'm filled to the brim.
Strong bones and teeth is what I give.
Drinking me makes you really live!
My vitamins make skin smooth as silk.
You should know me,
I'm Mr. Milk.

Puppets 63 Make puppets from construction paper and tongue blades   P
(Figs. 11-14 to 11-16). The puppet heads should be about 12
inches high with the following rhymes written on their backs:

Celery: "I'm Madam Celery
So much fun to eat
Serve me at your snacktime
Then you'll want no sweet."

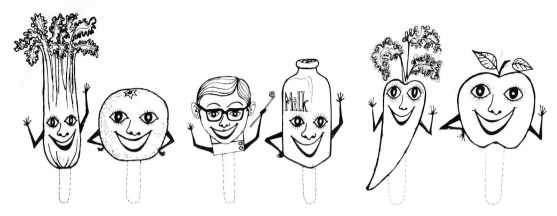

Fig. 11-14   Fig. 11-15   Fig. 11-16

NUTRITION—cont'd

Apple: "I'm Mr. Apple.
A juicy, swooshy bite
Eat me every day
To keep your teeth just right,"

Orange: "I'm Madam Orange
The sunshine color you see
I protect you from illness
Because I give you vitamin C."

Milk: "I'm your nice, sweet milk
I'll make your bones and teeth grow strong.
Drink and drink and drink some more
Then you'll be healthy your whole life long."

Carrot: "I'm Mrs. Carrot
So much fun to eat.
I go crunch, crunch, crunch, crunch
Between your strong, white teeth."

Dentist: "I am your friend the dentist
Come see me any day
I'll hunt out all cavities,
And fill them right away."

Grades

64 Have a puppet show centered around a boy visited by Mr. Candy and Mr. Pop, who persuaded him to eat these items as snacks instead of oranges and other fruits. Later the fruit (Mr. Orange) and vegetables (Mr. Carrot and Mr. Celery) come along and persuade the boy to try them as snack foods. — P, I

65 Use puppets or marionettes made in class to dramatize nutrition concepts, such as drinking milk daily, eating fruits and vegetables, importance of a good breakfast. — P, I

Riddle

66 Have children write such riddles as the following: — P, I

You find me in the garden,
I'm orange with long green hair,
You might find me on your table
So look for me there.
Who am I?

NUTRITION—cont'd

		Grades
Scrapbook	67 Locate pictures and information in magazines, newspapers, and pamphlets for making different kinds of sandwiches and preparing lunch boxes more attractively and put them into a booklet to be taken home.	P, I, U
	68 Prepare scrapbooks using pictures from magazines and other sources of such foods as fruits, vegetables, cheese, milk, butter, eggs, meat, fish, and poultry. Also organize these items into nutritious breakfasts, lunches, dinners, and snack foods.	P, I, U
Shadow box	69 Make shadow boxes depicting the Basic 4 foods as well as nutritious breakfasts, lunches, and dinners.	P
Speakers	70 Invite such resource people to class as nutritionists, school lunch managers, and others to discuss various aspects of nutrition.	U
Stories, songs, and rhymes	71 Write stories, songs, and rhymes as well as plays about nutrition.	P, I
Survey	72 Survey the number of children in class who are eating breakfast, as well as the nature of the food consumed.	I, U
	73 Survey the number of children purchasing plate lunches at school and compare this figure with the number who bring their lunch to school.	I, U
	74 Conduct a 1- to 3-day survey of snack foods eaten by pupils.	I, U
	75 Participate in a 3-day diet survey.	I, U
	76 Survey the number of children who eat candy or soft drinks at lunch time, as well as the amounts consumed.	I, U
Tasting party	77 Have a bunny party in which children make head bands with paper ears and all eat raw green vegetables and carrots.	P
	78 Participate in the eating of nutritious snack foods by having milk, fruit, fruit juices, nuts, celery, and carrot sticks instead of cake, candy, and soft drinks.	P, I, U
	79 Plan, prepare, and serve nutritious food items for parties and social gatherings at school.	U
Vegetable garden	80 Grow such vegetables as lettuce, tomatoes, and carrots in order to provide understandings of some of the foods needed for growth and development.	P, I

REST AND SLEEP

Bulletin board	1 Display pictures that children bring to class or draw showing sleep, work, play, and relaxation.	P, I
	2 Display humorous illustrations of the basic rules of sleep and rest.	P, I
Chart	3 Make a construction paper clock chart and put two sets of hands on it. Use red hands to indicate the time to go to bed and green hands to tell the time to get up.	P, I, U
	4 Construct a clock chart that shows children how to budget their time in order to get adequate amounts of rest, sleep, and exercise.	P, I, U

REST AND SLEEP—cont'd

		Grades
Demonstration	**5** Demonstrate a variety of exercises that can help one to relax.	P, I, U
Discussion	**6** Collect, show, and discuss pictures of animals at sleep and rest.	P
	7 Have children suggest ways to rest and relax and list these on the blackboard: warm bath, lying down, sit with head on desk, listening to music.	P
	8 Importance of sleep and rest and the amount needed.	P, I
	9 Rest, relaxation, and music.	P, I
	10 Children plan the work, play, and rest periods for the day.	P, I
	11 Discuss the following questions in class: What happens when we sleep? When did you get up this morning? Did you sleep well? Did you feel rested? What time did you go to bed last night?	P, I
	12 Discuss the best conditions for sleeping and include comments about air, bed, and the room itself.	P, I, U
	13 Discuss the meaning of the terms relaxation and tension. Demonstrate by having the pupils flex muscles in their bodies and then relax them.	I, U
	14 The causes of fatigue, the signs of fatigue, what to do when fatigued, and the effects of overfatigue.	I, U
	15 Sleep and rest in terms of their value, how one feels and acts when sufficiently rested, and the need for balance between sleep, rest, and exercise.	I, U
	16 Why we tire; how rest affects posture, work, and play; and how anxiety, fear, anger, and eating before bedtime may affect sleep.	I, U
Dramatization	**17** Children play house and devote part of their play to stressing sleep and rest.	P
	18 Children dramatize going to bed at night. One child stands in front of the class and makes suggestions while others pantomime the action during the singing of the tune "Mulberry Bush."	P
	19 Prepare a play emphasizing desirable habits of sleep and rest to be presented in class, to a school assembly, or to the Parent-Teachers' Association.	I
Drawings	**20** Draw pictures about sleep, rest, and relaxation.	P, I
Experience chart	**21** Prepare an experience chart or record of important points about sleep and rest.	P
Experiment	**22** Tie a weighted string near the tip of the left third finger of a pupil volunteer. Have the pupil raise and lower his finger as long as possible. Allow the child to rest for a minute and then repeat the procedure. Try this experiment using different fingers on both hands. The results show that exercise is fatiguing and there is need for rest and relaxation.	P, I, U

REST AND SLEEP—cont'd   Grades

Finger plays   **23** Have children participate in finger plays.   P, I

> This little boy is going to bed,
> As down on his pillow he lays his head.
> Tuck him in with the covers tight
> And this is the way he sleeps all night.

> *Rest and listen*
>
> I like to rest and listen.
> Let me listen while I rest.
> My eyes are closed so I can't see.
> I'll listen while you count for me.
> Sh—whisper, count to ten . . . . . .
> Now listen while I rest again.

> Time for us to take a rest.
> Lock the door up tight (lock lips).
> Pull the little window shades (close eyes)
> We'll play that it is night.

> *Let's play rag doll*
>
> Let's play rag doll.
> Dont't make a sound.
> Fling your arms and bodies
> Loosely around.
> Fling your hands!
> Fling your feet!
> Let your head go free!
> Be the raggediest rag doll
> You ever did see.

Individual and   **24** Pupils prepare oral and written reports on rest, sleep, fatigue,   I, U
  group   and relaxation.
  reports   **25** Write a story on the three R's, "Rest, relaxation, and recrea-   I, U
                  tion."

Music   **26** Play restful and relaxing music in class.   P, I, U

> Brahms' Lullaby
> Clair de Lune, Debussy
> Air from Suite No. 3 in D major, Bach
> The Swan from Carnival of the Animals, Saint-Saens
> The Lake from Adventures in a Perambulator, Carpenter
> White Peacock, Griffes

Poems   **27** Children listen to, participate in the reading of, and act out   P, I, U
                  poems on sleep, rest, and relaxation.

> I am a limp rag doll,
> I have no bones,
> My feet are flat and still,
> My hands are in my lap,
> My head is limp,
> Now my head rests on my knees
> And my hands hang at my sides.
> SARAH T. BARROWS

REST AND SLEEP—cont'd

Close your eyes, head drops down
Face is smooth, not a frown
Roll to left, head is a ball
Roll to right, now sit tall
Lift your chin, look at me
Deep, deep breath, one, two, three
Big, big smile, hands in lap
Make believe you just had a nap
Now you're rested from your play
Time to work again today.

I went into a circus town
And met a funny Bunny Clown,
He winked his eye, he shook his head,
"This is splendid exercise," he said.
He shook his head, he shook his feet,
He wobbled, bobbled, down the street,
He moved his jaw both up and down
This funny little Bunny Clown.

He played that he was a lazy man
And then sat down like a Raggedy Ann.
His head fell down and his arms fell, too,
And he went to sleep for an hour or two.

The stretching game*
Link your thumbs;
Raise your arms
Straight up and past your ears,
Stretch and pull;
Pull and stretch;
Try to touch the sky.
Pull and stretch;
Stretch and pull;
Pull—pull—pull!
Drop your arms, now sigh.
FRANCES C. HUNTER

			Grades
Posters	28	Make posters or pictures illustrating activities conducive to play, sleep, and relaxation.	P
Puppets	29	Make two puppets and call them "Sleepy Head" and "Wide Awake." Have children dramatize aspects of rest and sleep.	P, I
	30	Make paper-bag puppets and dramatize a problem, such as a boy who wants to stay up past his bedtime to watch television.	P, I
Scrapbook	31	Prepare scrapbooks of pictures showing restful and relaxing activities.	P, I
Stories	32	Read and create stories about rest, sleep, and relaxation.	P, I

*Los Angeles City School Districts, Calif.: Speech in the elementary school, pub. No. 479, 1949, Office of the Superintendent of Schools, p. 90.

SAFETY

BICYCLE SAFETY			**Grades**
Bulletin board	1	Display children's drawings on bicycle safety.	P, I, U
	2	Display bicycle safety posters and other printed materials available from the American Bicycle Institute and such organizations.	P, I, U
	3	A committee of pupils prepares a bulletin board display showing an outline of a bicycle labeled with its main parts and the safety rules. See Fig. 11-17.	I, U
Chart	4	Children prepare a chart listing the bicycles safety rules.	P, I, U
Checklist	5	Pupils prepare a checklist for use in the inspection of the mechanical safety of bicycles. The assistance of a bicycle repairman may be necessary.	I, U
	6	Organize a bicycle club in school.	I, U
Demonstration	7	Children demonstrate the following procedures correctly: getting on a bicycle, getting off a bicycle, guiding a bicycle, applying the brake, and stopping and parking the bicycle.	P, I, U
	8	Pupils demonstrate and practice the proper hand signals when riding bicycles.	P, I, U
	9	Demonstrate the mechanical inspection of a safe bicycle in class. It is advisable to bring a bicycle into the room.	P, I, U
	10	Have a demonstration of minor bicycle repairs. It may be necessary to invite a bicycle repairman to class.	I, U

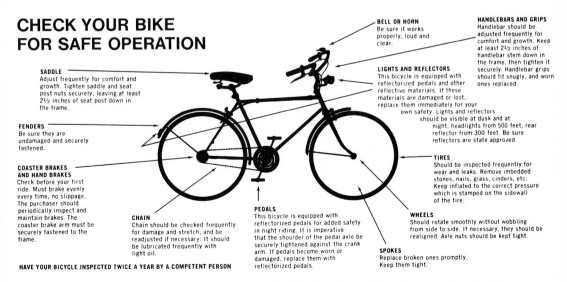

CHECK YOUR BIKE FOR SAFE OPERATION

SADDLE
Adjust frequently for comfort and growth. Tighten saddle and seat post nuts securely, leaving at least 2½ inches of seat post down in the frame.

FENDERS
Be sure they are undamaged and securely fastened.

COASTER BRAKES AND HAND BRAKES
Check before your first ride. Must brake evenly every time, no slippage. The purchaser should periodically inspect and maintain brakes. The coaster brake arm must be securely fastened to the frame.

CHAIN
Chain should be checked frequently for damage and stretch, and be readjusted if necessary. It should be lubricated frequently with light oil.

HAVE YOUR BICYCLE INSPECTED TWICE A YEAR BY A COMPETENT PERSON

PEDALS
This bicycle is equipped with reflectorized pedals for added safety in night riding. It is imperative that the shoulder of the pedal axle be securely tightened against the crank arm. If pedals become worn or damaged, replace them with reflectorized pedals.

BELL OR HORN
Be sure it works properly, loud and clear.

LIGHTS AND REFLECTORS
This bicycle is equipped with reflectorized pedals and other reflective materials. If these materials are damaged or lost, replace them immediately for your own safety. Lights and reflectors should be visible at dusk and at night; headlights from 500 feet, rear reflector from 300 feet. Be sure reflectors are state approved.

HANDLEBARS AND GRIPS
Handlebar should be adjusted frequently for comfort and growth. Keep at least 2½ inches of handlebar stem down in the frame, then tighten it securely. Handlebar grips should fit snugly, and worn ones replaced.

TIRES
Should be inspected frequently for wear and leaks. Remove imbedded stones, nails, glass, cinders, etc. Keep inflated to the correct pressure which is stamped on the sidewall of the tire.

WHEELS
Should rotate smoothly without wobbling from side to side. If necessary, they should be realigned. Axle nuts should be kept tight.

SPOKES
Replace broken ones promptly. Keep them tight.

Fig. 11-17. Bicycle safety check. (Courtesy the Bicycle Institute of America, Inc., New York.)

SAFETY—cont'd

		Grades
	11 Conduct a bicycle field day in which pupils participate in a variety of activities that show their ability and skill to ride bicycles safely. Automobile clubs and other organizations in the community often will provide assistance with this program.	I, U
	12 Pupils prepare a demonstration of bicycle safety to be presented to a school assembly.	I, U
Discussion	13 The motor vehicle laws and regulations in terms of licensing of bicycles, need to comply with rules, proper hand signals, parking, motor vehicle rules, and others.	P, I, U
	14 Safety factors involved in riding a bicycle to school.	P, I, U
	15 Pupils bring newspaper and magazine articles about bicycle safety or accidents to class.	I, U
	16 Pupils discuss the causes of bicycle accidents and how to prevent them. This could lead to a series of unanswered questions and start the problem-solving approach to bicycle safety.	I, U
Dramatization	17 Children dramatize riding a bicycle and demonstrate the necessary safe practices.	P, I, U
Excursion	18 Visit a bicycle repair shop to observe how bicycles are repaired.	I, U
Experience chart	19 Prepare an experience chart or record of bicycle safety rules.	P
Guest speaker	20 Invite a police officer to class to discuss bicycle safety traffic rules.	P, I, U
Individual and group reports	21 Prepare oral and written reports on the safest way to ride bicycles to and from school.	P, I, U
	22 Prepare oral and written reports on bicycle safety.	I, U
	23 Prepare school newspaper articles titled "Bicycle safety tips."	I, U
	24 Write a group letter to the police department or some other organization requesting a speaker to discuss bicycle safety.	I, U
	25 Children prepare a code of safety for bicycle riders. This can be posted on the bulletin board or may be printed in the school newspaper.	I, U
	26 Children write to the Bicycle Institute of America or other organizations for bicycle safety materials.	I, U
	27 Pupils prepare reports on the yearly accidents occurring on bicycles in the nation, state, county, and city.	U
Interview	28 Interview a police officer or some other authority on bicycle safety.	I, U
Scrapbook	29 Prepare a scrapbook containing newspaper and magazine articles, pictures, stories, and other obtainable materials on bicycle safety.	P, I, U
Self-test	30 Prepare a self-test or pretest on bicycle traffic safety.	I, U

SAFETY—cont'd

	Sample questions	YES	NO
1.	A bicycle can be ridden on the sidewalk in a business area.	☐	☐
2.	A bicycle rider should obey all traffic signs, lights, and devices.	☐	☐
3.	Pedestrians do not have the right-of-way in cross-walks.	☐	☐
4.	You should walk your bicycle across heavily traveled streets.	☐	☐
5.	Night riding without a light and reflector is unsafe.	☐	☐
6.	It is safe and proper to carry a passenger on a bicycle.	☐	☐
7.	Hitching to a moving truck is safe if you are careful.	☐	☐
8.	It is best to ride three abreast when riding in a group.	☐	☐
9.	You should give hand signals when turning at all times.	☐	☐
10.	On a country road you should ride on the left of the highway.	☐	☐

			Grades
Survey	31	Pupils conduct a survey of bicycle traffic violations noted on the way to and from school.	I, U

BUS SAFETY

Bulletin board	1	Display pictures, drawings, slogans, cartoons, and posters about bus safety.	P, I, U
	2	Make a bus out of construction paper and display this along with appropriate captions about bus safety.	P, I, U
Demonstration	3	With a small toy truck and blocks demonstrate why it is necessary to be seated at all times in the school bus. Show how blocks will fall when a sudden stop is necessary.	P, I
	4	Have children practice bus loading and unloading and discuss safe behavior while riding.	P, I, U
Discussion	5	The need to cooperate with the bus driver when riding the school bus.	P, I, U
	6	Discuss bus safety with children preparing a list of safe behavior rules.	P, I, U
Dramatic play	7	Make a bus out of large cardboard boxes and use dramatic play to practice safe bus rules.	P
Dramatization	8	Arrange chairs in classroom to represent a school bus and have children act out the right way and the wrong way to get on and off the bus.	P, I
	9	Dramatize getting on and off a bus safely and also safety on the bus.	P, I
Excursion	10	Visit a bus and have the driver discuss safe behavior while boarding and riding.	P, I
Experience chart	11	Prepare an experience chart or record of safe procedures on the bus.	P
Guest speaker	12	Invite the bus driver to discuss bus safety.	P, I
Mural	13	Prepare a mural depicting safety on the bus.	P, I

SAFETY—cont'd

			Grades
Scrapbook	14	Construct a scrapbook of pupil drawings about bus safety.	P, I
Songs and poems	15	Compose songs and poems about bus safety.	P, I

DISASTER SAFETY

Bulletin board	1	Display pictures, drawings, or diagrams of procedures to follow in the event of an atomic attack.	P, I, U
	2	Prepare an illustrated display of foods suitable for storing for emergency use.	P, I, U
Chart	3	Prepare a wall chart for each classroom, showing the floor plans, exits and entrances to the building, and the shortest route to the nearest shelter.	P, I, U
Demonstration	4	The signals in schools that signify alerts or attack and practice identification.	P, I, U
	5	Demonstrate and practice ways to protect the eyes, ears, nose, and mouth when under simulated attack.	P, I, U
	6	Demonstrate and practice thorough washing of hands, nails, face, and hair in order to decontaminate these areas.	P, I, U
	7	Demonstrate and practice emergency drills for evacuation or undercover.	P, I, U
	8	Have pupil committees prepare to demonstrate decontamination and other emergency procedures to children in school or to the community.	I, U
	9	Food pollution through the use of simple fungi and bacteriologic experiments.	I, U
	10	How and where to store foods safely at home during an attack.	I, U
	11	How to preserve perishable foods without refrigeration.	I, U
	12	How to properly dispose of polluted food.	I, U
	13	Demonstrate and display an appropriate first-aid kit for civil disasters.	I, U
	14	How to preserve and package foods for emergencies.	I, U
	15	First-aid procedures after civil disasters.	I, U
Discussion	16	What children may do (activities) while waiting in a shelter at school until the all-clear signal is sounded.	P, I, U
	17	The procedures to follow if caught outdoors during an attack or if an alert is on.	P, I, U
	18	The location of emergency shelters in the school and community.	P, I, U
	19	The meaning of civil defense and why it is necessary.	P, I, U
	20	The nature of radiation and its effect on human beings.	I, U
	21	The hazards from atomic, biologic, and chemical warfares.	I, U
	22	The procedures to follow if one has survived an atomic attack.	I, U
	23	The problems of emotions, panics, and other behaviors that will occur during an atomic catastrophe.	I, U
	24	First-aid procedures necessary in civil disasters.	I, U
	25	The contamination of food and water and ways to protect these items.	I, U
Dramatization	26	Dramatize proper conduct during disasters.	P, I, U

SAFETY—cont'd   Grades

Exhibit	27 Display pamphlets and other printed materials for pupil reference and use.	I, U
Guest speakers	28 Invite civil defense and Red Cross speakers to discuss aspects of atomic biologic, chemical, or other civil disasters.	I, U
Individual and group reports	29 Have individual or group oral or written reports on the civil defense recommendations for the protection of people in the event of atomic, biologic, or chemical warfare.	I, U
	30 Pupils write articles for the local newspaper or school paper on how individuals can protect themselves at home, at school, or when outdoors during an atomic attack.	U
Interview	31 Interview civil defense authorities and others about the feasibility of building home shelters or community shelters.	I, U
	32 Pupils interview local health officers and medical men about the availability of services and hospital facilities in the event of civil disasters.	U
	33 Pupils interview the health officer or a representative from the civil defense office on that person's role in civil defense.	U
Survey	34 Survey the school and community to locate the designated shelter areas.	I, U

FARM SAFETY

Bulletin board	1 Children obtain pictures or make drawings of tools and machinery found on the farm such as tractors, cotton pickers, cotton trailers, harvesters, plows, and discs and place caption "Dangerous equipment" below. Pictures may be obtained from pamphlets available from farm machinery companies or from farm organizations.	P, I, U
Discussion	2 Safe practices when riding on trucks and other farm machinery.	P, I, U
	3 The hazards of insect stings, poisonous sprays, canals, irrigation ditches, tools, and other unsafe places and equipment on the farm.	P, I, U
	4 The hazards of sharp implements such as pitchforks, hoes, saws, and axes used on the farm.	P, I, U
	5 Safety around horses, bulls, and other farm animals.	P, I, U
Experience chart or record	6 Children help to prepare an experience chart or record on farm safety rules.	P
Exhibit	7 Display a variety of sharp implements used in farm work and discuss the dangers of their improper use.	P, I, U
Individual and group reports	8 Children prepare oral and written reports on farm safety.	I, U

FIRE SAFETY		SAFETY—cont'd	Grades
Bulletin board	1	Prepare an illustrated bulletin board display about fire prevention using construction paper, real clothing materials, or crayons.	P, I, U
	2	Display pictures or news items about fires in the community.	P, I, U
	3	Use pictures and drawings to display the varieties of types of fire extinguishers.	I, U
	4	Display pictures of drop and roll and crawling in smoke-filled room procedures.	P, I, U
	5	Pictorially illustrate the action to be taken when fires occur or smoke appears at home and include escape plan and other procedures.	P, I
Chart	6	Prepare a list of illustrated fire safety rules.	P, I
	7	Make an illustrated chart listing the common causes of fires in the home.	P, I, U
	8	Make an illustrated chart of the fire exits in school.	P, I, U
Demonstration	9	Light two candles and fan one of them to show how moving air causes a flame to burn more vigorously.	P, I
	10	Sound the fire alarm bell and have children practice responding to it for fire drill.	P, I, U
	11	The way to report a fire using an alarm box and the telephone.	P, I, U
	12	Ways of putting out fires using a variety of fire extinguishers.	P, I, U
	13	How to put out a fire when someone's clothing is ablaze.	P, I, U
	14	How to use matches safely—use only safety matches and strike match with the cover closed; dispose of burned matches by breaking them and placing in a glass or tin container.	P, I, U
	15	Drop and roll and crawling low in smoke-filled room procedures.	P, I, U
	16	Demonstrate the making of a fire extinguisher by putting some vinegar in a bottle and adding some baking soda. (Wrap the soda in a tissue before adding it to the vinegar. This will delay the formation of the carbon dioxide gas.) Put a rubber stopper and a pipet in the bottle, turn it upside down and pour the fluid into a pail or sink.	P, I, U
	17	The combustibility of a variety of materials such as asbestos, glass, paper, water, cotton, cloth, wood, kerosene, and various types of clothing. Also discuss spontaneous combustion.	P, I, U
	18	Place a piece of cardboard against a small light bulb and show the brown spot that occurs. Explain in terms of the fire triangle.	P, I
	19	Teacher lights a candle in class, and pupils watch it burn. A glass is placed over the candle, and children attempt to explain action in terms of the triangle of fire why the flame was extinguished.	P, I, U
Discussion	20	Fire safety rules and reasons for fire drills.	P, I
	21	Beneficial and hazardous effects of fire.	P, I
	22	Fire hazards on special occasions, such as Christmas and the Fourth of July.	P, I, U
	23	Discuss and practice fire drills in school.	P, I, U
	24	Discuss these questions: What causes fires? How do fires start? What materials burn? Where should matches be kept? What should you do in case of fire? How should you put out a picnic fire? How can fires be prevented?	P, I, U

SAFETY—cont'd   **Grades**

25 The value of the home inspections conducted by firemen. In-   I, U
    troduce common electrical terms, such as wire, plug, socket,
    bulb, fuse, and fuse box.
26 Ways to prevent fires by good housekeeping procedures,   I, U
    proper disposal of rubbish and ashes, safe storage of fuel, cor-
    rect installation and care of stoves, electric equipment, and
    furnaces.
27 The types of fires and how they may be extinguished.   I, U
28 Pupils participate as members of the fire-safety patrol to in-   I, U
    form other pupils about fire prevention.
29 Baby-sitting.   I, U
30 Smoke detectors.   P, I, U
31 Fire escape plans from homes and other buildings.   P, I, U
32 First-aid procedures for burns.   P, I, U
33 Hazards and use of electricity and flammable materials.   I, U
34 Identity and proper storage of flammable liquids.   P, I, U
35 Fires reported in newspapers and magazines in terms of causes   I, U
    and prevention.
36 To whom and how to report fires and smoke discovered.   P, I
37 Combustibility and flammability of various types of clothing   I, U
    and other substances.
38 Importance of drop and roll and crawling low procedures.   P, I, U
39 False alarms.   I, U
40 Ways to call fire department.   P, I, U

Dramatization   41 Build a fire engine using large blocks, cardboard boxes, and   P
                    other items. Children participate in dramatic play by having a
                    corner in the classroom as a firehouse. Pupils bring their toy
                    telephones to practice reporting fires.
                42 Dramatize the procedures to follow when reporting a fire by   P, I, U
                    telephone.
                43 Dramatize fire safety through sociodramas, puppet shows, and   P, I, U
                    plays.

Drawings   44 Children make drawings of ways to prevent fires, escape from   P, I
                    fires, and signal when fire is discovered.
                45 Draw pictures of wires, plugs, sockets, electric appliances, and I, U
                    other items with descriptions placed below telling of the safe
                    ways to use these items.

Excursion   46 Visit the firehouse.   P, I, U
                47 Children walk around the school to locate fire hazards or be-   P, I, U
                    come familiar with the locations of extinguishers, exits, and
                    alarm boxes.
                48 Visit a fireboat.   P, I, U

Exhibit   49 Invite the fire department to display fire-fighting equipment   P, I, U
                    and its uses.
                50 Display a variety of combustible materials, such as paper,   P, I, U
                    wood, cloth, gasoline, and kerosene.
                51 Display books, magazines, pamphlets, and stories about fire   P, I, U
                    safety for pupil use.
                52 Show pictures and materials of fire hazards, such as overload of P, I, U
                    electrical circuits, trash accumulation, frayed electric wires,
                    and gasoline storage containers.

SAFETY—cont'd

		Grades
Experience chart or record	53 Prepare an experience chart or record about fire safety.	P
Experiment	54 Place a lighted candle on a table and let the class watch it burn. Cover the candle with a clear glass so that no air can enter. Have pupils note what happens to the candle—it goes out when the oxygen supply has been used. Relate this to extinguishing fires.	P, I, U
Flip chart	55 Prepare a series of illustrated flip charts for a discussion about fire safety. Include answers to these questions: how is fire helpful? What are the causes of fire? How many fires occur in our community? How can we prevent fires?	P, I
Games	56 Make crossword puzzles, riddles, and other games about fire prevention and fire safety.	P, I, U
Guest speaker	57 Invite a fire fighter to discuss fire safety.	P, I, U
	58 Invite the fire chief from your local fire department to discuss the junior fire marshall program and to encourage children to participate.	I
	59 Request the local fire department to conduct a demonstration of the types of fire extinguishers and smoke detectors.	U
	60 Invite a member of the National Board of Fire Underwriters Laboratory to discuss the work of this organization in fire safety.	U
Individual and group reports	61 Write stories about their experiences in fire safety.	P, I
	62 Write to insurance companies and others concerned with fire safety and request materials for display and class reading.	I, U
	63 Prepare oral or written reports on the causes, effects, and prevention of fires.	I, U
	64 Write articles for the school newspaper about fire safety.	I, U
	65 Student prepared report on baby-sitting and fire safety.	I, U
Inspection	66 Prepare checklist to search for fire hazards in home or school.	I, U
Map	67 Prepare a map of your community identifying the locations of firehouses, hydrants, alarm boxes, and other fire safety features.	I, U
	68 Students prepare home escape from fire plans in consultation with parents.	P, I
Models	69 Construct a fire alarm box, a firehouse, and fire prevention equipment for use in dramatic play.	P
	70 Make fire fighter hats out of construction paper.	P, I
	71 Draw or build a home that is free of fire hazards.	I, U
Mural	72 Prepare a mural of ways to prevent fires.	P, I
Poems and songs	73 Create and learn poems, songs, jingles, and stories about fire safety.	P, I
Posters	74 Conduct a contest for the best school poster on fire safety.	I, U

SAFETY—cont'd

		Grades
Scrapbook	**75** Pupils prepare scrapbooks containing pictures, photos, stories, poems, newspaper articles, and written reports about fires and fire prevention.	P, I, U
Self-test	**76** Give the following self-test:	I, U

Fire safety

Circle the correct answers to the right. If you do not know the answer, circle the letter "D."

1. A grease fire may be put out by pouring water on it.   T   F   D
2. One should run to extinguish flames when clothes are on fire.   T   F   D
3. A frayed wire on an electric appliance is a dangerous fire hazard.   T   F   D
4. Fire drills are not necessary at schools.   T   F   D
5. It is safe to run a lamp cord under a rug.   T   F   D
6. The leading causes of fire are matches and smoking.   T   F   D
7. A penny is good substitute for a blown-out fuse.   T   F   D
8. "EXIT" on a door means the door leads to the outside.   T   F   D
9. A wood fire may be put out by pouring water on it.   T   F   D
10. Gasoline can be stored safely in glass bottles.   T   F   D
11. Oily rags can catch fire without a match.   T   F   D
12. One should always close the cover of a safety match book before striking a match.   T   F   D

		Grades
Show and tell	**77** Children tell of their experiences with fire, fire engines, and fire fighters.	P
	78 Children identify names, addresses, and home telephone numbers.	P
Survey	**79** Pupils make survey forms to check their homes for fire hazards.	P, I, U
Television box	**80** Students make a movie with a title such as "The day Mary's house burned." Pupils draw pictures of the discovery of the fire and what they did.	P
Word lists	**81** Prepare a list of new words learned about fire prevention.	P, I, U

FIRST AID

		Grades
Bulletin board	**1** Show pictures and drawings that display first-aid procedures to be followed at school.	P, I, U
	2 Display pictures or drawings of poisonous snakes, insects, and plants.	P, I, U
Demonstration	**3** Have nurse or other person demonstrate how to cleanse a wound with soap and water, apply a sterile dressing and bandage, and stop a nosebleed and other bleeding.	P, I, U
	4 Demonstrate the correct procedure for removing foreign objects from the eye.	I, U
	5 Provide for a demonstration of the mouth-to-mouth procedure of artificial respiration.	I, U
Discussion	**6** What to do when injured at school, home, or when away from home.	P, I, U

SAFETY—cont'd

		Grades
	7 First-aid procedures for sunburn, chapped skin, poison oak or ivy, insect bites and stings.	P, I, U
	8 Discuss reasons for cleansing wounds and applying sterile dressings and bandages.	P, I, U
	9 First-aid procedures for minor cuts, burns, and bruises.	P, I, U
	10 Dog bites and the necessary first-aid procedures as well as other action that must be taken.	P, I, U
	11 First-aid procedures for bone fractures.	I, U
	12 The general first-aid procedures when accidents occur.	I, U
Dramatization	13 Children play doctor or nurse attending a child who has been injured.	P
	14 Dramatize the reporting of an accident at school, at home, and elsewhere.	P, I
	15 The procedure to follow in an emergency or when someone is injured.	P, I, U
	16 Dramatize a series of injuries and then permit the class to try to determine the first-aid procedures to be followed: A boy is using a penknife at school and whittling on some wood; a girl is running her hand along a wooden bench that is full of splinters; a boy is tackled playing touch football and falls, striking his wrist on the ground.	I, U
Drawings	17 Pupils prepare drawings of first aid being administered to injured children.	P, I
Exhibit	18 Display a variety of poisonous substances or containers that hold such materials.	P, I
	19 Display the contents of a simple first-aid kit. Nurse may be helpful in determining items to be included.	I, U
	20 Display an assortment of materials such as dressings, bandages, triangular bandages, and splints used in first aid.	I, U
Experience chart or record	21 Construct an experience chart or record that describes what to do when injured at school.	P
Guest speaker	22 Invite the school nurse to come to class to discuss first-aid procedures.	P, I, U
Individual and group reports	23 Children prepare reports on first-aid procedures for snake bites, epileptic seizures, frostbite, fractures.	I, U
	24 Children prepare a letter inviting a member of the Red Cross to come to class to discuss first aid.	I, U
Problem solving	25 Present a series of first-aid problems to individuals or committees and let them try to solve them. Such problems might include:	U

What would you do if your mother cut her finger while preparing dinner?

What would you do if your sister swallowed a poison, such as ammonia?

What would you do if a pupil at school fell from the horizontal bar that is 7 feet high?

	SAFETY—cont'd	Grades

Scrapbook	26 Make scrapbooks containing stories, pictures, magazine articles, and drawings about first aid.	I, U
Self-test	27 Prepare a self-test for use in the discussion on first aid.	I, U
Show and tell	28 Children tell of their experiences when injured.	P

HOME SAFETY

Bulletin board	1 Display pictures and magazine and newspaper articles on home accidents and safety.	P, I, U
	2 Pupils construct for display a graph or pie-shaped chart showing the numbers and types of home accidents.	U
Discussion	3 Children's prepared lists of hazardous conditions in and around the home.	P, I
	4 Student-planned "pick-up" day at home to remove hazards.	P, I
	5 Children's observations of safe and unsafe practices in the home and elsewhere.	P, I
	6 The causes and possible ways to prevent the accidents reported in newspaper articles brought to class by students.	I, U
	7 The safe handling of blasting caps and the procedures to follow when they are found.	I, U
	8 How to turn off the electricity and the gas at home.	U
	9 Prepare a list of responsibilities of baby-sitters and discuss the safety problems that sitters may have to handle.	U
Dramatization	10 Children play house the safe way by storing knives and matches properly, by using scissors carefully, by keeping stairs and closets clear of objects, and by putting away pins, needles, and other sharp objects when not in use.	P
	11 Children act out such situations as a stranger offering a ride, a cross dog barring the sidewalk, and one child double-daring another to do something reckless. Ask pupils to consider these questions: "What would you do?" "Why would this be a safe thing to do?"	P, I
	12 Dramatize an accident in the home, such as slipping on a scatter rug that has no rubber backing, and discuss how this could have been prevented.	I, U
	13 Prepare a play on home safety for presentation to the Parent-Teachers' Association or to a school assembly.	I, U
Drawings	14 Following a discussion on safe play areas at home, children draw pictures of where they play at home.	P
	15 Following a unit on home safety, each child draws pictures of what he or she does at home to make it a safer place.	P
Exhibit	16 Children bring some of the dangerous objects found in their back yards for display.	P, I
	17 Children construct a medicine cabinet using cardboard boxes and construction paper and have all items properly labeled.	P, I
	18 Prepare an exhibit of hazardous objects or materials found in the home such as metal toys with sharp edges, sharp knives improperly stored, rugs without rubber backing, and oily rags improperly stored.	P, I, U

SAFETY—cont'd Grades

| | 19 | Display pamphlets, booklets, and other resource materials on home safety for pupils' use. | I, U |

19 Display pamphlets, booklets, and other resource materials on home safety for pupils' use. — I, U

20 Display poisonous substances found in the home, such as ammonia, disinfectants, drugs, chocolate laxatives, moth balls, and crayons. — I, U

Experience chart or record
21 Prepare an experience chart on home safety containing such activities as walking carefully on polished floors, picking up toys when finished with them, and not playing with matches. — P

Flannelboard
22 Prepare home safety stories and use a flannelboard to illustrate them. — P

Game
23 Make a human train that must stop at railroad crossings before picking up full speed again. Signals to start and stop are given by the teacher. — P

Guest speaker
24 Invite a representative from the National Safety Council or the local safety council to come to class to discuss home safety. — I, U

Individual and group reports
25 Pupils use drawings or pictures to illustrate daily activities that will keep themselves safe. — I, U

26 Collect newspaper articles about accidents in the home and categorize them by types. Committees then do research and write reports about how they could have been prevented. — I, U

Model
27 Make a container for father's used razor blades. — P

28 Pupils construct a cross section of a house out of cardboard or wood and illustrate the possible hazardous places within. — I, U

Mural
29 Make a large cooperative mural of safe play areas in the neighborhood. — P, I

Newspaper
30 Pupils prepare a home safety newspaper to be published periodically containing stories about safety in the home. — I, U

Panel
31 Have a panel discussion on the topic, "Making a safe home." — I, U

Posters
32 Make posters showing how to correct hazardous conditions found in the home, such as not touching radio or electric light cords when bathing, proper position of cooking utensils on stove with handles turned in, and using a step-ladder rather than a chair to stand on. — I, U

Scrapbook
33 Children prepare a scrapbook with pictures, stories, and newspaper articles on "Safety at home." — P, I, U

Show and tell
34 Children tell about home accidents. — P

Songs and poems
35 Create home safety songs and poems. — P

Survey
36 Survey the neighborhood and prepare a report on the safe and unsafe places to play. — I, U

37 Conduct a survey of home hazards using a checklist prepared by children. Discuss how these problems can be changed. Emphasize specific areas such as unlighted, cluttered stairs; unscreened fire places; electric outlets and wiring; proper place to store garden tools, matches, nails, pins, sewing needles. — I, U

SAFETY—cont'd   Grades

	38 Prepare a home safety checklist for inspection of home work-shops.	U
Telephone card	39 Make a card to be hung by the telephone with the number of the fire and police departments, an ambulance, the family doctor, the nearest relative, and also the home address.	P, I
Telephone number	40 Children dial home telephone number and give the last name of parent, address, identity of road and street landmarks.	P, I

PEDESTRIAN SAFETY

Bulletin board	1 Prepare a display of student drawings about pedestrian safety.	P, I, U
	2 Develop pedestrian safety slogans for use on the bulletin board such as "Courtesy is safety," "Cross at the crosswalks," and "Wait for the traffic signal before crossing streets."	P, I
	3 Make a series of charts or graphs for display showing the number and kinds of pedestrian accidents.	U
Chart	4 Prepare a chart that lists the pedestrian safety rules.	P, I
Demonstration	5 Demonstrate and practice the proper way to cross streets.	P, I
	6 Prepare a table simulating a street corner using small cars, bicycles, policeman, and traffic lights and demonstrate safe pedestrian practices.	P, I
	7 Darken room and have students dressed in various colored clothes walk in front of the room. Be sure to have someone wearing white among these students. Children discuss which colors were more easily seen.	P, I, U
	8 In a darkened room have two lighted flashlights representing auto headlights. Have a student with dark clothes and one with white clothes walk in front of the lights to show the difference in the reflection of light.	P, I, U
Discussion	9 The importance of knowing names, addresses, and telephone numbers.	P
	10 What action to take if a stranger invites you to take a ride in an automobile.	P, I
	11 The school safety patrol and its role in helping children to cross streets safely.	P, I
Dramatization	12 Children bring small toy cars, trucks, and buses for use in dramatic play about pedestrian safety.	P
	13 Using a large space in the classroom or on the playground, lay out an intersection with strips of tape or chalk, including crosswalks, and have children cross the street properly. Prepare a number of crossing signal models, such as a traffic light with appropriate color, a walk-wait signal, and a stop sign.	P
Drawings	14 Children make drawings about pedestrian safety.	P, I
	15 Children draw pictures of how they come to school, pointing out safe practices.	P
Excursion	16 Visit the street corner nearest the school to see the traffic signals, the police officer, the yellow crossing lines, and other safety features.	P

SAFETY—cont'd   **Grades**

Exhibit	17 Display variety of traffic signs and discuss their meanings for traffic and pedestrian safety.	I, U
Experience chart and record	18 Prepare an experience chart or record of safety pedestrian rules that may include:	P

Red means stop.
Yellow means wait.
Green means go.
Cross at the crosswalks.

Flannelboard	19 Prepare illustrations to tell a story of pedestrian safety with emphasis on the danger of playing between parked cars.	P, I
Game	20 Write safety rules on strips of tagboard and cut them in half to form a simple puzzle. Children try to match the cut pieces and locate the correct safety rules.	P, I
Guest speaker	21 Invite a police officer to discuss pedestrian and traffic safety.	P, I, U
	22 Invite a member of the school safety patrol to discuss correct ways to cross streets.	P, I
Individual and group report	23 Record the number and type of pedestrian accidents listed in local newspapers for a designated period.	I, U
	24 Write letters to the National Safety Council, automobile clubs, and other community organizations requesting material on pedestrian safety for use in class.	I, U
	25 Pupils prepare oral or written reports on the number, kinds, and cause of pedestrian accidents.	U
Interview	26 Pupils interview a traffic police officer and a representative of the automobile club about pedestrian accidents and how to prevent them.	I, U
Map	27 Prepare a large map showing the route each child takes to school and discuss the safest ways to come to school.	P, I
Model	28 Make a traffic signal box with red, green, and yellow lights or signals for use in dramatic play.	P
Poems	29 Children create and learn poems about pedestrian safety such as the following:	P

Red says stop,
Green says go.
Yellow says wait,
You'd better go slow.
When I reach a crossing place,
To left and right I turn my face.
I walk, not run, across the street
And use my head to guide my feet.

Stop, look, and listen
Before you cross the street.
Use your eyes, use your ears
Before you use your feet.

Posters	30 Prepare posters and enter them in the school contest on pedestrian safety.	I, U

SAFETY—cont'd   **Grades**

Problem solving	31 Have children discuss this problem: "You come to a street corner that you must cross, but there is no signal. How will you get across?"	P, I
Puppets	32 Make puppets and dramatize ways to be a safe pedestrian.	P
Quiz	33 Have children write the five numbers listed below on a piece of paper and place yes or no answers beside the appropriate number.	P

1. We should cross streets at crosswalks.
2. We should cross streets when the traffic light is green.
3. We should look one way when crossing streets.
4. We should always go with the traffic when walking on highways.
5. We know the yellow light at a crosswalk means wait.

Riddle	34 Children make up riddles, such as the following:	P

It stands near the corner.
It turns red and green.
It helps keep us safe.
What is it?

Scrapbook	35 Make illustrated scrapbooks with pedestrian safety rules, slogans, rhymes, and limericks.	P, I, U
	36 Prepare a scrapbook of pictures and drawings showing safety as a pedestrian.	P, I
Self-test	37 Pupils take following self-test.	I, U

Do you   YES   NO

1. Cross streets only at intersections or marked crosswalks? ☐ ☐
2. Look left and right before crossing, making sure that the entire crossing can be made safely? ☐ ☐
3. Cross only on green light or "go" signals? ☐ ☐
4. Obey directions of traffic boys or officers? ☐ ☐
5. Walk on the left side facing traffic if walking on roadway and give way to approaching vehicles? ☐ ☐
6. Wear white at night or carry a light? ☐ ☐
7. Always get into and out of a vehicle on the side nearest the curb? ☐ ☐
8. Give the motorist the right of way where there are no signals? ☐ ☐
9. Stay out of streets when playing? ☐ ☐
10. Watch for oncoming traffic when catching or leaving a bus? ☐ ☐

Score ("yes" answers)

9-10—You may live to a ripe old age.
6-8—You may expect to get hurt before long.
5 or less—Stay in your own yard; you're living on borrowed time.

Show and tell	38 Children tell about pedestrian hazards they have seen.	P
Television box	39 Make a shadow box or television box and have students prepare a series of drawings about pedestrian safety. Include such illustrations as wearing white at night, crossing at street corners, and waiting for the green light.	P

RECREATION SAFETY	SAFETY—cont'd	Grades

Bulletin board   **1** Prepare displays of pictures and drawings of water skiing, hunting, camping, picnicking, fishing, skating, hiking, and vacation safety.   P, I, U

2 Display posters or drawings showing the correct and incorrect ways to get in and out of rowboats, canoes, and motorboats.   P, I, U

Chart   **3** Pupils prepare and complete charts of summertime safety for reference and use at home during vacation.   I, U

Summertime safety

My summer activities

1. _____

2. _____

3. _____

4. _____

What could hurt me

1. _____

2. _____

3. _____

4. _____

How to keep safe

1. _____

2. _____

3. _____

4. _____

Demonstration   **4** Have the Red Cross conduct a demonstration of swimming, boating, and beach safety at one of the local swimming pools, lakes, or rivers.   P, I, U

Discussion   **5** Safety on special occasions, such as Halloween and the Fourth of July.   P, I, U

6 The people who can help when you are injured or lost.   P, I, U

7 Safety on picnics and outings.   P, I, U

	SAFETY—cont'd	**Grades**
	8 Show pupils pictures of recreational equipment, such as a canoe, gun, skate, sled, ski, baseball bat, and fishhook, and have them tell of a good safety practice when using these items.	P, I, U
	9 Safe and unsafe features of swimming in lakes, rivers, oceans, canals, and other places. Learn how to choose a safe swimming area.	I, U
	10 The laws with which pupils should be familiar when hunting, fishing, and camping.	I, U
	11 Methods of protection while participating in various sports, such as football, baseball, basketball, and skiing.	I, U
	12 Safety in skin and scuba diving.	I, U
	13 Safe hunting procedures.	U
Dramatization	14 Children participate in dramatic play of safe practices while camping or picnicking.	P
	15 Prepare and present a skit on snow safety to an assembly, the Parent-Teacher's Association, or broadcast it over the local radio station.	I, U
	16 Pupils write a play ("Comedy of Errors") on how not to go on a camping trip.	I, U
Drawings	17 Make drawings of safe practices while boating, swimming, skiing, playing in the snow or at the beach.	P, I, U
Exhibit	18 Display the items of a "Lost" kit that may be usable when camping or out in the woods that contains such things as a single-edge razor blade, fishhooks, fish line and wet flies, pencil and notebook, Band-aids, soap and disinfectant, nail magnet and thread (for compass), sugar lumps, strong string (shoe laces), and matches water-proofed with paraffin. Seal the contents in a pipe tobacco can and attach with a belt strap.	P, I, U
	19 Display such hazardous objects as fishhooks, darts, sharp-pointed sticks, and blasting caps.	P, I, U
	20 Display the appropriate clothing to wear in various outdoor activities, such as hiking, camping, hunting, skiing, and boating.	P, I, U
	21 Display the equipment needed for skin and scuba diving and discuss safety features.	I, U
	22 Display safety items that give protection in various sports: football—mouth protectors; baseball—mask; skiing—safety binders.	I, U
Experience chart or record	23 Make an experience chart or record about safe procedures on vacations, when swimming, and at other times.	P
Game	24 Play the game "Little child lost." The teacher is a police officer and a student is lost. Have children determine what they would do, or should do, if this happens to them.	P
	25 Children collect pictures from magazines and newspapers of safe and unsafe ways of playing. Place all of these in a box and permit each child to select one item and tell whether it is a safe or unsafe procedure.	P, I, U

			Grades
		SAFETY—cont'd	
Guest speaker	26	Invite a member of the Red Cross or the school nurse to discuss first-aid procedures for possible recreation emergencies, such as sunburn, poisonous plants and insects, and blisters.	P, I, U
	27	Have a forest ranger discuss safe procedures in parks and playgrounds.	P, I, U
	28	Have a representative from the Red Cross or a skin and scuba diving club discuss the safety aspects of this sport.	I, U
	29	Invite guest speakers to discuss safety in such activities as football, basketball, skiing, tennis, and swimming.	I, U
	30	Have a member of the local rifle club demonstrate and discuss safety while hunting or the safe handling of guns.	U
Individual and group reports	31	Pupils prepare oral and written reports on the safety rules when camping, boating, hiking, fishing, swimming, hunting, skiing, and roller or ice skating.	I, U
	32	Pupils write report of their favorite recreational activities and include the safety rules that should be observed when participating.	I, U
Map	33	Prepare a map showing the safe swimming area in the immediate vicinity and within a comfortable driving distance from the local community.	I, U
Mural	34	Make a mural of safe places and safe ways to play while skiing, boating, swimming, hiking, skating, and others.	P, I, U
Puppet	35	Prepare a puppet show or dramatization of a safe camping or hiking trip.	P, I
Scrapbooks	36	Pupils prepare scrapbooks containing pictures, newspaper and magazine articles, stories, and other items on safety categorized into such areas as fishing, camping, swimming, boating, hunting, skiing, and skating.	I, U

SCHOOL SAFETY

			Grades
Bulletin board	1	Prepare a display of pictures and drawings showing safety at school.	P, I, U
Cartoon	2	Conduct a school safety cartoon or slogan contest.	I, U
Chart	3	Pupils prepare a chart or graph of the nature, number, and location of accidents that occur in school.	I, U
Demonstration	4	The safe use of tools, blocks, and other equipment.	P, I
	5	The safe way to use stairways, drinking fountains, and school equipment.	P, I
	6	The safe way to use playground apparatus and equipment, such as slides, swings, bats, and tetherballs.	P, I
Discussion	7	School safety helpers, such as the teacher, nurse, custodian, and bus driver.	P
	8	The dangers of throwing sticks, climbing fences, throwing balls improperly, and running in the hallf or crowded areas.	P, I
	9	The proper use of fountain pens, scissors, and other implements in class as well as the proper way to open doors and walk in the corridors.	P, I

	SAFETY—cont'd	**Grades**
	10 Prepare a list of safety rules for the classroom and the play- ground that may include:	P, I

I walk in the halls.
I use the slides properly.
I use scissors and pencils carefully.
I do not push when in line.
I do not throw rocks and other objects.

	11 What to do when injured at school.	P, I, U
	12 School and playground hazards and accidents.	P, I, U
Dramatization	13 Make puppets and dramatize safety practices at school.	P
	14 Dramatize safety precautions when playing softball, lining up in the cafeteria, waiting for the bus, and other situations.	P, I, U
Drawings	15 Make drawings of play areas and equipment and write cap- tions about school safety below.	P, I,
Excursion	16 Walk around the school and locate hazards to safety.	P, I
Exhibit	17 Children prepare drawings on safety in school, such as keep- ing feet under tables and desks, not pulling chairs away from others, and the incorrect way to use the drinking fountain.	P, I
Experience chart or record	18 Prepare an experience chart or record of safe practices in school.	P
Flannelboard	19 Make two children out of construction paper (or make draw- ings) and call them "Safety Sam" and "Silly Billy." Tell a story about school safety including these two characters and use drawings to illustrate their activities.	P, I

Safety Sam
  waits in line.
  stops the swing and gets off.
  uses pencils properly.

Silly Billy
  pushes in line.
  jumps off the swing.
  jabs pencils in his hand.

Guest speaker	20 Invite a physical education teacher or the supervisor of physi- cal education to discuss and demonstrate safety on the play- ground.	P, I, U
Handbook	21 A committee of pupils prepares an illustrated handbook of safe practices at school for distribution to all students.	I, U
Individual and group reports	22 Pupils or pupil committees prepare articles for the school newspaper on school safety.	I, U
	23 Pupils prepare written reports on the causes of school acci- dents and ways to prevent them.	I, U
Interview	24 A committee of pupils interviews the school nurse to find out how accidents occur in the school. After reporting their find- ings in class, they formulate a plan of prevention.	I, U

SAFETY—cont'd Grades

Map	25 Prepare a composite map of the neighborhood indicating the location of the traffic lights, stop signs, police officers, and sidewalks. Have students draw the safest way home using colored crayons or yarn. Children may also prepare individual maps to be taken home to parents.	P, I
	26 Draw map of the school grounds and illustrate safe and unsafe places to play.	I, U
	27 Plot locations of accidents on map of school and school grounds.	I, U
	28 Teacher prepares map of school showing drinking fountains, bicycle racks, incinerators, and other places. Place on bulletin board and children mark the hazardous places in school and locate accidents that occur.	P, I
Panel	29 Have panel discussion on "Safety at school."	I, U
Problem solving	30 Discuss solutions to these safety problems:	P, I

A boy runs from the cafeteria with an ice cream stick in his mouth.
Two groups walking in the corridor meet at a corner.
One student opens a door and bumps two boys standing in the corridor.
A boy throws his bat while playing in a softball game.
A girl steps in front of another girl who is using the swing.

	31 Form a school safety committee to locate hazardous school areas and to plan ways to prevent accidents.	I, U
Questionnaire	32 Prepare a "Do you remember?" questionnaire as a concluding activity to the unit on school safety. Include fifteen to twenty questions to be answered verbally by yes or no, such as, "Do I always walk down the halls and stairways properly?"	P, I
Songs and poems	33 Create songs, poems, stories, and drawings about school safety.	P
Survey	34 Children conduct a hazard hunt on school property and remove such objects as glass, rocks, wire, tacks, and nails.	P, I
	35 Children are "safety detectives" and locate examples of safety at school.	P, I
	36 Pupils prepare a safety checklist and then survey the school for hazards.	I, U

TOBACCO*

Buzz group	1 Conduct a buzz group discussion on the question, "Should teenagers smoke tobacco?"	U
Chart	2 Pupils prepare charts for bulletin board displays regarding the rise in death rates of major diseases associated with smoking; comparison of overall death rates of smokers and nonsmokers; location of disorders associated with smoking on an outline figure of the human body; computation of the cost of smoking one to two packages of cigarettes a day or a week for 1 year and listing of other uses of the same amount of money.	I, U

*Check the local lung association or the American Cancer Society for resources and material aids.

	TOBACCO—cont'd	**Grades**
Debate	**3** Have a debate on the use of tobacco by teenagers. Try to answer the questions: "Should teenagers smoke?" "Should tobacco advertising in newspapers and magazines be controlled?"	U
Demonstration	**4** Prepare materials as shown in Fig. 11-20. Open and close pinch clamp (acts as siphon—water may need to be replaced several times) to stimulate puffing on cigarette and observe (a) smoke collecting, (b) color of water after shaking flask, and (c) residue on walls of flask. Later discuss relationships to lung tissue in persons who smoke. Place pieces of cotton in glass tube between cigarette and flask without stopping up tube. After smoking several cigarettes (use siphon action previously mentioned), remove cotton and examine. Wipe tar-stained cotton on growing plants and observe results (abnormal growths will appear).	I, U
	5 Blow cigarette smoke through a clean handkerchief or paper tissue with and without inhaling. Observe difference in amount of residue and relate to lung tissue.	I, U
	6 Place a drop of solution containing paramecia on a microscopic slide and observe movement under the low-power lens of a microscope. Blow smoke on the slide and observe the effect on the paramecia.	I, U
	7 Wipe a cotton pellet that has been saturated with tobacco tars on the tongue of a live frog and note the frog's temporary collapse.	I, U
	8 Make a nicotine insecticide by soaking cotton pellets from a smoking machine or cigarette tobacco in water. Test and use as a spray on insects.	I, U
	9 Prepare a smoking machine, using materials shown in Fig. 11-18. Insert loosely packed cotton into the tubing and put a cigarette into the open end of tubing. Press firmly on the plastic container to force air out before lighting the cigarette, and then proceed with slow and regular pumping action. Later, cotton can be withdrawn from tubing to show the accumulation of tar.	I, U
	10 Prepare a smoking machine using materials shown in Fig. 11-19. Light the cigarette and pump the vacuum so as to draw smoke from cigarette into gallon jar and water until the cigarette is burned completely. Use additional cigarettes until tars can be seen in the water and around the jar. Cotton can be inserted in tubing behind the cigarette and examined later for tars.	I, U
Discussion	**11** The nature of tobacco smoke.	I, U
	12 The physiologic effects of tobacco on the human body.	I, U
	13 The relationship of the use of tobacco to lung cancer.	I, U
	14 Analyze the claims of several tobacco advertisements.	6, 7, 8
	15 Why people smoke.	6, 7, 8
	16 Laws related to smoking.	6, 7, 8
Dramatization	**17** Prepare a skit illustrating social pressures used by students to get others to smoke. Follow with a discussion regarding actions pupils should take to handle such situations.	U

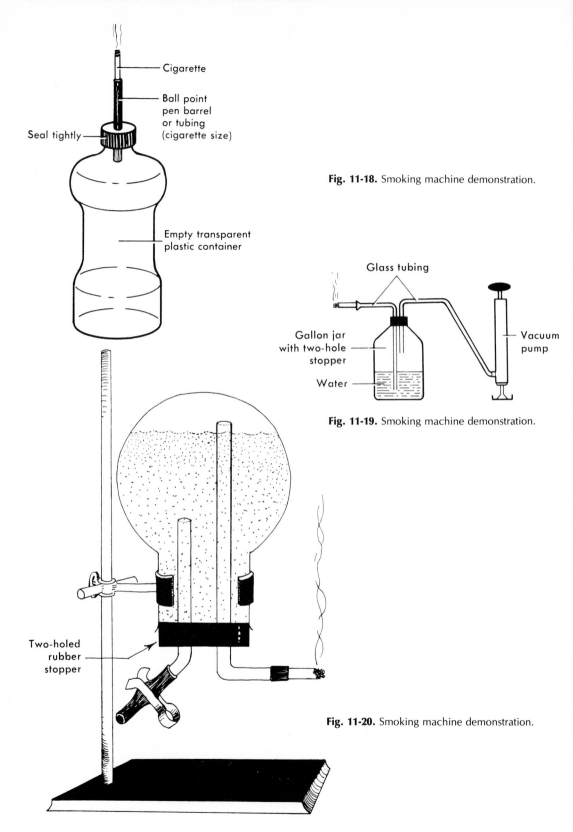

Cigarette

Ball point
pen barrel
or tubing
(cigarette size)

Seal tightly

Empty transparent
plastic container

Fig. 11-18. Smoking machine demonstration.

Glass tubing

Gallon jar
with two-hole
stopper

Water

Vacuum
pump

Fig. 11-19. Smoking machine demonstration.

Two-holed
rubber
stopper

Fig. 11-20. Smoking machine demonstration.

	TOBACCO—cont'd	Grades
Exhibit	18 Display a variety of brands and kinds of cigarettes. Break open several and show the types of filter tips.	6, 7, 8
	19 Display magazines, pamphlets, and other materials for student reference and use.	6, 7, 8
	20 Display newspaper and magazine articles on the use of tobacco.	6, 7, 8
	21 Display a variety of advertisements found in newspapers and magazines.	6, 7, 8
	22 Display a variety of charts and graphs available from the American Cancer Society on the extent and effect of smoking.	U
	23 Obtain samples of lungs of smoker and nonsmoker from the American Cancer Society.	I, U
Experiment	24 Obtain some nicotine and dissolve it in water in a fish bowl. Place a tadpole in the bowl and observe the results.	6, 7, 8
	25 Prepare two bowls or jars. One should contain plain water and a tadpole or small fish and the other should contain nicotine or tobacco smoke (Fig. 11-20) dissolved in water. After pupils observe the activity of the fish in the plain water, remove the fish and place it in the bowl with the nicotine and smoke. Have pupils observe results and draw conclusions. Promptly remove fish to plain water to revive soon after observations.	I, U
Graph	26 Pupils prepare graphs showing the incidence of heart disease, lung cancer, and emphysema among smokers and nonsmokers as well as the costs of smoking cigarettes yearly.	U
Guest speaker	27 Invite a physician to discuss and answer questions about the effect of tobacco on health.	6, 7, 8
Individual and group reports	28 Pupils investigate the laws regarding the sale of tobacco to minors.	U
	29 Pupils prepare oral and written reports on recent magazine articles about tobacco.	6, 7, 8
	30 Pupils prepare oral and written reports on emphysema, chronic bronchitis, lung cancer, effectiveness of filter tipped cigarettes, and the number of cigarettes sold.	6, 7, 8
	31 Students prepare individual notebooks on tobacco and health, including analysis of advertising, magazine article summaries, research data, and pictures.	I, U
Interview	32 Interview the local health officer for information about the incidence of lung cancer in the community.	U
	33 A committee of children interviews one or more physicians about the effect of tobacco on health.	U
	34 Ask people who smoke and do not smoke for their advice on making decision to smoke or not to smoke.	U
Newspaper	35 Prepare articles for the school newspaper as part of an antismoking campaign.	U
Parents	36 Involve parents in an antismoking campaign program with students writing letters against smoking, distributing pamphlets, or inviting them to see a film at school.	6, 7, 8
Self-test	37 Conduct a self-test on tobacco.	6, 7, 8

TOBACCO—cont'd

What do you know about smoking?

Circle the correct answers to the right. If you do not know the answer, circle the letter "D."

1. Smoking reduces the appetite.	T F D
2. Smoking irritates the throat.	T F D
3. Inhaling causes a smoker to absorb more nicotine.	T F D
4. Smoking may become a habit.	T F D
5. Teenagers frequently start smoking because they want to act like adults.	T F D
6. Some people smoke to relieve tension.	T F D
7. Smoke from tobacco may be annoying and unpleasant to other persons.	T F D
8. Smoking causes lung cancer.	T F D
9. Filter-tipped cigarettes prevent the absorption of nicotine into the body.	T F D
10. The use of tobacco causes a shortness of breath.	T F D

Grades

Survey

38 A committee of pupils conducts a survey of opinions of parents, friends, doctors, coaches, and teachers on the use of tobacco by teenagers. U

39 Conduct a survey of the smoking habits of pupils in the class. Have pupils post results on the bulletin board in the form of a bar graph. U

Smoking questionnaire

Check only one statement that best describes your smoking habits at present.

☐ 1. I smoke half a pack of cigarettes or more just about every day.

☐ 2. I smoke cigarettes just about every day, but less than half a pack a day.

☐ 3. I do not smoke cigarettes every day, but I do smoke them at least 1 day a week.

☐ 4. I have smoked cigarettes (including trying them to see what they were like) but do not now smoke them regularly, at least 1 day a week.

☐ 5. I have never smoked cigarettes at all.

Check one: ☐ Boy   ☐ Girl
Present school grade: ☐ 7   ☐ 8
Age: ☐ 11   ☐ 12   ☐ 13   ☐ 14   ☐ 15

SUMMARY

Methods and techniques of teaching health are extremely important in the instruction program that seeks the development of health practices and attitudes based on scientific information. Teachers who are familiar with the variety of activities described in this chapter and are competent in the selection of appropriate ones will have effective health education programs.

QUESTIONS FOR DISCUSSION

1. What is the role of the teacher in the learning process in health education?
2. What is the meaning of the terms "method" and "technique"?
3. What related factors to learning must receive teacher consideration?
4. What are the types of methods that contribute to effective health teaching and what are illustrations of each to health education?
5. What are the advantages and disadvantages of the various types of methods of teaching that may be used in the health instruction program?
6. What guidelines help the teacher determine the methods of health teaching to be used in the primary, intermediate, and upper grades?
7. What is meant by the term "incidents" or "incidental teaching" in health education with illustrations?
8. What are the limitations and possible problems in the use of incidents in health teaching?
9. How should the textbook be used when teaching health?
10. How can instructional materials be used effectively with methods in health teaching?
11. What are several ways students may be used in peer education programs?
12. What are the relationships between the objectives of health education and the techniques in teaching?
13. What factors should receive consideration when selecting activities and experiences for health teaching?
14. What are several activities or experiences suitable for health teaching in the primary, intermediate, and upper grades?
15. What are several health areas in which bulletin boards may be used in health teaching?
16. What are several demonstrations that are suitable for the primary, intermediate, and upper grades when teaching health?
17. In what grades is the use of buzz groups and self-tests probably most appropriate?
18. What are several experiments suitable for teaching fire safety, dental health, nutrition, and communicable disease control?
19. What are several illustrations of dramatic play that are usable in health teaching?
20. What are some examples of the use of the flannel-board in the health instruction program?
21. How can models, charts, and graphs be specifically used in the teaching of health?
22. What are several teaching techniques that may be used in the value clarification process?

SUGGESTED CLASS ACTIVITIES

1. Interview teachers to discover the kinds of health teaching methods used in the kindergarten-primary, intermediate, and upper grades.
2. Discuss the importance and relationships of methods in the teaching of health.
3. Discuss the types of methods used in health teaching.
4. Prepare a checklist of types of methods and have teachers rate them as to their importance in teaching health.
5. Discuss the criteria for the selection of methods in health teaching.
6. Prepare a sequence of questions for use in a question and answer session on some phase of health. Specify the grade level for which the questions are intended and where and why they should be used.
7. Prepare an outline to show how a field trip may be used effectively to introduce a unit on foods and nutrition, fire safety, or community health.
8. Discuss the use of incidents in health teaching.
9. Prepare an exhibit of teaching aids and discuss or prepare reports on ways to use these materials in health teaching.
10. Review a variety of health textbooks.
11. Prepare a series of strategies or procedures for teaching family health, drugs, and mental health using the value clarification approach.
12. Develop a venereal disease instruction program for use by junior high school students in peer education.
13. Prepare bulletin boards in specific health areas for the primary, intermediate, and upper grades.
14. Discuss occasions to use buzz groups, discussions, guest speakers, self-tests, and other teaching techniques.
15. Discuss the advantages and weaknesses of various types of teaching techniques.
16. Prepare reports on activities or experiences by subject area and include the following: grade for which suitable, concept or concepts emphasized in the lesson, detailed description of activities including illustrations, and the materials needed.
17. Create poems, songs, riddles, stories, and games for use in the teaching of health.
18. Collect poems, songs, riddles, finger plays, and games usable in health teaching.
19. Prepare several self-tests in a number of health areas to be used in the intermediate and upper grades.

20. Illustrate a variety of experiments usable in health teaching.
21. Collect stories suitable for use in teaching about mental health and other health areas.
22. Conduct several demonstrations and have pupils explore teachers' guides, textbooks, and other resources for additional ones.
23. Demonstrations of various types of activities and experiences.
24. Prepare models and materials for use on the flannelboard.
25. Collect pictures, photos, newspaper clippings, and pamphlets and discuss ways to use these materials in the teaching of health.
26. Discuss the use of films and filmstrips in health teaching.
27. Prepare reports on the plans for a field trip.
28. Prepare survey forms for use when teaching alcohol, tobacco, nutrition, and other health areas.
29. Discuss unit construction and the significance of health teaching techniques.
30. Develop problem-solving activities for specific health areas.
31. Survey in-service teachers to learn the kinds of teaching techniques they have found to be successful.
32. Select activities or experiences that may be appropriately used when teaching selected health concepts or problems and justify these choices.
33. Illustrate the use of activities or experiences when planning health lessons.
34. Prepare a checklist of teaching techniques and survey in-service teachers to learn the grades in which these activities should be used.
35. Prepare several value clarification teaching techniques for use in venereal disease, sex education, and drug education.
36. Conduct a health fair at a local elementary school.

REFERENCES

Alameda County, California: Dependency-producing substances; a teaching unit grades one through twelve, 1968, Office of the Superintendent.
American Association for Health, Physical Education, and Recreation: Drug abuse; escape to nowhere, 1967, Smith, Kline and French Laboratories.
American School Health Association: Health instruction; suggestions for teachers, Journal of School Health, revised, May, 1969.
American School Health Association: How to plan and present a school-community health fair, Journal of School Health 45: Dec., 1975.
Arrigoni, E. A.: Teenage antismoking campaign in elementary schools, School Health Review 3: March-April, 1972.
California Interagency on Cigarette Smoking and Health: Teachers resource kit on smoking and health, 1964.
Calsbeek, F.: Brainstorming health problems; a crea-
tive approach, Journal of School Health 38: Oct., 1968.
Canfield, J., and Wells, H. C.: One-hundred ways to enhance self-concept in the classroom, Englewood Cliffs, N.J., 1976, Prentice-Hall, Inc.
Clark, K. M.: A multimedia approach to mental health, School Health Review 3: March-April, 1972.
Cornacchia, H. J., Smith, D. E., and Bentel, D. J.: Drugs in the classroom; a conceptual model for school programs, ed. 2, St. Louis, 1978, The C. V. Mosby Co.
Dearth, F.: Construction and utilization of visual aids in dental health education, Thorofare, N.J., 1974, Charles B. Slack, Inc.
Dinkmeyer, D., and Ogburn, K. D.: Psychologists priorities; premium on developing understanding of self and others, Psychology in the Schools 11: Jan., 1974.
Ellensburg School District, Washington: Health instruction guides, grades kindergarten-6, 1968-1969, Office of the Superintendent.
Fitzgerald, J. A., and Fitzgerald, P. G.: Methods and curricula in elementary education, Milwaukee, 1955, The Bruce Publishing Co.
Fodor, J. T., and Dalis, G. T.: Health instruction; theory and application, ed. 2, Philadelphia, 1974, Lea & Febiger.
Griffith, M.: Techniques for relating health instruction to the real world, School Health Review 3: March-April, 1972.
Gross, R. E., and McDonald, F. J.: Classroom methods; the problem-solving approach, Phi Delta Kappan 39: March, 1959.
Henry, C. D.: Ideas that worked with black teenagers, School Health Review 4: Jan.-Feb., 1973.
Jones, H.: Smoke, choke, croak; teenagers fight back with a smoke out campaign, National Tuberculosis and Respiratory Disease Association Bulletin, March, 1970.
Kellam, S. G., and others: Mental health and going to school, Chicago, 1975, University of Chicago Press.
McClendon, E. J.: Innovations in health education practice; school and community, Journal of School Health 38: Nov., 1968.
McGuire, R.: Flintstones and Snoopy join the antismoking campaign, School Health Review 3: March-April, 1972.
McNeil, J. D.: Toward appreciation of teaching methods, Phi Delta Kappan 39: March, 1958.
National Clearing House for Smoking and Health: Smoking and health experiments, demonstrations and exhibits, 1968, U.S. Department of Health, Education, and Welfare, Public Health Service.
Osman, J. D.: Value growth through drug education, School Health Review 5: Jan.-Feb., 1974.
Raths, L. E., Harmin, M., and Simon, S. B.: Values and teaching; working with values in the classroom, Columbus, Ohio, 1966, Charles E. Merrill Publishing Co.
Rich, R.: Tests for acidity of the mouth in relation to

susceptibility to dental caries, Journal of School Health **33:** Feb., 1963.

Sasman, E. H.: Classroom methods; do laboratory and field experiences change behavior, Phi Delta Kappan **39:** March, 1958.

Scheer, J. K., and Williams, C.: Using children's stories to teach something we don't talk about (death education), Health Values **1:** May/June, 1977.

Schneeweis, S. M., and Jones, R.: Time-linked health problems; the monthly health specials calendar approach for use in grades K-6, Journal of School Health **38:** Oct., 1968.

Simon, S. B.: Promoting the search for values, School Health Review **2:** Feb., 1971.

Simon, S. B., Howe, L. W., and Kirschenbaum, H.: Value clarification; a handbook of practical strategies for teachers and students, New York, 1972, Hart Publishing Co., Inc.

Sleet, D. A.: The use of games and simulation in health instruction, California School Health **13:** Jan., 1975.

Stovall, T. F.: Classroom methods; lecture versus discussion, Phi Delta Kappan **39:** March, 1958.

Toohy, J. V.: Beatle lyrics can help adolescents identify and understand their emotional health problems, Journal of School Health **40:** June, 1970.

Valett, R. E.: Humanistic education; developing the total person, St. Louis, 1977, The C. V. Mosby Co.

Vincent, E. P.: Early safety education, Health Education **7:** July/Aug., 1976.

Wills, C. D., and Stegman, W. H.: Living in the kindergarten, revised, Chicago, 1957, Follett Corp.

12 Material aids in health teaching

As we have seen, the quality and value of health instruction depends largely on the classroom teacher's effective use of appropriate methods, techniques, and strategies—*and* the careful selection of the best available teaching aids. In wisely choosing and using material aids in health and safety, the teacher faces a challenging task.

Health instruction must be sensitive to the latest and most reliable research and information coming from the broad spectrum of the biologic, social, and physical sciences. Unlike some other areas of the elementary school curriculum, content and concepts in health and safety often change markedly and abruptly with new developments in medicine, public health, dentistry, nutrition, pharmacology, physiology, psychology, physical fitness, first aid and emergency care, and many other disciplines in the health sciences.

Hence, the classroom teacher—involved in a diverse range of subject matter areas—must keep abreast of the significant and applicable contributions of all those fields bearing on personal, family, and community health. To do this the busy teacher needs to know where to find, easily and quickly, scientifically sound information and appealing teaching aids.

Of course, resources and material aids are what the teacher makes of them. Even the best materials may be of little value when teachers use them improperly, ineffectively, or not at all. On the other hand, some teachers, especially those who may feel inadequately prepared in health science, may rely too heavily on certain material aids. This often results in the selection and overuse of mediocre or poor films.* The aware teacher

---
*Staton, W. M.: Monday morning at the movies, School Health Review **6:** Jan.-Feb., 1975.

will find that certain materials are stimulating and effective with some classes but not with others, that some materials are generally useful and others are not, and that there is a "best time" for introducing most material aids.

WHAT ARE MATERIAL AIDS?

The term "material aids to learning" is difficult to define because of its extent and breadth in the field of education. Learning material in the school program is said to be concerned with any material that is used directly with pupils. Moreover, it has been suggested that everything in the pupil's environment that contributes in any way to the learning situation may be considered as an aid to learning. Defined in these broad terms, material aids include all items that teachers and pupils use in enhancing the learning process.

Material aids—both visual and auditory—will be considered as *specific types of aids to learning used in addition to the standard traditional equipment* that is a part of almost every classroom. Consequently, such items as pencils, paper, chalk, chalkboards, and the like are in reality material aids, but they will not be discussed here.

The material aids to learning that we discuss in this chapter consist of a combination of various sensory aids and materials used either by pupils, teachers, or both. Those presented here are offered as examples and as a sampling of the numerous possibilities.

WHAT ARE THE AUDIOVISUAL MATERIALS IN HEALTH EDUCATION?

Various kinds of material aids to learning can be used in many ways. However, the general purpose is to aid the learning process by providing sensory experiences that clarify abstract concepts. These aids are also important motivational devices teachers will find useful.

Teaching aids include bulletin boards, cartoons, charts, pictures and photographs, maps, objects, specimens, models, posters, textbooks, workbooks, programmed instruction guides, newspaper and magazine articles, pamphlets, films, filmstrips, videotapes, cassettes, recordings, songs, radio and television, slides, transparencies, and exhibits.

Bulletin boards may present information using cartoons, charts, graphs, maps, posters, and other illustrative materials. Teachers should be constantly alert to potential bulletin board material relating to health and safety, which may appear in newspapers, magazines, pamphlets, and other printed materials. Students can actively participate in locating and preparing suitable materials for the bulletin board.

Cartoons relating to a wide range of current problems in child health and safety can be produced by the children or selected from newspapers and magazines. Cartoons often provide the qualities of humor and relevancy that can motivate pupils toward improved attitudes and behavior modification. Teachers should take care that the humor does not overshadow the message presented.

Charts and *graphs* and data for these visual aids are readily available from numerous sources and can be prepared by students, teachers, or both. They should not be too involved and complicated but rather should get across one or a few basic ideas or concepts that can be readily perceived and understood by pupils.

Objects, specimens, and *models* may be animate or inanimate. Hamsters may be used in classroom diet studies. On occasion children may bring a pet to class and talk about caring for its health and safety. Specimens, such as lung tissue (smoker and nonsmoker) or the heart of sheep or cattle, can provide realism in certain concept learning situations. Anatomic models—torso, ear, eye, or brain —can help students to better understand the remarkable working interrelationships of body organs and systems in maintaining good health. However, such models should *not*

be used as a medium for rote memorization of body parts.

Textbooks are increasingly available and serve as basic sources for both pupil and teacher. These aids are discussed in greater detail later in the chapter.

Newspaper items, magazine articles, and *books*—both popular paperbacks and reference—offer good sources of information for the teacher and students in connection with research projects, class discussion, and related assignments. Care should be taken to assure that these sources are up to date and scientifically sound.

Poems and *songs* are generally more effective with the younger children in kindergarten and the primary grades. Even with children in these grades the message should be clear and precise, not vague and trite.

Films, filmstrips, videotapes, transparencies, and *slides* are available in many topical areas. Most are commercially produced, though pupils and teachers can prepare some of their own transparencies and slides. Aids of this type can be effective in both the classroom and for parent educational programs.

Television and *radio* both at school and in the home now offer many opportunities for timely and worthwhile health education. "Specials" on both TV and radio deal with health and safety problems of children as well as adults. These are usually accurately presented and analyzed by the networks and many local stations. These two all-pervasive media also provide health news items and public service announcements, the latter usually bringing a message from an official or voluntary health agency or a professional society within the health professions.

Even commercials on TV and radio can be used as a teaching aid. Students can discuss the questions of the validity and reality of commercials promoting products and services for weight reduction, skin problems, nutritional value of foods, eye care, toy safety, beer and wine, motor vehicles (including motor bikes and mopeds), and other health-related items.

Two good examples of well-produced programs for TV and radio are the series "Inside

Out," produced under the direction of National Instructional Television,* and the long-time successful radio science series,† which presents stimulating discussions of up-to-date research in many aspects of the health sciences. These and other programs are available throughout the nation. Information regarding programming schedules is available from the National Instructural Television Center and the University of California, Los Angeles. Videotapes for use in schools can be obtained from the National Instructural Television Center, and printed copies of science edition scripts are available from the University of California, Los Angeles, for a nominal charge.

Exhibits may be the result of a pupil project or they may be bought, rented, or obtained free from commercial sources, health departments, voluntary health agencies, agricultural extension services, military organizations, and professional—medical, dental, nursing—societies. Exhibits should be timely and attractive, should offer a clear message, and should not be left on view for too long a period. They may serve in three ways: (1) motivating participating students, (2) peer education, and (3) parent education.

There is a growing need for a health education materials resource center in each school, or at least one centrally located for schools in small districts. Teachers individually or working together on a health education or overall audiovisual committee can rather easily build up a selected combination of useful material aids for each of the elementary grades. Such a center can provide teachers and students with easy access to stimulating and enriching materials. Another value of significance is the fact that a materials resource center can make an increasing number of special education teaching aids available. With new federal funds being committed to the education of children with certain health problems in the typical

*National Instructional Television Center, Box A, Bloomington, Ind. 47401.
†The Science Editor, University of California, Los Angeles, Calif. 90024.

elementary school setting, resource centers will be able to add more up-to-date materials and equipment to their holdings.

HOW ARE MATERIAL AIDS BEST USED?
What principles guide the teacher in using material aids?

In using material aids to learning in health teaching, teachers should consider certain basic procedures if the best results are to be obtained. In this regard the following suggestions are submitted to guide the teacher in the proper use of material aids.

1. The material aids should be readily accessible. There is nothing more disconcerting for a class than to have to wait for the teacher to locate materials that have been misplaced. When this occurs, continuity and interest in the lesson are often lost.

2. We should remember that the material aids are to be used and not just shown. The teacher must know just how a particular aid to learning fits into a specific situation. The material aids themselves will not do the teaching for the teacher. They should be used as tools in such a way that they will give the lesson more meaning.

3. If there are a number of different material aids to be used, it may be well to use them one at a time in sequence. When it is necessary to show relationships with graphs or charts, it is then feasible that more than one be displayed at a time.

4. Material aids, when used in a logical sequence, should be such that they complement each other. In other words, the teacher can use a psychologic approach within the logical limits of the unit.

The teacher of health education should think through and have clearly in mind the best and most logical approach to such factors as (1) the *selection* of audiovisual aids, (2) adequate *preparation* in the use of audiovisual materials, and (3) *evaluation* of audiovisual aids in health and safety education.

Selecting audiovisual aids. A consideration of the many visual aids available in health education indicates at once that there must be careful selection of the types to be used in the varying situations and circumstances arising in the educational process. Also, it is clearly perceptible that each type of aid has a particular function; that is, each aid usually can be used to the best advantage with some particular type of presentation. An example of this is that of the teacher or visiting instructor using the demonstration method in teaching artificial respiration or CPR (cardiopulmonary resuscitation). The actual demonstration along with the verbal description given by the teacher is a more logical and effective means of presenting this than through showing it on film or on television. One main advantage of an actual demonstration is that the teacher can stop at any point to answer questions, to retrace the steps, or to start over again. The selection and use of one type of audiovisual aid when some other would be more effective may be both inefficient and uneconomical.

Although it is highly important that the health education teacher give ample time and thought to the selection of the aid best adapted to a particular situation, selection of the best suited type of aid is only one phase of the process. The teacher must be able to use them intelligently, efficiently, and profitably after the selections are made. There are certain acceptable techniques and approaches in using the different types of sensory aids, as there are in other methods and procedures in teaching.

Another highly important point in the proper selection of any audiovisual aid is its suitability and appropriateness for the age, maturity, family and community background, and experience of the children with whom it is to be used. A teaching aid is most valuable only when it provides the maximum aid. Consequently, if an aid is unsuited to the level of maturity, background, experience, interest, and needs of a particular group, it cannot provide the maximum aid. If an aid is too advanced and difficult for a group, it use is not worthwhile and may be frustrating to pupils. If it is below the maturity level of a group, it may create adverse psychologic reactions and unfavorable attitudes as well as stifle interest.

Preparing to use audiovisual materials. For audiovisual materials to be used most efficiently and to get the most effective results, there must be adequate preparation on the part of both the teacher and the pupils. One undesirable tendency in the trial-and-error development of visual aid use was that of merely showing them without attempting to assure that the pupils derive the greatest benefit from their use. Some sensory aids, such as motion pictures and television, have often been used more for entertainment rather than for their contribution to the learning process. This does not mean to imply that aids should not be interesting and even entertaining. It does mean, however, that usually visual aids cannot be justified in health education solely on the basis of entertainment. The tendency to use some sensory aids and particularly motion pictures largely as entertainment has perhaps been greater in the teaching in health education—and particularly in drug education—than in most other fields. This has been caused in part by the comparative irregularity of the time schedule for health teaching in the school program and because elementary school classroom teachers and health education teachers often lack sufficient training in proper health teaching methods.

Most teaching aids are more or less abstract; that is, they deal with representation of reality rather than with reality itself. Consequently, teachers should have a very clear purpose in mind when aids are used, and they should convey this purpose to the children. There is usually a need to clarify some visual aids through the use of other aids and through discussions and demonstrations. In using health education aids particularly, there is a greater tendency for children to be unduly attracted by the comical, unusual, and morbid phases and thereby fail to gain the main points of the lesson or theme.

With some visual aids—motion pictures, videotapes, slides, and filmstrips—lesson plans and teachers' guides are often supplied. In most cases, though, it is necessary for teachers to make adaptations for their own specific use even though teachers' guides are provided. It is a good policy for teachers to develop gradually their own techniques and procedures in the use of audiovisual aids. The reason for this is that teachers vary greatly in their ways of teaching. Consequently, a teacher must fit the sensory aid to a unique personality and a particular style of presenting materials.

Proper preparation on the part of both teacher and pupils helps to avoid passive receptivity on the part of the children. As we have seen, in the past many aids have been used indiscriminately and as entertainment rather than primarily as an instrument of instruction. School children, to some extent, have come to accept this view, especially in the case of motion pictures and television. They are in the habit of viewing commercial entertainment films at the theater and seeing television at home. Consequently, the entertainment idea and attitude are likely to carry over into the school, especially when motion pictures and television are involved. Discussions, questions, reports, and tests covering the aids used help to develop a spirit and attitude of active participation in pupils.

What about evaluation? Two main reasons for evaluation of aids in health education are: (1) the aids should be evaluated in terms of their value and contribution to the educational process, and (2) the teacher should continually evaluate techniques and procedures in the use of the various aids in attempting to make them contribute most to the child's education. Reliable and objective means of evaluating the sensory aids program in health education are difficult to come by, so it is necessary for teachers to evaluate largely on a subjective basis. Yet both teachers and pupils can participate in the evaluation on the basis of interest, attitudes, general reactions, and tests of various kinds.

Other important phases of evaluation include such items as the accuracy and authenticity of the material; suitability in terms of the lesson involved; gradation in terms of age, background, and experience of the particular group; and value in view of the effort, expense, and time involved.

WHERE CAN TEACHERS FIND GOOD TEACHING AIDS?

A skilled surgeon without the latest proved operating instruments, a competent craftsman lacking high quality tools, a qualified engineer who does not have the modern devices he needs, a talented musician without an instrument of superior quality and tone—none of these people can perform at the top of his talent.

So it is with the classroom teacher. Unless teachers have materials that are educationally sound, scientifically accurate, stimulating, and up to date, they cannot possibly do an effective job of health education. Thus, one of the most important factors in determining the effectiveness of an elementary teacher in health education is the availability of and use of worthwhile teaching aids.

There are two main types of source materials available in the field of health education: (1) printed materials, such as textbooks, workbooks, and pamphlets, and (2) audiovisual aids, including motion pictures, television—closed circuit, educational, and commercial—filmstrips, photographs, transparencies, still pictures, slides, models, maps, posters, specimens, diagrams, graphs, museum exhibits, and anatomical charts. There are perhaps more teaching materials in health and safety education available to teachers from all types of organizations throughout the country than in any other area of the school program. One of the main reasons for this is that so many different types of organizations are interested in the health and safety of the school population. A great deal of the material available to teachers and children from organizations throughout the country are free or inexpensive. Therefore, just the very fact that so many groups are attempting to prepare study materials for the school child means that there is likely to be a great variation in the worth of the material in terms of modern educational values, objectives, and practices.

In the case of health and safety textbooks, as with other types of reading materials and textbooks used in the schools, there are usually criteria by which we can judge suitability. In some instances local communities as well as state groups have set up special criteria by which all textbooks and printed materials used in the schools are judged to make certain that desirable reading and study materials are finally selected. Although the criteria for all types of visual aids have not been as extensively developed and applied as for textbooks, nevertheless there is a great need in the field of health and safety education to apply certain criteria to the materials prepared and distributed by most of the organizations offering these to the schools.

Some criteria to keep in mind in selecting health and safety materials, both printed matter and visual aids, are the following:
1. They should be free from bias.
2. All factual materials should be accurate.
3. The vocabulary should be appropriate for the grade level, though this is difficult to apply too specifically because of the range of reading ability among pupils in the same grade.
4. Study materials should not be sensational.
5. Health and safety materials should be free from fear psychology.
6. All health and safety materials used should make a contribution in the areas with which they deal.
7. The size and style of type used in printed matter should be appropriate for the particular grade level.
8. The ideas expressed in both visual aids and printed matter should be appropriate for the grade level.
9. Health and safety materials should be designed to stimulate thought.
10. Health and safety study materials should be scientifically accurate.
11. All materials used should be attractive.

Teachers' questions concerning the sources of available satisfactory health education materials indicate that many, and especially elementary school classroom teachers, are not aware of the extensive amount of health and safety material available free or at very little cost. Because there are so many inquiries concerning sources of materials, this chapter has been devoted largely to listing those sources and to giving some indication of the material available from each. It is hoped that in this way teachers can obtain and make use of these study materials by directly contacting those organizations likely to have the kinds of material they want.

Textbooks

Textbooks on health science and safety are available for all grade levels in the schools. Several publishers offer series of textbooks that range from grades 1 through 8. Numerous schools throughout the country now provide one or more of the health series to encourage systematic progression of learning, beginning with the primary grades and progressing through the upper elementary grades.

Textbooks place in the hands of pupils and teachers the latest useful health science information, weighed and selected from many sources by health education specialists. Often, during the school day children have little opportunity to read, concentrate on, and comprehend health science concepts. For some, the text is the only readily available source of information so vital to their health and safety. Looking at it from the teacher's viewpoint, where else, in one convenient, compact source, can the teacher find the answers to the broad spectrum of children's health problems?

From time to time, questions are raised by some educators about the value of textbooks in elementary teaching. While a wide variety of supplementary printed materials—magazines, pamphlets, encyclopedias, newsletters, newspapers, almanacs, and reliable newspaper reports—are useful in enriching and updating health education, experienced teachers recognize the basic need for a good health text.

Turner, Randall, and Smith* have cited five major advantages in using a good health textbook:
1. It gives an accurate presentation of essential facts.

---

*Turner, C. E., Randall, H. B., and Smith, S. L.: School health and health education, ed. 6, St. Louis, 1970, The C. V. Mosby Co.

2. It presents an orderly and comprehensible arrangement of the material.
3. It furnishes a common core of content for the class.
4. It contains such teaching and learning aids as references, questions, summaries, reviews, exercises, pictures, maps, and diagrams.
5. It saves time.

Textbook series for elementary schools. Health and safety textbooks for elementary schools can be obtained from the following sources:

The Bobbs-Merrill Co., Inc., Indianapolis: *Health for Young America Series*, Wilson, Charles, and Wilson, Elizabeth.

    Grade 1 *Health at School*, 1968
        2 *Health Day by Day*, 1968
        3 *Health and Fun*, 1968
        4 *Health and Growth*, 1968
        5 *Health and Living*, 1968
        6 *Health and Happiness*, 1968
        7 *Men, Science and Health*, 1968
        8 *Health, Fitness and Safety*, 1968

Ginn & Co., Lexington, Mass.: Gallagher, J. Roswell, and Willgoose, Carl E.

    Grade K   *How About You?* 1965
        7-8 *Health for Life*, 1969

Houghton Mifflin Co., Boston: Miller, Benjamin F., Rosenberg, Edward B., and Stackowski, Benjamin L.

    Grades 7-8 *Investigating Your Health*, 1970
        Teacher's edition of above

Laidlaw Brothers, River Forest, Ill.: *The Healthful Living Program*, Fodor, John T., Glass, Lennin H., Gmur, Ben C., Moore, Virginia D., and Neilson, Elizabeth A.

    Grade 1 *Your Health*, 1974
        2 *Being Healthy*, 1974
        3 *Your Health and You*, 1974
        4 *Keeping Healthy*, 1974
        5 *Growing Up Healthy*, 1974
        6 *Health for Living*, 1974
        7 *A Healthier You*, 1974
        8 *Your Health and Your Future*, 1974

Lyons & Carnahan, Chicago: *Dimensions in Health Series*, Irwin, Leslie W., Farnsworth, Dana, Coonan, Caroline, Gavel, Sylvia, Fraumeni, Florence, and Shafer, Barbara.

    Grade 1 *All About You*, 1967
        2 *You and Others*, 1967
        3 *Growing Every Day*, 1967

        4 *Finding Your Way*, 1967
        5 *Understanding Your Needs*, 1967
        6 *Choosing Your Goals*, 1967
        7 *Foundations for Fitness*, 1967
        8 *Patterns for Living*, 1967

Scott, Foresman & Co., Glenview, Ill.: Richmond, Julius B., Pounds, Elenore T., Jenkins, Gladys G., Sussdorf, Dieter H., and Wesley, W. A.

    Grade 1 *Off to a Good Start*, 1971 (three activity tablets, combined under one cover, that make up a consumable junior primer)
        Teacher's booklet to accompany above

Health and Growth Series

    Grade 1 *Health and Growth:* 1, 1974
        Teacher's edition of above
        2 *Health and Growth:* 2, 1974
        Teacher's edition of above
        3 *Health and Growth:* 3, 1974
        Teacher's edition of above
        4 *Health and Growth:* 4, 1974
        Teacher's edition of above
        5 *Health and Growth:* 5, 1974
        Teacher's edition of above
        6 *Health and Growth:* 6, 1974
        Teacher's edition of above
        7 *Health and Growth:* 7, 1972
        Teacher's edition of above
        8 *Health and Growth:* 8, 1972
        Teacher's edition of above

Most of these books are accompanied by teachers' manuals either bound with the text or as a separate booklet. Some publishers provide free and inexpensive materials for health education, including charts that outline the concepts to be taught at the various grade levels.

Some 90% of all elementary textbooks used in this country are produced by publishers of textbooks. Most states and the District of Columbia provide free textbooks to all elementary school pupils. These are paid for by the state, the state and local school district, or the local district alone. Less than one half of all elementary pupils are required to buy or rent their own texts. Often publishers make available specially trained consultants to visit elementary schools and help teachers use textbooks more effectively. Textbooks are used universally in elementary schools with the modern emphasis on using the book as a source of information for discussion and problem solving rather than simply as a basis for pupil recitation.

Most of the newer elementary school health series are written by experts in the fields of health science and education, are geared to the vocabulary and comprehension level of each grade, are concerned with the health needs and interests of each age group, and are presented in a format that appeals to children. Teachers and administrators must seek constantly to keep textbooks up to date, replacing old texts periodically. Table 12-1 contains books for students from which teachers and administrators may choose.

Table 12-1. Books for students*

Subject	Resource information	Grades†
Alcohol		
FICTION	The long ride home, Summers, Philadelphia, 1966, The Westminister Press (alcoholic father).	U
	The pit, Maddock, Boston, 1968, Little, Brown & Co. (home drinking).	U
NONFICTION	Alcohol and you, Lee and Israel, New York, 1975, Julian Messner.	I
	Alcohol; proof of what? Lee, New York, 1976, Julian Messner.	U
	You and your alcoholic parent, Hornik, New York, 1973, Association Press.	U
Anatomy/physiology		
FICTION	The kitten who is different, Saunders, Minneapolis, 1966, T. S. Denison & Co., Inc.	P, I
	Who's in that mirror? Berends, New York, 1968, Random House, Inc.	I
	Your body and how it works, Lauber, New York, 1962, E. M. Hale & Co.	I, U
NONFICTION	A is for anatomy, Cosgrove, New York, 1965, Dodd, Mead & Co. (inside body).	I
	The armor within us, Samachson, Skokie, Ill., 1966, Rand McNally & Co.	I, U
	Drop of blood, Showers, New York, 1967, Thomas Y. Crowell Co., Inc.	P, I
	Hear your heart, Showers, New York, 1968, Thomas Y. Crowell, Co., Inc.	P, I
	How we hear, Fryer, Minneapolis, 1968, Lerner Publications Co.	I
	Human body; the heart, Elgin, 1968, New York, Franklin Watts, Inc.	P, I
	Human skeleton, Schuman, New York, 1965, Atheneum Publishers.	I
	Me mighty, Kidder, Minneapolis, 1964, T. S. Denison & Co., Inc.	I
	Mr. Wonderful, Kidder, Minneapolis, 1964, T. S. Denison & Co., Inc.	P
	The story of brain and nerves, Weart, New York, 1961, Coward, McCann & Geoghegan, Inc.	I
	The story of respiratory system, Weart, New York, 1964, Coward, McCann & Geoghegan, Inc.	I, U
	The story of your blood, Weart, New York, 1960, Coward, McCann & Geoghegan, Inc.	I, U
	The story of your bones, Weart, New York, 1966, Coward, McCann & Geoghegan, Inc.	I
	Wonders of the human body, Keen, New York, 1966, Grosset & Dunlap, Inc.	I
	Your wonderful body, Chicago, 1961, Follett Corp.	I
Consumer health		
FICTION	How hospitals help us, Meeker, Westchester, Ill., 1962, Benefic Press.	I
	See the first star, Simon, Chicago, 1968, Albert Whitman & Co. (eye exam).	P
NONFICTION	Doctors and nurses; what do they do? Greene, New York, 1963, Harper & Row, Publishers, Inc.	P

*Adapted from Library books; resources for health instruction, 1970, Olympia, Wash., State Superintendent of Public Instruction.
†Grades: U = upper; I = intermediate; P = primary.

Continued.

Table 12-1. Books for students—cont'd

Subject	Resource information	Grades
	Doctors' tools, Lerner, 1960, Medical Books for children.	P, I
	The first book of hospitals, Coy, New York, 1964, Franklin Watts, Inc.	I
	A visit to the doctor, Berger, New York, 1960, Grosset & Dunlap, Inc.	P
Dental health		
FICTION	The alligator's toothache, Dorian, New York, 1962, William Morrow & Co., Inc.	P
	The tooth fairy, Feagles, Provo, Utah, 1962, Young House.	P
NONFICTION	Dentist's tools, Lapp, Minneapolis, 1961, Lerner Publications Co.	I, U
	A visit to the dentist, Garn, New York, 1959, Grosset & Dunlap, Inc.	P
Disease control		
FICTION	Betsy-back-in-bed, Udry, Chicago, 1963, Albert Whitman & Co.	P
NONFICTION	Karen gets a fever, Gilbert, Chicago, 1961, Children's Press.	P
	Medicine in action; today and tomorrow, Hyde, New York, 1964, McGraw-Hill Book Co.	I, U
	Microbes in your life, Schneider, New York, 1966, Harcourt Brace Jovanovich, Inc.	U
	The true book of bacteria, Frahm, Chicago, 1963, Children's Press.	P
Drugs		
FICTION	Danger beats the drum, Madison, New York, 1966, Holt, Rinehart & Winston.	U
	Tuned out, Wojciechowski, New York, 1968, Harper & Row, Publishers, Inc.	U
NONFICTION	About Jerry and Jimmy and the pharmacist, Thompson, 1964, Melmont.	P
	Basic concepts of drugs, Summer and others, River Forest, Ill., 1972, Laidlaw Brothers.	U
	Drugs; facts on their use and abuse, Houser and others, Glenview, Ill., 1971, Scott, Foresman & Co.	U
	Drugs and people, Read, Boston, 1970, Allyn & Bacon, Inc.	I, U
	Drugs and you, Madison, New York, 1971, Julian Messner.	I
	Drugs for young people, ed. 2, Leech and Jordan, Elmsford, N.Y., 1974, Pergamon Press, Inc.	U
	What you should know about drugs, Gorodetsky and Christian, New York, 1970, Harcourt Brace Jovanovich, Inc.	I, U
Family health		
FICTION	Amy and the new baby, Brown, New York, 1965, Franklin Watts, Inc.	P
	Half-breed, Lampman, New York, 1967, Doubleday & Co., Inc.	I
	Time of understanding, Ferris, New York, 1963, Burt Franklin & Co., Inc.	U
	Willy is my brother, Parish, Provo, Utah, 1963, Young House.	P
NONFICTION	A baby starts to grow, Showers, New York, 1969, Thomas Y. Crowell Co., Inc.	P
	Chicken ten thousand, Jackson, Boston, 1968, Little, Brown & Co.	P
	Growing up; how we became alive, are born, and grow, De Schweinitz, New York, 1965, The Macmillan Co.	P, I
	The human story, Hofstein, New York, 1969, William Morrow & Co., Inc.	I
	Love and facts of life, Duval, New York, 1967, Association Press.	U
	Love and sex in plain language, Johnson, Philadelphia, 1967, J. B. Lippincott Co.	U
	Sam, Scott, New York, 1967, McGraw-Hill Book Co.	P
	The story of a baby, Ets, New York, 1969, The Viking Press.	I
	What's happening to me, Lerrigo, New York, 1969, E. P. Dutton & Co., Inc.	I, U
	The wonder of life, Levine, Racine, Wis., 1964, Western Publishing Co., Inc.	I
	The wonderful story of you, Gruenberg, 1960, Garden City Books.	I, U

Table 12-1. Books for students—cont'd

Subject	Resource information	Grades
Mental health		
FICTION	The hidden lookout, Brown, New York, 1965, McGraw-Hill Book Co.	I
	It takes all kinds, Means, Boston, 1964, Houghton Mifflin Co.	U
	Laugh and cry, Beim, New York, 1955, William Morrow & Co., Inc.	I
	The loner, Wier, New York, 1963, David McKay Co., Inc.	I, U
	Mr. Tall and Mr. Small, Brenner, Provo, Utah, 1966, Young House.	P
	My book of the ugly duckling, Anderson, 1960, Maxton.	P
	The quarreling book, Zolotow, New York, 1963, Harper & Row, Publishers, Inc.	P, I
	The scary thing, Bannon, Boston, 1956, Houghton Mifflin Co.	P
NONFICTION	Happiness is a warm puppy, Schulz, 1962, Determined Production.	P, I
	Looking at you, Smaridge, Nashville, Tenn., 1962, Abingdon Press.	I, U
	Nobody said it's easy, Smith, New York, 1965, The Macmillan Co.	U
	Red man, white man, African chief, Lerner, 1960, Med. Books Children.	P
	Why did he die? Harris, Minneapolis, 1965, Lerner Publications Co.	P
Tobacco		
NONFICTION	About you and smoking, Houser and others, Glenview, Ill., 1971, Scott, Foresman & Co.	I, U
	Basic concepts of tobacco and smoking, Needle, River Forest, Ill., 1970, Laidlaw Brothers.	I, U
	Smoking and you, Madison, New York, 1975, Julian Messner.	I

Library sources

A variety of printed matter dealing with health science information is available in both school and community libraries. Although most of these sources are more suitable for intermediate and upper grade students—as well as for teachers, some are prepared for younger pupils. Here are some of the more readily available sources:

1. Library books*—especially the more recent paperbacks—in various areas of the health sciences.

2. A rather large number of general, or popular, magazines provide well-written articles on new developments in the health sciences. However, they must be carefully evaluated for scientific authenticity. Here are some of the popular magazines which regularly include significant health articles and reports:

Changing Times
Consumer Reports
Ebony

Family Circle
Family Health
Newsweek
New York Times Magazine
Parent's Magazine
Psychology Today
Reader's Digest
Science
Science Digest
Scientific American
Time
U.S. News & World Report
Woman's Day

More technical articles are to be found in the professional journals in the health sciences and education. These are listed later in this chapter.

3. Encyclopedia and almanacs.

4. Newspapers, some of which carry regular articles by health authorities and science writers, provide almost daily news items on health and safety. Most of these are accurate. Others can be used to help pupils develop the ability to critically analyze material from newspapers.

In many cases the school library is used as a place for concentrating books, charts, leaflets, bulletins, and health materials of a

---

*See the guidelines for accuracy and truthfulness in Chapter 2.

similar nature. In this way all persons who teach health are able to benefit from all that is acquired.

A major advantage of using the various current materials in health education is that, from an early age, children may be taught to become discriminating and careful in their evaluation of sensational, unsubstantiated, and inadequately documented reports.

Departments of education and health

Both education and health departments are included in this category because of their close relationship in matters of school health. In many cases education and health departments at city, county, and state levels constitute a major source of health teaching materials and information. A primary function of both groups is to provide information, audiovisual aids, and other materials for educational purposes. Pamphlets, filmstrips, motion picture films, study guides, reference lists, and audiovisual handbooks, or guides are only a part of the usual offering.

In a growing number of school systems, school health education coordinators are employed to assist teachers with information and guidance relating to curriculum, unit content and objectives, methods, material aids, and community resource people, facilities, and services. The health educator usually has a major, or at least a minor, concentration in school health education at the undergraduate or graduate level. Such a person can be of inestimable assistance to the harried, hurried, and very busy classroom teacher.

Certain personnel and programs of health departments may be regarded as especially valuable sources for health materials and information. Often the resource person closest to the teacher is the school nurse, who is usually of great assistance in bringing the offerings of the health department within the teacher's reach. Moreover, in some instances the nurse is qualified to make competent presentations to classes and parent-teacher groups on certain subjects. Some teachers have found nurses to be especially valuable for teaching some of the functions and problems of public health work in their own cities.

It is sometimes possible to arrange for other health department personnel to assist in health instruction in the classroom. For example, physicians may be invited to talk about their specialty, answer questions, or demonstrate and teach the meaning of the physical examination. They, along with dentists, mental health workers, and statisticians, may also serve as consultants on current health information.

Federal government

Various branches of the federal government provide a considerable amount of worthwhile health materials. Outstanding among these are the Office of Education, the Public Health Service, and The Children's Bureau under the U.S. Department of Health, Education, and Welfare. The Office of Education has consultative services in health education; the individuals in charge of this program will provide information as to desired source materials and current practices in the nation. The U.S. Public Health Service's various organizations, including the National Institutes of Health, will provide a great deal of valuable information and research on the major diseases; the Public Health program in general; the relationship between the national public health service and local health departments; and statistics on various aspects of public health (the National Center for Health Statistics is a division of the Public Health Service).

Other governmental organizations that are important in this connection include the Human Nutrition Research Division of the U.S. Department of Agriculture, Food and Drug Administration, the Bureau of Narcotics and Dangerous Drugs, the Institute of Alcohol Abuse and Alcoholism, and the United Nations' World Health Organization.

Professional and voluntary health organizations

A large number of professional organizations are excellent sources for materials and information on many health topics. They may be utilized as major sources for a wide variety of audiovisual aids, including charts, models, slides, exhibits, filmstrips, and motion pictures. Some furnish free or inexpensive literature on a wide variety of health topics and, in some cases, teaching plans to aid the teacher. Many professional organizations may be called on to furnish speakers and demonstrators who can add materially to the success of teaching units and of informing citizens' gatherings.

Many professional organizations are included among the sources of free or inexpensive materials listed later in this chapter. However, some of the organizations most useful in providing information and guidance to teachers are as follows:

American Alliance for Health, Physical Education, and Recreation, Health Education Division, 1201 16th St., N.W., Washington, D.C. 20006

American Cancer Society, 777 Third Ave., New York, N.Y. 10017

American Dental Association, 211 Chicago Ave., Chicago, Ill. 60611

American Heart Association, 7320 Greenville Ave., Dallas, Tex. 75231

American Medical Association, 535 N. Dearborn St., Chicago, Ill. 60610

American National Red Cross, 17th and D Sts., N.W., Washington, D.C. 20006

American Public Health Association, 1015 18th St., N.W., Washington, D.C. 20036

American School Health Association, 515 E. Main St., Kent, Ohio 44240

American Social Health Association, 1790 Broadway, New York, N.Y. 10019

American Speech and Hearing Association, 9030 Old Georgetown Rd., Washington, D.C. 20014

National Association for Mental Health, 1800 N. Kent St., Arlington, Va. 22209

National Foundation, 800 Second Ave., New York, N.Y. 10017

National Lung Association, 1790 Broadway, New York, N.Y. 10019

National Safety Council, 425 N. Michigan Ave., Chicago, Ill. 60611

National Society for the Prevention of Blindness, Inc., 16 E. 40th St., New York, N.Y. 10016

Teachers of health science should be aware of the many services and materials available from these sources.

Business and commercial groups

Although it is true that health materials distributed for public relations and advertising purposes by business and commercial groups must be scrutinized carefully for bias and distortion (frequently teachers are required to submit films and certain other audiovisual aids to some school authority for approval), many of these groups distribute materials of excellent quality, sometimes free and sometimes at a very low price. In many instances advertising is restricted to a single identifying label or statement. Some concerns have banded together to promote the sales of all presenting a particular product. For example, the Cereal Institute, the Florida Citrus Commission, and the Athletic Institute do not advertise particular brands but rather devote their efforts to improving the general market involved. Thus, the Cereal Institute identifies itself as "A research and educational endeavor devoted to the betterment of national nutrition" and has a number of individual cereal companies as its supporting membership. Similarly, much of the health information provided by the large life insurance companies is only indirectly related to their business interest. Organizations of these kinds usually do not deal in objectionable advertising, and on the contrary, they sometimes go to considerable expense for personnel and research to provide factually sound and colorful supplementary materials.

FREE OR INEXPENSIVE MATERIALS FOR ELEMENTARY SCHOOL TEACHERS AND PUPILS

Many organizations make available free and inexpensive pamphlets, charts, posters, and other printed matter on health and safety. A majority of the materials are at the teacher's level, although a substantial number have been prepared for pupil use at various grade levels. In most instances the materials are free; others are provided at a moderate cost. Some national organizations distribute their materials from state or local offices.

The listing of a business or commercial

organization should not be construed as an endorsement of its products or services by the authors or the publisher. Yet some of the best materials are provided by such organizations, generally with a minimum of advertising. However, it is desirable for teachers to submit such materials to school administrators for approval before use or viewing by pupils.

Although teaching and learning materials from listed sources provide worthwhile and up-to-date information, they are *not* intended to serve the purpose of textbooks or other regular study materials. Free or inexpensive materials in health and safety are most effectively used as (1) sources of more detailed or more recent data than is provided in the textbooks; (2) examples of health and safety education services of governmental agencies, professional associations, private (voluntary) organizations, and commercial groups; and (3) reference materials or media (posters and charts) for student projects.

Requests should be made three or four weeks before the material is needed. Often it is best to first write for a catalog listing specific materials. Topic, age level, and quantity desired should be specified in the request. Here are major sources of free or inexpensive health materials.

Sources of free or low cost health and safety materials*

Abbott Laboratories
14th and Sheridan Rd.
North Chicago, Ill. 60064
 (pharmacy, nutrition, and drugs)

Aetna Life and Casualty Companies
Public Relations and Advertising
151 Farmington Ave.
Hartford, Conn. 06115
 (health and safety)

Al-Anon Family Group Headquarters
P.O. Box 182
Madison Square Station
New York, N.Y. 10010
 (alcoholism and family)

Alcohol, Drug Abuse, and Mental Health
 Administration
5600 Fishers Lane
Rockville, Md. 20852
 (alcohol and drugs)

Allstate Insurance
Safety Director, Allstate Plaza
Northbrook, Ill. 60062
 (motor vehicle safety)

American Academy of Pediatrics
1801 Hinman Ave.
Evanston, Ill. 60201
 (child health and safety)

American Alliance for Health, Physical
 Education, and Recreation
1201 16th St., N.W.
Washington, D.C. 20006
 *(school health, physical education, and
 recreation)**

American Automobile Association
Traffic Engineering and Safety Department
Falls Church, Va. 22042
 (highway and pedestrian safety)

American Camping Association
Bradford Woods
Martinsville, Ind. 46151
 *(camping health and safety)**

American Cancer Society, Inc.
777 Third Ave.
New York, N.Y. 10017
 (cancer)

American Chiropractic Association
2200 Grand Ave.
Des Moines, Iowa 50312
 (chiropractic medicine)

American Dental Association
Bureau of Dental Health Education
211 Chicago Ave.
Chicago, Ill. 60611
 (dental health)

American Diabetes Association, Inc.
1 E. 45th St.
New York, N.Y. 10017
 (diabetes)

---

*Following each source citation the general or specific subject matter of available materials is indicated in parentheses. An asterisk (*) means that there is a charge for some or all of the materials provided by a given organization.

American Dietetic Association
18 W. 48th St.
New York, N.Y. 10020
 (*nutrition and diet*)*

American Dry Milk Institute, Inc.
130 N. Franklin St.
Chicago, Ill. 60601
 (*nutrition*)

American Fire Insurance Companies
Engineering Department
80 Maiden Lane
New York, N.Y. 10007
 (*safety*)

American Foundation for the Blind
15 W. 16th St.
New York, N.Y. 10011
 (*blindness and rehabilitation*)*

American Heart Association
Inquiries Section
44 E. 23rd St.
New York, N.Y. 10010
 (*heart*)

American Hospital Association
840 N. Lake Shore Dr.
Chicago, Ill. 60611
 (*hospital care*)*

American Institute of Baking
Consumer Service Department
400 E. Ontario St.
Chicago, Ill. 60611
 (*nutrition*)

American Institute of Family Relations
5287 Sunset Blvd.
Los Angeles, Calif. 90027
 (*family living and mental health*)

American Lung Association
1740 Broadway
New York, N.Y. 10019
 (*tuberculosis, respiratory diseases, and
  smoking*)

American Medical Association
Bureau of Health Education
535 N. Dearborn St.
Chicago, Ill. 60610
 (*health and safety*)*

American National Red Cross
17th and D Sts., N.W.
Washington, D.C. 20006
 (*contact local chapter first*)
 (*first aid, safety, and nutrition*)

American Optometric Association, Inc.
Department of Public Information
700 Chippewa St.
St. Louis, Mo. 63119
 (*eye health*)

American Osteopathic Association
212 E. Ohio St.
Chicago, Ill. 60611
 (*health and career information*)

American Podiatry Association
3301 16th St., N.W.
Washington, D.C. 20010
 (*foot care*)

American Public Health Association
1015 18th St., N.W.
Washington, D.C. 20036
 (*community health*)*

American School Health Association
515 E. Main St.
Kent, Ohio 44240
 (*school health program*)*

American Social Health Association
1790 Broadway
New York, N.Y. 10019
 (*sex education*)*

American Veterinary Association
600 S. Michigan Ave.
Chicago, Ill.
 (*pet health and career information*)

Arthritis Foundation
1212 Avenue of the Americas
New York, N.Y. 10036
 (*arthritis and quackery*)

Association for Family Living
6 N. Michigan Ave.
Chicago, Ill. 60602
 (*family health*)

Association of American Publishers
1 Park Ave.
New York, N.Y. 10016
 (*health texts*)

---

*Following each source citation the general or specific subject matter of available materials is indicated in parentheses.
An asterisk (*) means that there is a charge for some or all of the materials provided by a given organization.

Association of American Railroads
School and College Service
Transportation Building
Washington, D.C. 20006
  (railroad safety)

Association of Casualty and Surety Companies
Accident Prevention Department
Publications Division
60 John St.
New York, N.Y. 10038
  (safety)

Better Vision Institute, Inc.
230 Park Ave.
New York, N.Y. 10017
  (glasses and eye care)

Bicycle Institute of America
122 E. 42nd St.
New York, N.Y. 10017
  (bicycle safety)

The Borden Co.
Consumer Services
350 Madison Ave.
New York, N.Y. 10011
  (nutrition, weight control, and health inventory)

Bureau of Health Education Center for
  Disease Control
U.S. Public Health Service
Atlanta, Ga. 30333
  (health education programs)

California Fruit Growers Exchange
Educational Division
Box 5030 Met. Station
Los Angeles, Calif. 90055
  (nutrition)

Carnation Milk Co.
Home Service Department
5045 Wilshire Blvd.
Los Angeles, Calif. 90036
  (nutrition)

Cereal Institute, Inc.
Home Economics Department
135 S. LaSalle St.
Chicago, Ill. 60603
  (nutrition)

Channing L. Bete, Inc.
45 Federal St.
Greenfield, Mass. 01301
  (nominally priced health booklets)

Child Study Association of America
9 E. 89th St.
New York, N.Y. 10028
  (special education and mental health)

Chiffon Consumer Center
Anderson Clayton Foods
1 Main Place
Dallas, Tex. 75250
  (nutrition)

Ciba Pharmaceutical Co.
556 Morris Ave.
Summit, N.J. 07901
  (health science)

Colgate-Palmolive Co.
300 Park Ave.
New York, N.Y. 10010
  (skin care and dental health)

Community Health Service
Health Services and Mental Health
  Administration
U.S. Public Health Service
Rockville, Md. 20852
  (medical care)

Consumer and Food Economics Institute
Agricultural Research Service
U.S. Department of Agriculture
Hyattsville, Md. 20782
  (nutrition and food economics)

Consumer Center Information
Pueblo, Colo. 81009
  (health products and services, safety)

Consumer Reports
P.O. Box 1111
Mount Vernon, N.Y. 10550
  (health and safety products, reprints)

Environmental Protection Agency
401 M St., S.W.
Washington, D.C. 20460
  (pollution)

Epilepsy Foundation of America
1828 L St., N.W.
Washington, D.C. 20005
  (epilepsy)

---

*Following each source citation the general or specific subject matter of available materials is indicated in parentheses. An asterisk (*) means that there is a charge for some or all of the materials provided by a given organization.

Federal Food and Drug Administration
200 C St., S.W.
Washington, D.C. 20204
 (food, drug, and cosmetic standards)

Florida Citrus Commission
Institutional and School Marketing Department
P.O. Box 148
Lakeland, Fla. 33802
 (citrus fruits and nutrition)

Ford Motor Co.
Research and Information Department
The American Rd.
Dearborn, Mich. 48127
 (traffic safety and seat belts)

General Mills, Inc.
Public Relations Department
Educational Services
9200 Wayzata Blvd.
Minneapolis, Minn. 55426
 (nutrition and synthetic foods)

Gillette Toiletries
Box 3431
Chicago, Ill. 60654
 (grooming)

Health Information Foundation
Public Relations Director
420 Lexington Ave.
New York, N.Y. 10017
 (health and medical economics)

Health Insurance Council
488 Madison Ave.
New York, N.Y. 10022
 (health insurance)

Health Insurance Institute
277 Park Ave.
New York, N.Y. 10017
 (health insurance)

Health Services and Mental Health
 Administration
Office of Information
Public Inquiries
Rockville, Md. 20852
(health services and mental health)

Heart Disease Control Program
Division of Special Health Services
U.S. Public Health Service
Department of Health, Education, and Welfare
Washington, D.C. 20025
 (heart diseases)

Heart Information Center
National Heart Institute
U.S. Public Health Service
Bethesda, Md. 20014
 (heart diseases and heart research)

Highway Safety Foundation
Box 5900
Cleveland, Ohio 44101
 (motor vehicle safety)

The Hogg Foundation for Mental Health
University of Texas–Austin
Austin, Tex. 78710
 (mental health)

IDEA
C. F. Kettering Foundation
Box 446
Melbourne, Fla. 32901
 (drug abuse)

Institute of Makers of Explosives
420 Lexington Ave.
New York, N.Y. 10017
 (blasting cap safety)

International Cellucotton Products Co.
919 N. Michigan Ave.
Chicago, Ill. 60611
 (menstrual hygiene)

Joint Commission on Accreditation of Hospitals
200 E. Ohio St.
Chicago, Ill. 60611
 (hospital accreditation)

Kellogg Co.
Home Economics Service
235 Porter St.
Battle Creek, Mich. 49017
 (nutrition)

Kemper Insurance Companies
4750 Sheridan Rd.
Chicago, Ill. 60640
 (traffic safety)

Kimberly-Clark Corporation
Life Cycle Center
Neenah, Wis. 54956
 (menstrual hygiene and colds)

Lead Industries Association
292 Madison Ave.
New York, N.Y. 10017
(lead poisoning)

Lederle Laboratories Division
American Cyanamid Co.
Public Relations Department
Pearl River, N.Y. 10965
(child health, immunizations, and nutrition)

Lever Brothers Co.
Public Relations Division
Consumer Education Department
390 Park Ave.
New York, N.Y. 10022
(cleanliness)

Liberty Mutual Insurance Co.
175 Berkeley Square
Boston, Mass. 02116
(safety and rehabilitation)

Licensed Beverages Industries, Inc.
155 E. 44th St.
New York, N.Y. 10017
(alcohol)

Mental Health Materials Center
104 E. 25th St.
New York, N.Y. 10010
*(family life, mental health, and health interests)**

Metropolitan Life Insurance Co.
School Health Bureau
Health and Welfare Division
One Madison Ave.
New York, N.Y. 10010
(health, safety, and first aid)

Muscular Dystrophy Association of America, Inc.
Public Information Department
1740 Broadway
New York, N.Y. 10019
(muscular dystrophy)

Narcotics Anonymous
Box 2000
Lexington, Ky. 40501
(drug addiction)

National Academy of Sciences
National Research Council
Washington, D.C. 20025
*(food and nutrition)**

National Association for Mental Health
1800 N. Kent St.
Roslyn, Va. 22209
(mental health)

National Association of Hearing and Speech
  Agencies
919 18th St., N.W.
Washington, D.C. 20006
(speech and hearing defects)

National Board of Fire Underwriters
85 John St.
New York, N.Y. 10038
(fire prevention)

National Clearinghouse for Alcohol Information
National Institute on Alcohol Abuse and
  Alcoholism
Box 2345
Rockville, Md. 20852
(alcohol and health)

National Clearinghouse for Drug Abuse
  Information
5454 Wisconsin Ave.
Chevy Chase, Md. 20203
(drugs and drug abuse)

National Commission on Safety Education
National Education Association
1201 16th St., N.W.
Washington, D.C. 20036
(safety)

National Congress of Parents and Teachers
700 N. Rush St.
Chicago, Ill. 60611
*(child health and safety)**

National Coordinating Council on Drug Abuse
  Education
1346 Connecticut Ave., N.W.
Washington, D.C. 20036
(drug education)

National Coordinating Council on Drug Abuse
  Information
Box 19400
Washington, D.C. 20036
*(materials list on drugs)**

National Council on Alcoholism
2 Park Ave.
New York, N.Y. 10016
(alcoholism)

---

*Following each source citation the general or specific subject matter of available materials is indicated in parentheses. An asterisk (*) means that there is a charge for some or all of the materials provided by a given organization.

National Council on Drug Abuse
8 S. Michigan Ave.
Chicago, Ill. 60603
  (drug education)

National Council on Family Relations
1219 University Ave., S.E.
Minneapolis, Minn. 55414
  (teacher's kit on family living, $2.50)

National Dairy Council
111 N. Canal St.
Chicago, Ill. 60606
  (nutrition and health education workshops)*

National Epilepsy League
203 N. Wabash Ave.
Chicago, Ill. 60610
  (epilepsy)

National Fire Protection Association
60 Batterymarch St.
Boston, Mass. 02110
  (fire prevention)

National Foundation
Division of Scientific and Health Information
P.O. Box 2000
White Plains, N.Y. 10602
  *(poliomyelitis, arthritis, birth defects, and
    disorders of the central nervous system)*

National Health Council
1740 Broadway
New York, N.Y. 10019
  (health careers)

National Highway Traffic Safety Administration
U.S. Department of Transportation
400 Seventh St., S.W.
Washington, D.C. 20590
  (motor vehicle safety)

National Institutes of Health
Department of Health, Education, and Welfare
U.S. Public Health Service
Building 8
Bethesda, Md. 20014
  *(allergy and infectious diseases; arthritis and
    metabolic diseases; cancer; child health and
    human development; dental research; general
    medical sciences; heart; mental health,
    including drugs and alcohol; neurological
    diseases and blindness; specific diseases and
    preventive medicine)*

National Interagency Council on Smoking and
  Health
8600 Wisconsin Ave.
Bethesda, Md. 20014
  (smoking)

National Kidney Foundation
116 E. 27th St.
New York, N.Y. 10016
  (kidney disease)

National Livestock and Meat Board
Nutritional Department
36 S. Wabash Ave.
Chicago, Ill. 60603
  (nutrition)*

National Medical Association
2109 East St., N.W.
Washington, D.C. 20037
  (health and medical careers)

National Multiple Sclerosis Society
257 Fourth Ave.
New York, N.Y. 10010
  (multiple sclerosis)

National Nephrosis Foundation, Inc.
143 E. 35th St.
New York, N.Y. 10016
  (kidney disease)

National Nutritional Foods Association
708 Catherine Dr.
Montebello, Calif. 90640
  (nutrition)

National Safety Council
425 N. Michigan Ave.
Chicago, Ill. 60611
  (safety and accident statistics)*

National Science Teachers Association
1742 Connecticut Ave., N.W.
Washington, D.C. 20009
  (related health science materials)*

National Society for the Prevention of Blindness,
  Inc.
10 E. 40th St.
New York, N.Y. 10016
  (eye care)*

---

*Following each source citation the general or specific subject matter of available materials is indicated in parentheses.
An asterisk (*) means that there is a charge for some or all of the materials provided by a given organization.

Nationwide Insurance
Safety Department
246 N. High St.
Columbus, Ohio 43216
 (traffic and child safety)*

Nutrition Foundation, Inc.
99 Park Ave.
New York, N.Y. 10016
 (nutrition)

Office of Civil Defense
Public Information
The Pentagon
Washington, D.C. 20310
 (first aid)

Oral Hygiene Publications
911 Perin Ave.
Pittsburgh, Pa. 15222
 (dental health)*

Ortho Pharmaceuticals
Raritan, N.J. 08869
 (sex education)

Pennsylvania Insurance Commission
Office of the Commissioner
Harrisburg, Pa. 17120
 (consumer health)*

Pepsodent
Division of Lever Brothers Co.
390 Park Ave.
New York, N.Y. 10022
 (dental health)

Personal Products Corporation
Education Department
Milltown, N.J. 08850
 (menstrual hygiene)

Pet Milk Co.
Director of Home Economics
400 S. Fourth St.
St. Louis, Mo. 63101
 (nutrition)

Pharmaceutical Manufacturers' Association
Department NW-601
1155 15th St., N.W.
Washington, D.C. 20005
 *(over-the-counter and prescription drugs, drug
  abuse, consumer health)*

Planned Parenthood Federation of America, Inc.
810 Seventh Ave.
New York, N.Y. 10019
 (sex education)

Preservation
Box 2800
Washington, D.C. 20013
 (environment)

President's Council on Physical Fitness and Sports
400 Sixth St., S.W.
Washington, D.C. 20202
 (physical education and fitness)

Proprietary Association
1700 Pennsylvania Ave., N.W.
Washington, D.C. 20006
 (proprietary drugs)

Prudential Insurance Company of America
Public Relations and Advertising
Newark, N.J. 07102
 (safety)

Public Affairs Committee
381 Park Ave. S.
New York, N.Y. 10016
 (health, safety, consumer health)*

Public Health Service
Public Inquiries Branch
U.S. Department of Health, Education, and
 Welfare
Washington, D.C. 20025
 (health)*

Ralston Purina Co .
P.O. Box 9092
St. Paul, Minn. 55190
 (pet health care)*

Rutgers Center of Alcohol Studies
Box 560, Rutgers University
New Brunswick, N.Y. 08903
 (alcohol education)*

G. D. Searle and Co.
Chicago, Ill. 60680
 (gastrointestinal health)

Schering Corporation
Kenilworth, N.J. 07033
 (sports health information)

---

*Following each source citation the general or specific subject matter of available materials is indicated in parentheses.
An asterisk (*) means that there is a charge for some or all of the materials provided by a given organization.

Science Research Associates, Inc.
259 E. Erie St.
Chicago, Ill. 60611
  (health)*

Sex Information and Education Council of the
  U.S.
1855 Broadway
New York, N.Y. 10023
  (sex education)

Smith, Kline and French Laboratories
1500 Spring Garden St.
Philadelphia, Pa. 19101
  (pharmacologic and legal drug abuse)

State Farm Insurance Co.
Bloomington, Ill. 61701
  (safety)

Superintendent of Documents
Government Printing Office
Washington, D.C. 20402
  *(request free price lists; PL 31, education; PL 51,
  health and medical services; 51A, diseases
  and physical conditions; PL 71, child
  development; PL 84, atomic energy and civil
  defense; and PL 88, ecology)**

Spenco Medical Corp.
P.O. Box 8113
Waco, Tex. 76710
  (pamphlets, posters, audiovisual materials)*

Tampax, Inc.
P.O. Box 271
Palmer, Mass. 01059
  (menstrual hygiene)

The Toni Co.
Merchandise Mart Plaza
Chicago, Ill. 60654
  (grooming)

Travelers Insurance Companies
Public Information and Advertising Department
One Tower Square
Hartford, Conn. 06115
  (health and safety)

United Cerebral Palsy
369 Lexington Ave.
New York, N.Y. 10017
  (cerebral palsy)

U.S. Children's Bureau
Department of Health, Education and Welfare
Washington, D.C. 20025
  (child health and safety)

U.S. Coast Guard
Department of Transportation
Washington, D.C. 20590
  (boating safety)

U.S. Department of Agriculture
Food and Nutrition Service
14th St. and Independence Ave., S.W.
Washington, D.C. 20250
  (nutrition and school information)

U.S. Office of Education
Department of Health, Education and Welfare
Washington, D.C. 20025
  (health)*

The Upjohn Co.
Trade and Guest Relations Department
Kalamazoo, Mich. 49003
  (vitamins)

Wheat Flour Institute
309 W. Jackson Blvd.
Chicago, Ill. 60606
  (nutrition)

World Health Organization
Office of Public Information
Pan American Sanitary Bureau
525 23rd St., N.W.
Washington, D.C. 20037
  (international health)

Since some organizations move, change policy, or go out of business each year, it is virtually impossible to prepare a list of sources of free and inexpensive materials that will not require revision periodically. Teachers can keep up to date on such changes by consulting the guides and catalogues listed among references at the end of this chapter. The same problem applies to film sources, and references to these are also provided. A current yearly almanac is also helpful. Many of the better teacher's manuals that accompany health textbooks furnish the teacher with accurate and selective lists of

---

*Following each source citation the general or specific subject matter of available materials is indicated in parentheses. An asterisk (*) means that there is a charge for some or all of the materials provided by a given organization.

printed materials, films and filmstrips, and their sources.

Periodicals

Teachers should have access to a number of professional periodicals that make available sound information on children's health problems, content, methods, and materials for health education. Although the classroom teacher cannot be expected to subscribe to more than a few of these, most or all of them should be available in the school library or teachers' reading room.

Accident Facts, published annually, National Safety Council, 425 N. Michigan Ave., Chicago, Ill. 60611

Childhood Education, Association for Childhood Education International, 3615 Wisconsin Ave., N.W., Washington, D.C. 20016

Health Education Monographs, Society of Public Health Educators, 419 Park Ave. S., New York, N.Y. 10016

Journal of Drug Education, published quarterly, Baywood Publishing Co., 43 Central Drive, Farmingdale, N.Y. 11735

Journal of Health, Physical Education, and Recreation, American Alliance for Health, Physical Education, and Recreation, 1201 16th St., N.W., Washington, D.C. 20006

Journal of School Health, American School Health Association, P.O. Box 416, Kent, Ohio 44241

Medical World News, McGraw-Hill, Inc., 1221 Avenue of the Americas, New York, N.Y. 10020

Parents' Magazine, Parents' Magazine Press, 52 Vanderbilt Ave., New York, N.Y. 10017

Psychology Today, Communications Research Machines, Inc., Carmel Valley Rd., Del Mar, Calif. 92014

Health Education, American Alliance for Health, Physical Education, and Recreation, 1201 16th St., N.W., Washington, D.C. 20006

School Safety, National Safety Council, 425 N. Michigan Ave., Chicago, Ill. 60611

Science News, 1719 N Street, N.W., Washington, D.C. 20036

Social Hygiene News, American Social Health Association, 1790 Broadway, New York, N.Y. 10019

Today's Education, The National Education Association, 1201 16th St., N.W., Washington, D.C. 20006

World Health, World Health Organization, 777 United Nations Plaza, New York, N.Y. 10017

This is a selected list of some publications that have proved to be especially helpful to elementary school classroom teachers and to school health coordinators. In addition to these and other nationally circularized periodicals, there are health journals and newsletters that are published by state departments of public health and by some state departments of education.

Health films

It is always somewhat misleading to list individual health films by topics since distributors are continually changing films in their library as new ones become available and old ones become outdated. Moreover, some motion pictures are available throughout the country while others have limited state or regional circulation. Hence, only the major centralized sources are cited here.

College film libraries—Local or nearby college film libraries generally have good films on health and safety. Check with the film librarian or the library nearest to you.

Departments of health—City, county, or state health departments usually maintain a health film library. Many of these relate to health problems of elementary students. Write or call for a film catalogue.

Voluntary health agencies—Many voluntary health organizations produce and distribute excellent films, usually dealing with those diseases with which the agency is mainly concerned. Consult your local telephone directory or that of the major city in your state for information on the location of the leading voluntary agencies. Write or call for a film catalogue.

Commercial organizations—A large number of commercial firms prepare and distribute films on health and safety. Many of these are listed previously in this chapter in the section "Sources of free and inexpensive materials in health and safety." They, too, provide catalogues of health films.

State departments of education—Most state departments of education maintain a film library, usually containing some good health films. However, since their chief interest is in both elementary and secondary schools, it is important to check carefully to determine the grade level for which a particular film is designed.

Professional organizations—Some local and state medical or dental societies have films suitable for showing to nonprofessional young people. Contact them through listings in the local or big city telephone directory.

In addition to these centralized general sources, the following distributors and film information centers can be most helpful in keeping up with the latest useful films. Write for catalogues or other information to:

Agency for Instructional Television, Box A, Bloomington, Ind. 47401

AIMS Instructional Media Services, Inc., P.O. Box 1010, Hollywood, Calif. 90028

Association Films, Inc., 600 Grand Ave., Ridgefield, N.J. 07657

Bailey Films, Inc., 6509 DeLongpre Ave., Hollywood, Calif. 90028

BFA Educational Media, 2211 Michigan Ave., Santa Monica, Calif. 90404

Carousel Films, 1501 Broadway, New York, N.Y. 10036

Churchill Films, 662 N. Robertson Blvd., Los Angeles, Calif. 90069

Columbia Broadcasting System, 51 W. 52nd St., New York, N.Y. 10019

Columbia University, Center for Mass Communication, 562 W. 113th St., New York, N.Y. 10023

Coronet Films, 65 E. South Water St., Chicago, Ill. 60601

Encyclopedia Britannica Films, Inc., 425 N. Michigan Ave., Chicago, Ill. 60611

Guidance Associates, 757 Third Ave., New York, N.Y. 10017

Indiana University, Audiovisual Center, Bloomington, Ind. 47401

International Film Bureau, Inc., 332 S. Michigan Ave., Chicago, Ill. 60604

Medical Arts Productions, P.O. Box 4042, Stockton, Calif. 93203

National Film Board of Canada, 680 Fifth Ave., New York, N.Y. 10019

National Information Center for Educational Media, University of Southern California, University Park, Los Angeles, Calif. 90007 (computerized updated lists of films in specific subject areas)

National Instructional Television, Bloomington, Ind. 47401

Narcotic Educational Foundation of America, 5055 Sunset Blvd., Los Angeles, Calif. 90027

Serena Press, 70 Kennedy St., Alexandria, Va. 22305 (up-to-date film lists by subject)

Guidelines for selecting health education films. It seems desirable to evaluate films in terms of their contribution to a specific learning situation. Like any other instructional technique, film values depend on whether they increase the individual's knowledge of a particular subject and his awareness of the uses and significance of that knowledge.

A basic consideration in the evaluation of a film is whether it materially assists the pupils in progressing toward the desired learning goals. Of course, technical matters of film making and mechanical matters of visibility, sound, and the condition of the film should be taken into account in determining the value of a motion picture.

Following are some questions that should be considered when selecting a health educational film:

1. Is it interesting and appropriate to the age, grade level, community locale, and racial and ethnic background of students?
2. Does it convey the desired facts and concepts, and is it likely to contribute to the formation of desirable attitudes?
3. Is it accurate and up to date?
4. Can it be correlated with and integrated into the course of study at the particular grade level?
5. Is the language well suited to the intended audience?
6. Is it likely to be understood by pupils?
7. Does it meet reasonable standards of technical excellence in terms of good quality pictures, satisfactory sound, and natural acting?
8. Is the film suitable length?

One group of teachers developed the following film evaluation report for use in their classes. It is shown here to illustrate how the basic information may be modified to meet the needs of particular individuals.

Film evaluation report

Name of school _____

Film title _____

Sound _____ Length _____ min.

Year produced _____ B&W _____

Silent _____ fast _____

Color _____

Description of content _____

Intended teaching purpose(s) _____

Main ideas and/or skills presented _____

Production rating	ENCIRCLE	
Photography	Good	Bad
Sound	Good	Bad
Vocabulary	Good	Bad
Acting	Good	Bad

Contents rating	ENCIRCLE	
Accurate and authentic	Yes	No
Correlated with the curriculum	Yes	No
Presents needed facts	Yes	No
Stimulates pupil activity	Yes	No

Types of learning   CHECK
Developing concepts   ☐   Critical thinking   ☐
Values clarification   ☐   Behavior modification   ☐
List particular strengths or weaknesses:

Of course, much more extensive and detailed evaluation devices may be employed, but to most teachers brevity is important. A short evaluation card is usually ample to recall the film and to refresh your memory on the essential factors.

Games for health education*

PRIMARY GRADES

Nutrition
Breakfast U.S.A.—Kellogg Co. (free)
Nuts to you—basic facts, Nutrition Dynamics Inc. ($29)

Mental health
Blockhead—balancing skill of persistence, Safield Publishing Co. ($2)
Don't Blow Your Top—problems build up tension, Schaper Manufacturing Co. ($3.49)
DUSO Kit No. 1—feelings, goals, values, American Guidance Service, Inc. ($100)
Jack Straws—develop manual dexterity, deal with frustration, Parker Brothers ($1.99)

---

*Adapted from Packer, K.: Peer training through game utilization, Journal of School Health **45:** Feb., 1975.

Jigsaw puzzles—stimulate cooperation or lack of cooperation
Tension—feelings of tension, Kohner Brothers, Inc. ($4.49)
Threads—human relations, Kopy Kat Printing ($4.50: book)
Trouble—reasons students get in trouble, Kohner Brothers, Inc. ($4.49)

Tobacco
Smoker's Roulette—diseases associated with smoking, Spenco Medical Corp. ($44.50)

INTERMEDIATE GRADES

Anatomy
Operation Skill Game—identify body parts, Milton Bradley ($4.39)

Drugs
Trip or Trap Playing Cards—drug identification, Spenco Medical Corp. ($2.95)

First aid
Help—decisions in simulated emergencies, Educational Manpower, Inc. ($15)

Heart
Coronary Tic-Tac-Toe—heart attack factors, Spenco Medical Corp. ($2.95)

Nutrition
Soup's On—balanced diet bingo, Dietor ($12)
Stay Alive—nutritional breakfast, Milton Bradley ($12)
Wheels—vitamin/mineral game, Dietor ($12)

Mental health
Aggravation—student feelings, Lakeside Games ($1.99)
Blockhead—balancing skill of persistence, Safield Publishing Co. ($2)
Chaos—student confusion feelings, Lakeside Games ($4.39)
Don't Blow Your Top—problems build up tension, Schaper Manufacturing Co. ($3.49)
DUSO Kit No. 2—self-concept, interpersonal relations, feelings, beliefs, and so forth, American Guidance Service, Inc. ($100)
Generation Rap—parent-children reversal of roles, Educational Manpower, Inc. ($8)
Happiness—keys to and need for happiness, Milton Bradley ($5.39)
Headache—reasons for, Kohner Brothers, Inc. ($4.49)
Jigsaw puzzles—stimulate cooperation or lack of cooperation
Tension—feelings of, Kohner Brothers ($4.49)

Threads—human relations, Kopy Kat printing ($5.50: book)

Trouble—reasons students get in trouble, Kohner Brothers, Inc. ($4.49)

The Ungame; Tell It Like It Is—feelings, attitudes, motives (such as hopes, fears, joys, sorrows), Contemporary Design ($7.95)

Values in Action—role playing in social situations, Holt, Rinehart & Winston ($103.95)

Tobacco

Smoker's Roulette—diseases associated with smoking, Spenco Medical Corp. ($44.50)

UPPER GRADES

Alcohol

Drinking Clock—drinking and driving, Spenco Medical Corp. ($39.50)

Innocent Until—role play drunk driving, ABT Associates, Inc. ($30)

To Drink or Not to Drink—peer pressure situations, Educational Manpower, Inc. ($25)

Drugs

Cutting Grass—peer group pressure tactics, Instructional Simulations, Inc. ($35)

Downer's Roulette—do not mix drugs, Spenco Medical Corp. ($44.50)

The Social Seminar—community response to drug abuse, National Institute of Mental Health ($13.75)

Youth Culture Game—positive/negative of subculture, Urbandyne ($15)

Heart

Coronary Tic-Tac-Toe—heart attack factors, Spenco Medical Corp. ($2.95)

Mental health

Agenda—decision-making simulation, Educational Manpower, Inc. ($15)

Chaos—student confusion feelings, Lakeside Games ($4.39)

Games People Play—child-parent-adult role play, MASCO ($12.50)

Generation Gap—parent-children interactions, Western Publishing Co. ($15)

Generation Rap—parent-children reversal of roles, Educational Manpower, Inc. ($8)

Hang-Up—pantomime in stress situations, Synectics Education Systems ($16)

Happiness—keys to and need for happiness, Milton Bradley ($5.39)

Headache—reasons for headache, Kohner Brothers, Inc. ($4.49)

Search for Meaning—life choices review, Pflaum/Standard Publishing Co. ($33.95)

Search for Values—life choices review, Plaum/Standard Publishing Co. ($44.95)

Values—values clarification processes, Friendship Press ($5.95)

Woman and Man—war between sexes, Educational Manpower, Inc. ($8)

Nutrition

Good Loser—weight control, Dietor ($12)

Soup's On—balanced diet bingo, Dietor ($12)

Wheels—vitamin/mineral game, Dietor ($12)

Death education stories*

PRIMARY GRADES

Borack, B.: *Someone Small*, New York, 1969, Harper & Row, Publishers, Inc.

de Paola, T.: *Nana Upstairs and Nana Downstairs*, New York, 1973, G. P. Putnam's Sons.

Dobrin, A.: *Scat*, New York, 1971, Four Winds Press.

Harris, A.: *Why Did He Die?* Minneapolis, 1965, Lerner Publications Co.

Lee, V.: *The Magic Moth*, New York, 1972, The Seabury Press, Inc.

Miles, M.: *Annie and the Old One*, Boston, 1971, Little, Brown & Co.

Stull, E.: *My Turtle Died Today*, New York, 1961, Holt, Rinehart & Winston.

Tresselt, A.: *The Dead Tree*, New York, 1972, Parents' Magazine Press.

Tresselt, A.: *Johnny Maple Leaf*, New York, 1948, William Morrow & Co., Inc.

Viorst, J.: *The Tenth Good Thing about Barney*, New York, 1971, Atheneum Publishers.

Warburn, S. S.: *Growing Time*, Boston, 1969, Houghton Mifflin Co.

White, E. B.: *Charlotte's Web*, New York, 1952, Harper & Row, Publishers, Inc.

Zolotow, C.: *My Grandson Lew*, New York, 1974, Harper & Row, Publishers, Inc.

INTERMEDIATE GRADES

Abbott, S.: *The Old Dog*, New York, 1972, Coward, McCann & Geoghegan, Inc.

Courlander, H.: *Terrapin's Pot of Sense*, New York, 1964, Holt, Rinehart & Winston.

---

*Adapted from Scheer, J. K., and Williams, C.: Using children's stories to teach "something we don't talk about" (death education), Health Values 1: May/June, 1977.

Engle, M.: *Meet the Austins*, New York, 1960, Vanguard Press, Inc.

Smith, D. B.: *A Taste of Blackberries*, New York, 1973, Thomas Y. Crowell Co., Inc.

Zinn, H. S.: *Life and Death*, New York, 1970, William Morrow & Co., Inc.

UPPER GRADES

Armstrong, W.: *Sounder*, New York, 1969, Harper & Row, Publishers, Inc.

Engle, M.: *Meet the Austins*, New York, 1960, Vanguard Press, Inc.

Ottley, R.: *No More Tomorrow*, New York, 1971, Harcourt Brace Jovanovich, Inc.

QUESTIONS FOR DISCUSSION

1. What are the main sources of health instruction materials and information available to you?
2. Why are textbooks of great importance in health education? How should other materials and information be used in relationship to the textbook?
3. In what ways can your library be most fully utilized as a source of health materials and information?
4. What are some cautions to be taken into account when considering materials provided by commercial and industrial sources?
5. What are the various kinds of audiovisual aids useful in health education?
6. What principles may be helpful to the teacher in the use of material aids?
7. Why should teaching aids in health education be evaluated?
8. What are five specific sources of health teaching aids?

SUGGESTED CLASS ACTIVITIES

1. Prepare a list of the various materials provided by your education and health departments.
2. Examine the lists of sources presented in this chapter. Select those that seem to offer most useful materials for your particular needs, and write to them for their catalogues and sample materials.
3. Select a unit in health education that you may be teaching in the near future (for example, dental health). Make a list of sources of materials and information on this subject. Send for free and inexpensive materials and evaluate them for possible use in teaching.

REFERENCES

American Alliance for Health, Physical Education, and Recreation: Health concepts; guides for health instruction, Washington, D.C., 1967, The Alliance.

American Educational Research Association: Instructional materials, educational media and technology, Review of Educational Research **32:** April, 1962.

American Medical Association, AMA publications list; health education materials, Chicago, published annually, The Association.

Beyrer, M. K., Nolte, A. E., and Solleder, M. K.: A directory of selected references and resources in health instruction, ed. 3, Minneapolis, 1975, Burgess Publishing Co.

Cornacchia, H. J., Smith, D. E., and Bentel, D. J.: Drugs in the classroom; a conceptual model for school programs, ed. 2, St. Louis, 1978, The C. V. Mosby Co.

Educator's guide to free health, physical education, and recreation materials, Randolph, Wis., 1969, Educators Progress Service.

Elementary teachers guide to free curriculum materials, Randolph, Wis., published annually, Educators Progress Service.

Harris, W. H.: Suggested criteria for evaluating health and safety teaching materials, Journal of Health Physical Education, and Recreation **35:** Feb., 1964.

Joint Committee of the National Education Association and the Association of American Publishers: Selecting instructional materials for purchase; procedural guidelines, Washington, D.C., 1972, The National Education Association.

National Information Center for Educational Media (computerized up-to-date references on films), Los Angeles, Calif., University of Southern California.

Olsen, E. A.: Format and hardware of programed instruction. In American Alliance for Health, Physical Education, and Recreation: Programed instruction in health and physical education, Washington, D.C., 1970, The Alliance.

Osborn, B. M., and Sutton, W.: Evaluation of health education materials, Journal of School Health **34:** Feb., 1964.

Publications and films on health and safety, New York, published annually, Metropolitan Life Insurance Co.

Staton, W. M.: Monday morning at the movies, School Health Review **5:** Nov./Dec., 1974.

Superintendent of Documents, Price lists PL 31, PL 51, PL 51A, PL 71, PL 84, and PL 88, Washington, D.C., Government Printing Office.

PART SIX

Evaluation

13 Evaluating the school health program

Sooner or later teachers find that evaluating—and the testing, measuring, appraising, assessing, and other forms of data collecting that go with it—can be a complex and sometimes frustrating task. Some teachers gear their teaching almost entirely toward the goal of preparing students to take a test. Others teach toward objectives that are empirically selected, poorly defined, and vaguely stated; then they test for specific facts, often of little real significance, that fail to provide any measure of real learning and understanding. A few teachers try to function without any attempt to base their teaching on written objectives of any kind.

There has recently been a growing alarm and dissatisfaction with reports that many students cannot read, write, or do simple arithmetic. There can be little doubt that such is the case based on results of specified national and state examinations. Yet one must wonder about the validity of such tests, that is, does the test measure what it is designed to measure? And are we sure that we want these types of learning outcomes in the first place?

Not too long ago Dr. S. I. Hayakawa,* former President of the University of California at San Francisco and later California's United States Senator cited what he considered to be the *basic goals* of all education:

1. To learn to understand, appreciate and take care of the natural world we live in . . . civilized people need to know not only what the environment is like, but how to keep it habitable.
2. To understand, appreciate and learn to live with the fellow inhabitants of our planet. Every child must learn about the races and peoples of the world and the rich variety of the world's cultures . . . that there are many people in the world who differ from him profoundly in habits, ideas and ways of life.
3. Every student should have an area of esthetic experience . . . the esthetic experience is the organization of our feelings—the search for and the creation of order in our affective life.
4. Everyone should be capable of earning a living. This can be learned in school or out, and at any level from humble work to highly paid, professional skills.
5. I have saved for the last that which I regard as the most important of all, namely the learning of some kind of critical or intellectual method . . . we live in the age of an information explosion. But we are also in the middle of a misinformation explosion. With the proliferation of mass communications media, we are surrounded by hawkers, pitchmen, hard and soft sells, persuaders hidden and overt. It [propaganda] cannot always be analyzed by scientific method, since propagandistic statements are rarely capable of proof; but it can be approached with a scientific attitude.

Although all educators would not necessarily agree with this list of priority goals, most would probably admit that evaluating pupil progress toward these goals is not an easy task.

So too in the broad spectrum of health education—embracing facts, partial truths, theories, attitudes, values, skills and behavior modifications—the productive use of valid and reliable tests and other evaluative procedures poses a challenge to the classroom teacher.

We shall try in this chapter to clarify some of the conceptions and misconceptions regarding evaluation in health instruction as well as in the areas of health services and healthful school environment.

---

*From Hayakawa, S. I.: The Hayakawa column, El Paso (Texas) Times, Sept. 5, 1972.

In any venture in which progress is desired, there must be plans for taking stock of how well a program is achieving its objectives. We need to assess and know the nature and value of *what* we are doing, the *direction* we are taking, and the degree to which we are attaining program *aims* and *goals*. Beyond this, we need to know *how* to evaluate, *when* to evaluate, and *who* shall evaluate.

WHAT IS ACCOUNTABILITY?

Today there is an increased emphasis on what school administrators, teachers, school board members, and other interested persons refer to as accountability. Accountability means responsibility and liability for something. This usually means a responsibility for a mission or program, funds, goals, facilities, equipment, materials, or activities. Beyond this, accountability depends on not only what is done but also how it is done.

With regard to schools, accountability usually implies that educators and parents want some tangible evidence of progress in attaining educational *objectives*. Such evidence may be quantitative or qualitative, easy to collect or difficult to collect, value-independent or value-dependent.

Of course, the concept of accountability means different things to different people, but it can be carried to extremes. Some school boards and administrators are hypersensitive to the presumed right of the public to an accounting. Some parents are aggressively inquisitive about school programs and pupil progress or lack of it. On the other hand, some parents appear to have little interest in what their children do in or out of school.

Yet the majority of educators and parents have a sincere, more realistic view of the value of evaluating pupils and programs in the schools. They realize both the need for and the problems involved in objectively assessing all learning outcomes and school health activities and environment.

WHO IS ACCOUNTABLE?

Teachers, principals, administrators, school nurses, guidance counselors, health coordinators, school boards, and other school personnel may be held accountable for the school's health program.

In view of recent research on variance in pupil achievement at schools in different communities where educational programs were considered equal and recognizing the repeated difficulty of securing correction of pupils' health defects, accountability of parents must not be overlooked. We have seen in earlier chapters that informal parent education can be a valuable aid in improving various phases of the school health program.

Since the pupils' health attitudes and practices are substantially influenced by the availability and quality of medical and dental care, public health services, psychologic counseling, recreational leadership and facilities in the community, as well as by such negative environmental factors as pollution, poor housing, prostitution, and drug trafficking, the *community* must also be considered accountable.

And so we see that not only teachers and schools but also parents and the community are accountable for the successes and failures of the school health program.

WHAT IS EVALUATION?

Evaluation in school health is concerned with planned and organized efforts to assess how well we are conducting our program and how much progress we have made in improving pupil performance. Some of our measures are objective (statistically organized data); others are, of necessity, subjective (opinions, observations). Some appraisals can be made here and now; others must wait for the clock to run. We can test today for what pupils know and understand and for what attitudes they now hold. Though some of their behaviors are observable during the current term, some will not change or be visible for months or years. This is true, too, of certain attitude changes that may be characterized by a time-bomb effect. These delayed alterations in health practices and attitudes may be the result of additive effects of reinforcing information, new life situations, psychologic maturation or a changed environment.

How do measurement and evaluation differ?

Teachers are often confused by the variable uses and interpretations of the terms "measurement" and "evaluation." For our purposes here, measurement involves the use of techniques and instruments to collect quantitative evidence concerning the degree of progress toward stated objectives in health teaching, health services, and healthful school environment; evaluation is a broader concept that includes quantitative measurement as well as qualitative assessment of the products or outcomes of the three phases of the school health program. To illustrate, quantitative measurement may include a score on a test, the number of nurses provided, or whether a lunch service is available. Qualitative assessment may refer to the extent of behavioral changes in pupils, the effectiveness of school nurses, and the nutritional value of foods in the lunch program.

General and specific evaluation

Two rather broad aspects should be considered in evaluation and appraisal of the school health program. For purposes of discussion here, we refer to these aspects arbitrarily as general evaluation and specific evaluation. General evaluation is concerned with an appraisal of a school's entire health program, whereas specific evaluation refers to the appraisal by classes and individual pupils. Both approaches may include quantitative and qualitative evaluative aspects.

General evaluation. A general evaluation of a health program may be carried on in a number of ways. A committee within the school system may be charged with the responsibility for evaluation. This group may consist of a subcommittee of an overall curriculum committee, or it may be made up of faculty members appointed directly by an administrator or supervisor who has primary responsibility for the overall school health program.

Some state courses of study and curriculum guides set forth recommendations in the form of a checklist to be used in evaluating the total elementary school health program. An example of an evaluative criteria checklist is given in Appendix C. On some occasions the services of outside evaluating committees may be obtained. All the general evaluation methods presented here have been used with varying degrees of success. When properly applied, any of them can be useful in the evaluation of the school health program. However, it is sometimes advisable for an individual school to develop methods and instruments for general evaluation of its own health program.

Specific evaluation. Specific evaluation is concerned with the appraisal of learning and estimate of educative growth of individual pupils and groups of pupils in a class. This procedure calls for valid and reliable measures, not only of health knowledge but also of health attitudes and health practices.

Various techniques for estimating educative growth in knowledge, attitudes, and practices are presented and discussed later. At this point, we need to remember the important relationships between and among health knowledge, attitudes, and practices.

Although a pupil may have accumulated a certain amount of knowledge regarding a given health topic, there still remains the important consideration of his assuming an attitude that will influence the development of proper health practice. It is obvious that "knowing is not doing." Empiric evidence bears this out in cases where people are fully aware of the importance of certain health practices but fail to observe them. For example, millions of people know about the health hazards of smoking, yet they continue to smoke cigarettes. Nevertheless, if cognitive learning experiences are *not* provided, pupils will have little desirable knowledge to use as a basis for developing scientifically sound attitudes. Consequently, it is unlikely that favorable health practices will be developed.

As we have seen, health knowledge accumulated may not be put to immediate use. Pupils may not gain full insight into the values to be derived from a certain health practice even though they may have a fairly complete knowledge of it. However, it is possible that the knowledge may eventually be reflected in desirable behavior. Therefore, when evaluating for attitudes and practices, results may be discouraging in situations where pupils show satisfactory growth in factual knowledge but are not inclined to immediately formulate health attitudes and practices commensurate with that knowledge.

In substance, the point of importance is that although the ultimate goal is in the direction of desirable health practices, pupils must acquire certain knowledge that will favorably influence these practices. Therefore, there are inherent values in placing an estimate on the pupils' educative growth in health knowledge.

Why evaluating in school health?

At this point let us review the reasons for evaluating in school health. *First*, we need to continually assess our objectives in the instructional, services, and environmental aspects of the program to assure that we keep up with new developments in education and in the health sciences. An example of this need can be seen in the state-by-state immunizational chart in Appendix B. A few states and school systems continue to require or recommend students to be vaccinated against smallpox. Yet as for back as 1971 both the U.S. Public Health Service and the World Health Organization recommended that this immunization should no longer be given routinely.

Second, we have the responsibility—more recently referred to as accountability—to pupils, parents, school health coordinators, and other concerned persons to measure, evaluate, and report on policies, procedures, and learning outcomes. Understandably, teachers and parents are most interested in the latter.

Third, evaluation is an essential part of good teaching. While testing and other evaluative techniques may be overdone in some classes, they are part and parcel of the teaching-learning process. Both teacher and pupil can function more efficiently when they are periodically apprised of where they are, where they are going, and how much progress they have made.

What are the specific uses of evaluation in health education?

The specific uses of evaluation include the following:

1. As diagnostic devices. These tests can be given at the beginning of a subject or unit of study. Both teacher and pupils benefit from knowing what they know—and, perhaps more importantly, what they *do not* know—how they feel, and what they do with respect to certain health and safety problems.

2. To appraise changes in understandings, attitudes, and practices resulting from learning experiences in health education. In this way pupil progress may be directly assessed —though it should be kept in mind that important changes in attitude and behavior often may not occur for months or years as a result of the time-bomb effect of some learning—and the effectiveness of health teaching methods may be indirectly evaluated.

3. To motivate pupils by stimulating their curiosity about specific health issues. Then one can observe the way they react to such problems in thought and practice.

4. To provide a basis for grading. Whether a grading system of A-B-C-D-F; pass-fail; or O (outstanding), S (satisfactory), and U (unsatisfactory) is used, the results of sound tests will help to provide information for grading and reports of pupils progress. Knowledge tests are most valuable for this purpose since attitudes and behavior are more difficult to measure reliably, particularly if pupils know that their responses to questions about feelings and behavior will be employed for grading. Today there is a trend away from the use of categorical grades to the use of a more descriptive procedure in elementary schools. This approach is worthy of consideration in health education.

5. To provide data useful in continual revision of course and curriculum content. Testing affords an objective approach to curriculum improvement in terms of better meeting the pupil needs.

6. To develop good public relations for the health instruction program. Students and parents alike tend to place a higher value on those subjects or courses in which they are

tested and assigned a grade. Then, too, reports of status and progress in specific units of study help to communicate the idea that modern health science is significantly more comprehensive and sophisticated than the old "narrow-gauge" hygiene course that was centered around anatomy and physiology.

What are evaluative techniques for health education?

Evaluative techniques for health education may be placed arbitrarily in several different classifications. Some of these classifications include (1) teacher-prepared techniques, (2) standardized tests, (3) pupil records, and (4) pupil evaluation. It may be noted that a certain amount of overlapping occurs in these classifications. However, delineation of the evaluative techniques in this manner is proposed for the purpose of giving a clearer understanding of and insight into the procedure of estimating growth of pupils with regard to those factors that influence their health.

Teacher-prepared techniques. Teachers in health education may use various ways of collecting evidence of pupil growth. Such factors as individual ability, resourcefulness, and ingenuity of teachers will influence, to a large extent, the successful application of these techniques. The following generalized list indicates some data-gathering devices that have met with varying degrees of success:

1. Teacher-prepared objective tests
2. Teacher-prepared essay-type tests
3. Oral questioning
4. Demonstrations
5. Dramatization
6. Teacher observations

Standardized tests. There are a number of standardized tests used to gather information regarding health knowledge, attitudes, and practices. The standardized test is one that has been previously administered to large number of pupils to establish norms for specific grade levels or combinations of grade levels. When this type of measuring device is used, it is generally recommended that the test be given before and after health teaching takes place so that specific changes in health knowledge, attitudes, and practices may be noted.

Teachers should keep in mind that, though there are many published standardized tests, most are out of date and omit certain critical current health problems. Hence, teachers may build better tests if they use the textbook teacher's manual, up-to-date material aids, information gleaned from health science sources, and current health and safety problems in the school and community.

As we have learned, most published health knowledge tests are out of date for much of their content. This is because of the lag time between test construction and publication. Even today most published tests still available were developed and published in the 1950s and 1960s. We all know that some of the more significant health problems have come to public attention since then.

There are more unpublished useful tests that have been developed than there are those that have been published in books or professional association publications. The best of the unpublished health tests are usually the subject of a master's thesis or doctoral dissertation. These are difficult for elementary teachers to locate. However, with the help of your school or community librarian, theses or dissertations on elementary health tests can be borrowed through the interlibrary loan service.

Still another source of more up-to-date tests is the professional periodical. These include the *Research Quarterly* of the American Alliance for Health, Physical Education, and Recreation; the *Journal of School Health; Health Education;* and the *American Journal of Public Health.* Occasionally articles on test construction for school health tests are included in these journals.

Though they are somewhat dated, the following tests for elementary school students are included in an official publication of the American Alliance for Health, Physical Education, and Recreation*:

---

*Adapted from Solleder, M. K.: Evaluation instruments in health education, Washington, D.C., 1969, American Alliance for Health, Physical Education, and Recreation.

Adams, G. S., and Sexton, J. A.: California tests in social and related sciences, Part III, Related sciences, Test 5, Health and safety, Monterey, Calif., 1953, California Test Bureau. *For grades 4 through 8, this 75-item test is composed of true-false and multiple-choice items designed to measure knowledge in the health and safety areas. Norms and a manual of directions are available. This test is one of a battery of subject matter tests in the sciences for the upper elementary grades.*

Crow, L. D., and Ryan, L. C.: Health and safety education tests, revised, Brookport, Ill., 1960, Psychometric Affiliates. *For grades 3 through 6, this 90-item multiple-choice test was constructed to measure a student's knowledge, application of rules, understanding of cause and effect, and ability to select the best habits in health and safety areas. Norms and teacher's directions are available.*

Dzenowagis, J. G.: Self-quiz of safety knowledge, Chicago, 1956, National Safety Council, School and College Department. *This test, consisting of 40 safety misconceptions, is designed to measure safety preparedness at the fifth- and sixth-grade levels. See What's your safety I. Q.? Safety Education 36:6-7, Nov. 1956, for a description of the test.*

Klein, W. C., *A Health Knowledge and Understanding Test for Fifth Grade Pupils*, La Crosse, Wis., 1960, Northern Engineering and Manufacturing, Co. *This test has two forms and is composed of 60 best-answer type items. Norms and T-scores are developed. Refer to Klein, W. C.: Development of a health knowledge and understanding test for fifth grade pupils, Research Quarterly, 32:530-537, Dec., 1961.*

National Safety Council: Bicycle safety information test, Chicago, (no date), National Safety Council. *This is a 20-item true-false test suitable for use at the elementary level.*

Speer, R. K., and Smith, S.: Health test, Brookport, Ill., (Form A revised 1960, Form B revised 1957), Psychometric Affiliates. *This test, for grades 3 through 8, has two forms and was designed to test the student's judgment, understanding, and knowledge of health facts. Multiple choice and problem-type questions are used. Norms and teacher's directions are available.*

Yellen, S. (Edward B. Johns, Consulting Editor): Health behavior inventory; elementary, Monterey, Calif., 1962, California Test Bureau. *This 40-item picture-question inventory is designed for grades 3, 4, 5 and 6. Personal health habits, nutrition, safety, rest and relaxation, dental health, cleanliness, and disease prevention are some of the areas included.*

Pupil records. In arriving at a valid estimate of educative growth of pupils, teachers of health should attempt to use all of the materials that are available. In this respect pupil records of all kinds may be explored with the idea in mind of gathering evidence of changes in behavior. For example, anecdotal accounts, case study outlines, and behavior records have been found to be very useful for this purpose.

Pupil evaluation. One very important aspect in the appraisal of learning concerns the procedure that gives pupils an opportunity to determine those things that were learned through the study of a certain health topic. This procedure not only serves as a means of estimating educative growth but also helps the teacher to determine the extent to which a health teaching unit needs revision for use in a subsequent teaching situation.

EVALUATING FOR HEALTH KNOWLEDGE

Appraising the educative growth of pupils in the cognitive domain may take place in a number of ways. The discussion that follows includes some commonly used methods as well as others that have been successfully applied in practical situations.

Teacher-prepared paper and pencil tests. The teacher-prepared test is by far the most universal means of collecting evidence related to health knowledge. This is perhaps partially because paper and pencil testing has been one of the most traditional methods of appraising learning in virtually all of the subject matter areas.

The two kinds of paper and pencil tests perhaps most often prepared by teachers include the objective test and the written essay or subjective-type test. In general, the objective test items may be placed in the two broad categories of *recognition* and *recall*. The recognition type of test item requires that the pupil recognize and select the correct answer that occurs among other answers in the test item. The recall type of test items requires that the pupil supply the correct answer that has been omitted in the test item.

There are several variations of the recognition test item. Some of these include (1) true-false, (2) multiple-choice, and (3) matching. In testing for health knowledge, it is recommended that the teacher use a variety of the recognition test items rather then relying on one type. The purpose is to help offset some limitations involved in the various recognition items.

TRUE-FALSE. The true-false test item may have little diagnostic value since the correct response may be merely an indication that the pupil guessed correctly in selecting the answer. When true-false items are used, extreme care should be taken in constructing the false items so that they will not leave a fixed false idea with the pupils, particularly the slow-learning pupils. False ideas in this way may develop into erroneous concepts. For instance, it has been shown that statements, such as the following, frequently fix themselves as misconceptions in the minds of some children who eventually remember only the false statements:

1. A good way to give first aid for a burn is to put iodine on it.
2. If your clothing catches fire, you should run for water.
3. Oil, grease, and rag fires should be put out with plenty of water.
4. Everyone with weak feet should wear arch supports.
5. Milk is pasteurized to make it easy to digest.
6. A pain in your right side usually means you have appendicitis.
7. Spring water that is clear and cold is always safe for drinking.
8. Most fat people are healthy.

MULTIPLE-CHOICE. The multiple-choice recognition test item is not as widely used because of the amount of time and difficulty involved in its construction. When carefully prepared, the multiple-choice item can be very thought-provoking, and it is an excellent way of determining whether pupils have achieved the desired health knowledge and information that the test covers. In the multiple-choice test item there are usually from three to five possible responses. Five responses are preferred because as the number of possible answers is increased, the possibility for guessing the correct answer is reduced. Some samples of multiple-choice items in health knowledge testing follow:

Instructions: Place the letter of the best answer in the space provided.
1. _____ Persons who do not perspire readily may be especially subject to (a) colds, (b) heat stroke, (c) sun tan, (d) tonsillitis, (e) sinusitis.
2. _____ Volume of blood in the body may be reduced by (a) dehydration, (b) anemia, (c) hemorrhage, (d) all of the above, (e) none of the above.
3. _____ A new sedative-hypnotic drug that is falsely reported to have sex-stimulating effects is (a) Seconal, (b) methaqualone, (c) cocaine, (d) brandy, (e) hashish.
4. _____ The span of life expectancy today is approximately (a) 48 years, (b) 58 years, (c) 71 years, (d) 78 years, (e) 88 years.
5. _____ The leading cause of death for elementary-age pupils in the United States is (a) tuberculosis, (b) heart disease, (c) accidents, (d) polio, (e) drug overdose.

MATCHING. Matching test items have the obvious limitation of being the type of items used for the collection of mere factual information. However, when properly constructed, this type of test item can be useful in measuring achievement and educative growth. The following is a sample of matching test items in health knowledge testing. Note that the two columns present an unequal number of items. The purpose of this is to prevent the possibility of getting a free answer through the process of elimination.

Instructions: Match the following items by placing the letter of the correct answer in the space provided.

1. _____ liver cirrhosis	(a) social problems
2. _____ protein	(b) citrus juice
3. _____ calcium	(c) gonorrhea
4. _____ vitamin B_1	(d) narcotic
5. _____ drug abuse cause	(e) milk
6. _____ iodine	(f) hypertension
7. _____ food tube	(g) glycogen
8. _____ high blood pressure	(h) thiamine
	(i) alcoholism
9. _____ sexual promiscuity	(j) nitrogen
10. _____ heroin	(k) thyroxin
	(l) calorie

COMPLETION. The recall test item that requires the pupil to supply the correct answer takes the form of a completion or fill-in item. One of this test item's chief disadvantages is that it may place a premium on mere rote memorization of health facts. Another possible limitation is that the test item may be such that more than one correct answer can be given. For example, in a recall test item, such as "Exercise generally shows an increase in _____ development," a correct answer may be either "muscular" or "organic." On the contrary, a recall item such as "_____ makes up the greatest part of the body" has only one possible correct answer, which is "water." When there is a possibility of more than one correct answer the teacher should include each one in the test scoring key.

ESSAY. The written essay or subjective-type test of health knowledge, although somewhat lacking in objectivity, may help the teacher determine evidence of achievement and educative growth that frequently cannot be measured through the purely objective test. For example, the teacher can formulate questions in such a way as to provide for better problem-solving situations than is usually possible in straight objective-type tests. Then, too, the teacher may ask pupils to write a summary of what has been learned through the study of a certain health unit. If this procedure is undertaken, the teacher should analyze the summaries to determine how closely they are related to the objectives of the unit. In this way the teacher should be able to ascertain to a reasonable degree whether pupils have gained insight into the understanding and concepts that formed the basis for the unit objectives.

Teacher's criteria for reviewing test questions. Teachers should keep the following criteria in mind what they review test questions:

General

1. Do questions provide hints to answers?
2. Is space at right provided for answers?
3. Is space allowed for legible writing?

Multiple-choice

1. Are there four or five answers with all but one distractor?
2. Are distractors reasonably plausible?
3. Is there grammatical consistency?
4. Does the introduction contain most of the items?
5. Are choices of answers brief?
6. Are there ambiguities?

True-false

1. Are statements true or false without additional qualifications?
2. Are statements expressed simply and clearly?
3. Are items relatively short and each restricted to one central idea?
4. Are statements ambiguous?
5. Are there an equal number of true and false questions?
6. Do statements contain determiners? False—only, never, all, always, none, every, no; true—usually, severally, sometimes, constantly, often.

Matching

1. Are lists of comparative items as homogeneous as possible?
2. Are some items included that cannot be matched?
3. Can questions be easily scored?
4. Are lists of responses relatively short?

Completions

1. Are these indefinite answers?
2. Are key words and phrases omitted?

Essay

1. Are questions carefully written with clarity—no ambiguities?
2. Are written instructions explicit?

Oral questioning. One good way to find out what pupils know and think is by oral questioning. When this method is used the teacher should devise a technique suitable for keeping satisfactory records. Otherwise, there will be no documentary evidence of growth when final evaluation and appraisal are made. Some teachers find it desirable and helpful to keep a log where results of oral questioning can be quickly recorded.

Oral inquiry may be formal or informal in nature. In any event, questions should be such that the teacher can actually tell whether pupils are accumulating satisfactory health knowledge. In this respect, certain types of questions usually should be avoided. For example, questions that require only a yes or no answer may have little value in that the pupil has a 50% chance of guessing the correct answer. On the other hand, questions necessitating critical thinking and judgment can be phrased in such a way that the teacher should be able to immediately detect evidence of correct and accurate health knowledge. Perhaps one of the main disadvantages that teachers have found in using the oral questioning technique is that it may be difficult to appraise the achievement of all pupils if classes are large. The chief advantage in this means of evaluation, however, lies in the fact that the teacher may get a more valid estimate of the individual who expresses himself best through the spoken word.

Demonstrations. Evaluation of health knowledge through demonstrations can be carried out by either teacher-demonstratons or pupil-demonstrations. When the teacher demonstrates, the pupils are required to identify those items that are demonstrated. When pupils perform a demonstration, they show the health knowledge they have gained as well as their interest in the topic.

The efficacy of this approach to health knowledge evaluation is obvious because it tests pupil knowledge in a real and lifelike situation that could be carried over and applied in a practical way, such as helping in the selection of proper foods while shopping with the family.

Asking pupils to demonstrate certain procedures that were developed in a health unit is a valid way of evaluating health knowledge. The chief disadvantage of this is in the amount of time required for such an evaluation procedure. As in the case of oral questioning, evaluation of health knowledge through pupil-demonstration may provide for a better estimate of educative growth in those pupils who do not express themselves well on written tests.

Evaluation of pupil projects. Appraisal of learning in terms of health knowledge need not always take the form of testing. For example, the teacher can evaluate scrapbooks, notebooks, and other materials prepared by pupils. This can be done for the purpose of determining whether pupils have gained insight into certain health concepts necessary for the satisfactory preparation of these materials.

Dramatization. Another way to assess health knowledge is through dramatization. Original health plays, skits, and sociodramas provide another form of dramatization that is useful in evaluating health knowledge. When pupils write a health play, skit, or sociodrama, evidence of health knowledge is shown in terms of the degree of validity of the dialogue of the play. That is, the teacher should determine whether the dialogue written by the pupils shows that they understand the health concepts that the original health play intended to convey.

Still another possibility of health knowledge evaluation through dramatization consists of having pupils act out some of the understandings that were developed during the study of a health unit. This procedure is most useful at the elementary school level and can be accomplished through pantomime or play acting. In pantomime the teacher might ask pupils to show the correct way of brushing the teeth. In a playacting situation pupils might show the correct procedure to take in crossing a street bearing heavy traffic. In this type of evaluation the teacher can see the extent to which educative growth has taken place with regard to health and safety knowledge and attitudes.

Teacher observation. While we generally think of teacher observation as one of the best techniques in health *appraisal*, it can be a primary measure in the assessment of pupils' progress in the affective and action domains of health *education*. Teachers know their pupils. They see them day in and day out. Probably no one except parents are better able to evaluate a child's attitudes and practices. Again, communication between

---

STUDENT FIRE SAFETY ATTITUDES

Please circle the numbers to the right that best express your feelings about each of the following statements:

	Strongly agree	Agree	Don't care	Disagree	Strongly disagree
1. The stop, drop, and roll procedure should be used when clothes are on fire.	5	4	3	2	1
2. In smoke-filled rooms people should crawl low to get out.	5	4	3	2	1
3. Fire drills at school are important.	5	4	3	2	1
4. Smoke detectors are needed in homes.	5	4	3	2	1
5. Fire and smoke discovered should be promptly reported to fire departments.	5	4	3	2	1
6. Fire fighters are community protectors.	5	4	3	2	1
7. Home escape plans are necessary in case of fire.	5	4	3	2	1
8. Fire burns may be dangerous to people.	5	4	3	2	1
9. Fire inspection of buildings should take place on occasions.	5	4	3	2	1
10. Improper storage of flammable materials is hazardous.	5	4	3	2	1
11. Matches, flammable substances, and electrical appliances should be used safely.	5	4	3	2	1
12. Lightning may cause fires.	5	4	3	2	1
13. Overloaded electrical circuits are hazardous.	5	4	3	2	1
14. Baby-sitter fire safety plans protect individuals.	5	4	3	2	1
15. Electrical equipment that has been tested for fire and safety hazards should be used.	5	4	3	2	1

Fig. 13-1. Student fire safety attitudes.

teacher and parent is most helpful in evaluating pupil progress.

APPRAISING HEALTH ATTITUDES

Although it is highly important that we try to determine changes in pupils' attitudes toward health, they are difficult to measure and appraise objectively. This is because attitudes are concerned with one's feelings and emotions and are involved in behavior modification (Fig. 13-1). Consequently, the teacher is confronted with the problem of evaluating in an area that is more or less intangible. In other words, it may be relatively easy to determine what an individual knows about health, but it is a much more difficult matter to arrive at valid conclusions concerning that person's feelings toward the subject even though knowledge and attitude may be related to a certain extent. A pupil may display an undesirable attitude about a certain phase of health because of past experiences, invalid concepts, or home and community environment. In some cases a lack of knowledge can contribute to this condition. An indifferent or negative attitude may be synonymous with ignorance. For example, a child may display a negative attitude toward a certain kind of food simply because he has been in a family environment where parents have had a dislike for that particular kind of food. If proper learning experiences are provided, the child's attitude toward the food may be reflected in various ways. Let us see how the teacher can make an appraisal in terms of change of attitude.

Some methods of assessing health knowledge may also be used to measure health attitudes. However, the limitations of these techniques should be recognized. The obvious disadvantage in using the teacher-prepared paper and pencil test is that the pupil has the opportunity to write down the answers that are correct but that may not portray the child's true feelings. When the paper and pencil test for health attitudes is used, it may be less difficult to secure an entire class attitude than an individual's health attitudes by administering a test without requiring pupils to place their names on the test paper in a public opinion type of procedure. In this way it is more likely that a valid estimate of health attitudes will result.

The limitations indicated in the written test as a health attitude measuring device necessitate a consideration of other methods that will yield more valid results. In this connection, teachers will perhaps be likely to arrive at a more accurate measurement of health attitudes by using procedures that involve casual actions and expressions of pupils.

Such techniques as dramatizations, individual conferences, and observation have been used with varying degrees of success as aids to teachers in determining attitudes toward health. The zeal some children show in dramatizing health situations can furnish the teacher with clues indicating the differences in attitudes some pupils may have. Informal conferences and conversations with pupils likewise reflect their health attitudes. Observation on the teacher's part is another desirable instrument in determining attitudes. For example, pupils' eating habits in the school cafeteria may be observed to find how they feel about certain kinds of foods.

Although these techniques are necessarily subjective in nature, they seem to contain a certain degree of validity as health attitude measuring devices. They can be reduced to a more or less objective basis when the teacher keeps an anecdotal record of the actions and expressions of pupils. Periodically, these records can be analyzed to see if favorable changes in attitudes have taken place as a result of health teaching.

Evaluating values

Every decade or two sees education add to or subtract from its ideas about how learning best takes place. Often we see philosophies from the past come full circle and receive new welcome and emphasis in the academic community. William Shakespeare referred to it as "old wine in new bottles."

In recent years this truism has shown itself in the attention accorded humanistic education, including values clarification. Values clarification has distinct and significant potential for health education in our elementary schools as evidenced in Chapters 7, 9 and 11 under mental health. One illustration of the use of this procedure is to have students complete these sentences:

> I am cool when I. . . .
> I am happiest when I. . . .
> I feel best when people. . . .
> The one thing I want most. . . .
> I feel important when. . . .
> I'd like my friends to. . . .

This method can be used as a diagnostic tool or to measure progress toward goal achievement.

Raths, Harmin, and Simon* in their pioneer writing point out that traditional strategies in helping children develop values—such as persuading and convincing, limiting choices, appealing to conscience, moralizing, establishing firm rules, and inculcating—do not always work and sometimes are counter productive in behavior modification. Since values in students need clarification and identification, they are considered as deepseated attitudes and can be closely identified with the positive objectives of health education.

ASSESSING HEALTH PRACTICES

One of the most important factors to consider in evaluation of health learning experiences concerns the extent to which pupils put health knowledge into actual practice. In other words, are they performing those actions that have been accepted as valid procedures for the maintenance and improvement of health?

Some techniques used to measure health knowledge and attitudes may be employed to a limited extent in making a valid appraisal of health practices. However, many methods previously mentioned for the appraisal of health attitudes have similar limitations when used to assess health practices. For example, in the case of the paper and pencil test as a possible means for evaluation of

---

*Raths, L., Harmin, M., and Simon, S. B.: Values and teaching, Columbus, Ohio, 1966, Charles E. Merrill, Publishing Co.

health practices, there arises the problem of whether pupils actually practice what they have indicated as the correct answers on the test. The survey below illustrates this process as applied to the use of drugs applicable to grades 5 to 8.

Drugs I have used the past 12 months

Check the appropriate box below for these drugs.

	NUMBER OF TIMES				
	0	1-2	3-9	10-49	50+
Alcoholic beverages	☐	☐	☐	☐	☐
Tobacco	☐	☐	☐	☐	☐
Marijuana	☐	☐	☐	☐	☐
LSD	☐	☐	☐	☐	☐
Amphetamines (meth, speed, bennies, pep pills)	☐	☐	☐	☐	☐
Barbiturates (downers, reds, yellow jackets, blues)	☐	☐	☐	☐	☐
Heroin	☐	☐	☐	☐	☐
Cocaine	☐	☐	☐	☐	☐
Solvents	☐	☐	☐	☐	☐

Perhaps one of the most effective ways of determining those favorable health practices in which pupils should engage is through alert observation. Such observations can be made by teachers, nurses, parents, and physicians.

Parents may report to teachers and other school personnel changes in pupils' behavior at home in terms of such practices as brushing teeth after meals, eating nutritious foods, and pedestrian safety.

Although the technique of observation may be subjective in nature, it can be reduced to a more or less objective basis. As such, observation becomes a fairly reliable instrument for the evaluation of health practices.

TEACHER COMPETENCIES IN EVALUATING HEALTH INSTRUCTION

Because evaluation and appraisal of learning is an essential phase of a valid teaching-learning cycle, teachers should develop certain competencies necessary for successful evaluation. Some of these basic abilities include the following:

1. The ability to construct and use the results of objective-type health tests suitable for use at the particular grade level

2. The ability to select and use those standardized tests best adapted to the local situation
3. The ability to use oral questioning in such a way that it becomes an effective means of evaluation
4. The ability to construct written essay-type questions of a problem-solving nature
5. The ability to interview pupils through conferences and casual conversations to appraise learning that has accrued
6. The ability to employ the technique of observation in matters that concern pupil health so as to make the best possible valid estimate of growth in health attitudes and practices

Health education objectives and evaluation

Chapter 9 has indicated the importance of clear and concise identification of objectives in the *cognitive, affective,* and *action* domains of learning in health education. Teachers must specifically know the purposes of their teaching. Our efforts in measurement and evaluation in the school health program, therefore, should be focused on the extent to which these goals have been achieved. The information in this chapter should provide the guidance necessary to learn what has happened to pupils in terms of their understandings, attitudes, and behaviors.

REPORT CARDS AND EVALUATION IN HEALTH INSTRUCTION

Pupils and parents alike show great interest in report cards. Pupils generally like to be rated in comparison with their classmates and with their own previous marks. In other words, the typical elementary school child is anxious to get a report on his status and progress. Often the report card provides the parents with their only information about what is taught in the school. The report card, therefore, reflects school philosophy and serves as one important medium in public relations. Although many elementary schools continue to use the letter system (A-B-C-D-F) in reporting pupil progress and performance, the trend toward more functional

and descriptive methods of reporting continues.

Many elementary schools today attempt to assess a pupil's progress in the light of his own capacities and abilities. Such an approach usually means that a pupil is marked as *O* for outstanding progress, *S* for satisfactory progress, and *U* for unsatisfactory progress. The emphasis is on the progress, or educational growth, of each child as an individual. At the elementary school level, progress reports are usually supplemented by teacher-parent conferences that should bring about a sharing and comparing of knowledge and observation that contributes to a better understanding of the child and his performance in school.

The parent-teacher conference should use the report card simply as a point of departure in analyzing the pupil's strong and weak points. Usually, if parents are objective, they can provide the teacher with significant information on a child's health attitudes and health practices in and around the home. Good teachers make the most of these all-too-brief conferences.

PROBLEMS IN EVALUATING HEALTH INSTRUCTION

Appraising the outcomes of health education in terms of knowledge and understanding offers little in the way of difficult problems. Yet teachers often face the task with hesitance and reluctance because they feel they have neither the background nor the time to prepare valid and reliable tests for pupils. While the educational literature continues to exhort teachers to prepare their own paper and pencil test, the hard fact is that most classroom teachers have some difficulty in doing this. Since the health problems for a specific grade level are fairly consistent throughout the country, and since teachers are already hard pressed for time, it would seem obvious that teachers should use every available worthwhile aid in measuring pupil status and progress.

Thus, teachers should utilize textbooks, teachers' editions, teachers' manuals, and standardized tests, if in print, as resource material. Often measurement activities provided in these sources will need only slight revision to fit effectively the needs and purposes of individual teachers and classes. Where available, the health coordinator can offer expert consultant service in test construction.

Appraisal of health attitudes and practices is much more difficult than measuring knowledge and understanding. The dual question "Do they know, and will they tell?" is a major deterrent to consistently valid and reliable testing for these learning outcomes. It is extremely difficult to construct test items of the "What do you think?" and "What do you do?" type without betraying some telltale clue that helps pupils decide which response is desired by the teacher. Children have become so conditioned to the use of tests for marking purposes that they hesitate to give frank answers to attitude and practice items for fear that a low grade or other penalty may result. However, teachers can at least partially overcome this problem by making it clear to pupils that responses will not be used for marking purposes and that the chief value of such testing is to improve the worth of health teaching.

To the specific items for measuring health attitudes and behavior can be added the many opportunities for teacher observation of boys and girls. Although essentially a subjective technique, teacher observation can be systematized and sharpened to provide one of the most significant sources of information on attitudes and behavior. Pupil diaries, health record data (especially immunization and correction of defects), routine inspections, and teacher conferences with pupils and parents all may afford additional information regarding a child's progress in the development of desirable health attitudes and health practices.

Data on the product, or outcomes, of health education are vital to judicious assessment of the worth of the instructional program in terms of teaching methods, subject-matter emphasis, and fundamental objectives. Thus, many of our efforts in measuring pupil knowledge, skills, attitudes, and prac-

tices help us to carry on a continuing evaluation of our health teaching. If changes in pupils have not taken place as we expected, perhaps we need to revise our plans somewhat. Perhaps our goals have been set too high. Perhaps our methods have not been psychologically sound. Perhaps curricular emphasis has been misplaced. Perhaps we have been looking at health problems through the eyes of the adult rather than those of the inexperienced child. In any case, true evaluation of the elementary school health instruction program is not an easy task.

CRITERIA FOR EVALUATING HEALTH TEACHING

Evaluative criteria for judging the quality of the school's health instruction program are available from several sources. Evaluative instruments usually take the form of score cards or checklists by which schools can be rated in terms of what is considered desirable for good health teaching. Factors that appear prominently in such evaluative criteria include (1) philosophy and objectives, (2) organizational policies, (3) curriculum development, (4) scope and sequence of learning experiences, (5) scheduling and time allotment, (6) size of classes, (7) teaching methods, (8) quality and quantity of supervision, (9) teacher preparation, (10) teaching-learning materials, and (11) library services.

To the extent that it provides guidelines for better health teaching as well as sample units and scope and sequence guides, this book might be considered a source of evaluative criteria.

EVALUATING SCHOOL HEALTH SERVICES

Health services are more easily evaluated than is health instruction. This is so because health services either exist or they do not. Checklists for school health services usually include questions relating to health examinations, dental inspections or examinations, screening tests for vision, hearing, and growth, and teacher observation of pupil health, communicable disease control, follow-up program, and first aid. One of the more recent useful checklists has been developed by the California State Department of Education. An adaptation of this evaluative form for elementary schools is cited in Appendix C.

EVALUATING HEALTHFUL SCHOOL ENVIRONMENT

Healthful school living, like health services, is much easier to appraise than is health education and its outcomes. Either the water supply is checked periodically, or it is not; the sewerage system meets state standards, or it does not; the school has an automatic fire alarm system, or it does not. Of course, it is more difficult to assess the emotional environment since the interpersonal relationships involving teacher-pupil, pupil-pupil, teacher-principal, and community-school are rather subjective and elusive of objective measurement. Nonetheless, it is both feasible and desirable to evaluate continually the elementary school environment in terms of its contribution to the health of pupils and school personnel. Anderson* has prepared an outstandingly practical scale for evaluating the quality of healthful school living and school health services.

CRITERIA FOR THE ELEMENTARY SCHOOL HEALTH PROGRAM

As we have seen there are a variety of sources for sound evaluative scales and checklists for the elementary school health program. One of the most recent has been published by the California State Department of Education† and is partially reproduced in Appendix C as a guide for teachers and administrators. This is an exceptionally comprehensive and detailed checklist, and teachers may find it more convenient to cull those items that are most applicable to their school situation.

---

*Anderson, C. L.: School health practice, ed. 5, St. Louis, 1972, The C. V. Mosby Co.
†California State Department of Education: Elementary school health education program inventory, Sacramento, 1962, Bureau of Health Education, Physical Education, and Recreation.

QUESTIONS FOR DISCUSSION

1. What is the difference between measurement and evaluation?
2. Why is evaluation important to the school health program?
3. What is meant by *general* evaluation in health education?
4. What is meant by *specific* evaluation in health education?
5. What special problems can you foresee for the teacher who attempts to evaluate for health values clarification?
6. How can individual ("one-on-one") talks with pupils help teachers evaluate learning in terms of concepts (cognitive), attitudes (affective), and behavior modification (action)? Which of these would seem best suited to such teacher-pupil conferences?
7. What do you think of parent-teacher conferences as aids in assessing pupil learning in halth? What if the parent refuses or cannot come to your school?
8. Is there a difference between oral questioning of the teacher by pupils and a group discussion involving both teacher and students? Which would you prefer? Why?
9. What are the most effective kinds of recall and recognition items for a health science test? To what extent would you use such items? Why?
10. What are the specific uses of evaluation in health science evaluation? Which of these do you consider most important? Why?
11. Can a student's health values be realistically and reliably evaluated? How?
12. How are behavioral objectives, such as those described in Chapter 9, related to the evaluative procedures and techniques a teacher uses?
13. Which of the health education learning outcomes —cognitive, affective, and action—is most difficult to evaluate? Why? Which is the easiest to evaluate? Why?
14. As a classroom teacher would you prefer to use (1) a test you constructed yourself, (2) a test you got from a textbook or published test, or (3) a combination of the two? Why?
15. Do you think evaluative checklists (criteria) used to assess the three aspects of the elementary school program should be applied and recorded by school health coordinators, school administrators, community health authorities, teachers, state department of education personnel, the school health council, parents, the school nurse, or a combination or some of these persons and groups? Give reasons for your preferences.

SUGGESTED CLASS ACTIVITIES

1. Prepare a checklist for evaluating a school health program with which you are familiar.
2. Conduct a round-table discussion on the relationships among health knowledge, health attitudes, and health practices.

3. Write a report indicating how pupil records could be used for evaluation in health education.
4. Prepare a general report card for elementary pupils showing how status and progress in health knowledge, attitudes, and behavior could be included.
5. Prepare five true-false items on a specific health topic.
6. Prepare five matching test items on a specific health topic.
7. Prepare five completion or fill-in questions on a specific health topic.
8. Referring to the illustrative units in Chapter 9, prepare tests for knowledge (cognitive domain), attitudes (affective domain), and practices (action domain).
9. Prepare a checklist to evaluate the attitudes of a fourth-grade group of pupils toward nutrition.
10. Prepare a health behavior inventory for first-grade pupils.

REFERENCES

Ahmann, J. S., and Glock, M. D.: Evaluating pupil growth, Boston, 1963, Allyn and Bacon, Inc.

Allen, R. E.: Evaluation of the conceptual approach to teaching health education, Journal of School Health, May, 1973.

Alschuler, A., and Ivey, A.: Internalization; the outcome of psychological education, Personnel and Guidance Journal, May, 1973.

Baker, B., and others: A new approach in determining health misconceptions, Journal of School Health, June, 1964.

California State Department of Education: Elementary school health education program inventory, Sacramento, 1962, The Department.

Charles, C. M.: Individualizing instruction, St. Louis, 1976, The C. V. Mosby Co.

Cornely, P. B., and Bigman, S. K.: Some considerations in changing health attitudes, Children, Jan., 1963.

Department of Health and Medical Services: Fifty-second annual report, 1976-1977, Denver, Colo., 1977, Denver School Press and The Department.

Dalis, G.: Effect of precise objectives upon student achievement in health education, Journal of Experimental Education, Winter, 1970.

Foder, J. T., and Dalis, G. T.: Health instruction; theory and application, ed. 2, Philadelphia, 1974, Lea & Febiger.

Hastings, J. T.: Evaluation in health education, Journal of School Health, Oct., 1970.

Hochbaum, G. M.: Behavior modification, School Health Review, Sept., 1971.

Hochbaum, G. M.: Measurement of effectiveness of health education activities, International Journal of Health Education, 1972.

Kilander, H. F.: Evaluating health teaching, Journal of Health, Physical Education, and Recreation, Nov., 1961.

Knapp, R. R.: The measurement of self actualization and its theoretical implications, San Diego, 1971, California, Educational and Industrial Testing Services.

National Society for the Study of Education: Educational evaluation; new roles, new means, Chicago, 1969, University of Chicago Press.

Oberteuffer, D., Harrelson, O. A., and Pollock, M. B.: School health education, New York, 1972, Harper & Row, Publishers, Inc.

Rosenshine, B.: Evaluation of instruction, Review of Educational Research, April, 1970.

Shaw, J. H.: Evaluation in the school health instruction program, American Journal of Public Health, May, 1957.

Sinclair, R. L.: Elementary school environment survey, Amherst, Mass., 1969, University of Massachusetts.

Sliepcevich, E. M.: School health education study; a summary report, Washington, D.C., 1964, School Health Education Study.

Solleder, M. K.: Evaluation instruments in health education, Washington, D.C., 1969, American Alliance for Health, Physical Education, and Recreation.

Veenker, H. C.: Evaluating health practice and understanding, Journal of Health, Physical Education, and Recreation, May, 1966.

Wilhelms, F. T., editor: Evaluation as feedback and guide, Washington, D.C., 1967, Association for Supervision and Curriculum Development.

Willgoose, C. E.: Providing for change; new directions. In Read, D. A., editor, New directions in health education, New York, 1971, The Macmillan Co.

Young, M. A. C.: Review of research and studies related to health education practice (1961-1966); what people know, believe, and do about health, Health Education Monographs, No. 23, San Francisco, 1967, Society for Public Health Education.

Appendices

A Communicable disease summary for teachers

COLORADO STATE DEPARTMENT OF PUBLIC HEALTH, EPIDEMIOLOGY SECTION, 1969*

Many communicable diseases are as contagious before the start of symptoms as afterwards. For this reason parents should be instructed to keep their children at home whenever they appear to be ill, even with a common cold.

Teachers should observe each child as he comes into the schoolroom and during the day for signs of illness. If a child becomes ill, he should be isolated from the other children, and parents notified to remove him from school.

Teachers should watch for the appearance of a rash, for a child with cold symptoms, including a cough—common symptoms of infectious diseases.

When children are exposed to communicable diseases in the classrooms, the parents should be notified so that those children who have not had the disease can be observed for symptoms at the end of the incubation period.

*This entire communicable disease summary for teachers has been quoted from Colorado State Department of Health Communicable Disease Summary, Epidemiology Section, 1969.

CHICKENPOX

Chickenpox is a very contagious but not a serious disease. It is caused by a virus. There are few, if any, complications.

What to look for	When cases are occurring in school or community, watch for symptoms of a "cold" or a rash. The rash of chickenpox resembles small blisters and usually appears on body, chest, or upper back 14-21 days after exposure. Child may have no sign of rash when he comes to school and by midmorning it may begin to appear.
How disease is spread	By contact with case, often before symptoms appear in the case. Spread by droplets from the nose and throat. Scabs are not infectious.
How to prevent	No immunization. Child who has chickenpox should be kept away from others until no new "spots" appear (usually 6-7 days). Examine household contacts for symptoms before sending to school during incubation period.
Regulations	*Case:* Exclude from school for 7 days after symptoms appear. *Contact:* None.

COMMON COLD

The common cold is easily spread from one person to another. It is due to a number of different viruses. Everyone is susceptible to common colds. Complications may occur and parents should be urged to keep children at home at the first sign of a cold. Many times symptoms of colds are early signs of other childhood illnesses.

What to look for	Common symptoms are runny nose, sneezing, general tired feeling. There is usually no fever unless complications have developed.
How disease is spread	By contact with a person who has a cold. The discharges from the nose and mouth are infectious and the disease is spread by sneezing or coughing.
How to prevent	No immunizing agent. Avoid people who have colds if possible. Urge parents to keep children with colds at home.
Regulations	None.

DIARRHEAL DISEASES

Diarrhea and/or vomiting may occur as sporadic cases or in epidemics and are caused by a number of different viruses and bacteria.

How disease is spread	The most common method is probably by person-to-person spread in cases of viruses, and by improperly washed hands in case of bacteria. In rare instances, food contaminated with bacteria or virus by an infected person or faulty sanitation may result in food poisoning.
Prevention	It is probably unlikely that all cases can be prevented with presently available methods. However, by educating children in good personal hygiene the spread of these illnesses can be kept to a minimum. Ill children should be excluded from school until symptoms subside or a physician's advice is obtained.

DIPHTHERIA

Diphtheria is a dangerous disease both during the illness and because of complications. A child should be seen by his doctor immediately if symptoms suggestive of diphtheria occur. It is caused by a bacterium.

What to look for	It begins with a sore throat and signs of fever. The symptoms rapidly become more severe. A person may develop diphtheria within a few hours to 4 to 5 days after being exposed.
How disease is spread	By contact with a case or with a person who "carries" the germ in his throat but is not sick. The discharges from the nose and throat carry the germs.
How to prevent	All children should be immunized against diphtheria in first year of life. When cases occur in a community, school children should be given booster shots.
Regulations	*Case:* Exclude until released by health department or private doctor. *Contacts:* Household and other intimate contacts—same as case.

DOG BITES

If a child is bitten by a dog or other animal while at school, the parents must be notified. A child with an animal bite should have immediate medical treatment. The school is also responsible for notifying the health department of any dog bite. Most animal bites are provoked and a person is not exposed to rabies unless the animal has rabies.

Prevention	1. Immunize all dogs and cats.
	2. Report all cases of animal bites to local health department.
	3. If there is any delay in getting patient to a physician, wash wound with soap and rinse thoroughly.
	4. Treatment as recommended by a physician after bite by rabid animal.
	5. Any animal biting a person must be *confined* for a period of *10 days* from the date of the bite. Should the animal become ill or die during the observation period, the doctor should be promptly notified. Never destroy an animal that is being observed for rabies.

GERMAN MEASLES

German measles is a very contagious but very mild disease. It is due to a virus. When a pregnant woman develops it during the first three months of her pregnancy, her child may be born with certain defects.

What to look for	It may begin with mild symptoms of a cold, but usually the first symptom is a rash. The rash is fine and faint and appears on the face and chest. Glands are usually swollen along the hairline in the back of the neck and below the ear. These symptoms occur between 14 and 21 days after exposure.
How disease is spread	By contact with a case. The droplets from the nose and throat are infectious, especially before the rash appears.
How to prevent	All children should receive rubella vaccine before school age. A child developing the disease should be kept home until the rash disappears, 2-3 days usually.
Regulations	*Case:* Exclude from school until symptoms are gone. *Contacts:* None.

HEAD LICE (PEDICULOSIS)

Pediculosis means being infested with head lice. It is common in areas where people live under crowded conditions or where children are in close contact as in school.

What to look for	Itching is the main sign. One does not always see the lice; one sees the eggs which the louse lays on the hair—they look like tiny beads strung along the hair.
How disease is spread	By close contact with an infested person or by using their caps, scarves, or combs.
How to prevent	By the application of an effective insecticide promptly to the head of a case to prevent spread. Children should not be in school so long as they have lice. They can be in school if they are under treatment.
Regulations	None.

IMPETIGO

Impetigo is a contagious skin infection caused by bacteria. It spreads easily if neglected. A child with impetigo must be excluded from school until the sores receive medical attention.

What to look for	The first sign of impetigo is the appearance of crusty sores, often around the nose and mouth. The sores start as a small blister that soon breaks open and forms a brownish crust.
How disease is spread	The discharge from the sores of impetigo is infectious. Articles used by person who has the infection (towels, washcloths, etc.) can also carry the germs.
How to prevent	No immunizing agent. Prompt separation of cases from other children is important. When treated, impetigo clears up in two or three days.
Regulations	*Case:* Exclude from school until physician advises return. *Contacts:* None.

EPIDEMIC MENINGITIS

Epidemic meningitis, caused by a bacterium, is not a highly contagious disease. If there is a case in school, parents should be notified so that they may contact their physician.

What to look for	This illness develops suddenly with fever, intense headache, nausea or vomiting, 3-7 days after exposure.
How disease is spread	By direct contact with persons who are sick with this disease. It is also spread through the nose and throat droplets of people who carry the disease but are not sick (carriers).

How to prevent	No specific preventive measure except chemoprophylaxis that may be prescribed by a physician.
Regulations	*Case:* Exclude from school until released by private physician or health department. *Contacts:* None.

MEASLES

Measles is a very contagious disease, especially in the first few days before the rash appears. This disease is dangerous for young children or children ill with some other condition. Complications can be severe. It is caused by a virus.

What to look for	This disease begins with cold symptoms; sneezing, inflamed eyes, a hard, dry cough. The fever is high and a rash develops after several days of fever—blotchy, dusky red in color. Symptoms develop 7-14 days after exposure.
How disease is spread	By contact with a person who has it. Discharges from the nose and throat are infectious, especially early in the illness before symptoms appear.
How to prevent	By vaccination with live measles vaccine, preferably at one year of age. Gamma globulin can be given to very young or to ill children after exposure. This serum will prevent a case or make it mild. Children in the family of a case who have not had measles or vaccine should be observed closely for symptoms of illness during the second week after exposure.
Regulations	*Case:* Exclude from school for 5 days following appearance of rash. *Contacts:* None.

INFECTIOUS HEPATITIS

Infectious hepatitis is a disease caused by a virus, which produces inflammation of the liver. Often occurs in epidemics in schools and among members of households of cases.

What to look for	Early signs of this disease are nausea, possibly vomiting, extreme fatigue, and often pain in the upper abdomen. Following these symptoms some cases develop jaundice—a yellow color in the skin and whites of the eyes. Many cases excrete dark (coffee-colored) urine and light (clay-colored) stools. Symptoms develop 2 to 6 weeks following exposure.
How disease is spread	By person-to-person contact. The virus causing hepatitis is found in the human bowel and spread by dirty hands to the mouth. It can be spread by water if contaminated with human excretions.
How to prevent	Gamma globulin may be given to the members of the family of a case. This serum is too limited to give in mass programs. Careful handwashing, after using the toilet and before meals, will help control the spread.
Regulations	*Case:* Exclude from school for one week or until symptoms are gone. *Contacts:* None.

MUMPS

Mumps, due to a virus, is highly contagious, but so mild that one third of all cases are unrecognized. Mumps is usually not dangerous except in teen-agers or adults.

What to look for	In a young child, the first sign is a swelling under the ear lobe. Symptoms appear 12-26 days after exposure, commonly 18 days.
How disease is spread	By contact with a person who has it. Droplets from the nose and mouth are infectious from two days before the swelling appears until the swelling has subsided.
How to prevent	A live mumps vaccine will be available shortly.
Regulations	*Case:* Exclude from school until the swelling is gone. *Contacts:* None.

PINK EYE (CONJUNCTIVITIS)

Conjunctivitis is not a single disease like mumps or measles. It is an eye infection and can be caused by a number of germs.

What to look for	The whites of the eyes are reddened and drain matter. Sometimes the lids are swollen and stuck together. Usually develops 48-72 hours after exposure.
How disease is spread	By direct contact or contact with articles used by an infected person (towels, washcloths, etc.).
How to prevent	No immunizing agent. A child should not be in school with an eye infection.
Regulations	None.

POLIOMYELITIS

Poliomyelitis, caused by a virus, like many other illnesses, causes headache and pain in the back. However, in polio, this pain is often followed by paralysis.

What to look for	Headache or stiffness of the neck or back. If a child has these symptoms he should see his family doctor.
How disease is spread	This is not clearly understood. The virus is present in the throat secretions and stools of cases, unrecognized cases, and especially carriers. No way is known to prevent the virus from spreading.
How to prevent	By immunization. Everyone should be immunized beginning at 6 weeks to 2 months of age. Schools should urge that all children be immunized before entry into school.
Regulations	*Case:* Exclude case from school until released by health department or physician. *Contacts:* None.

RINGWORM

Ringworm is a skin infection that appears as a circular dry spot on the skin or as bald spots on the scalp that contain short, whiskery-like hairs.

What to look for	Dry, circular patches on the skin and bare spots on the scalp.
How disease is spread	By direct contact with children or animals who have it. By the use of caps, combs, towels of infected persons.
How to prevent	Cases must be under treatment, including wearing a cap if the ringworm is on the scalp. When ringworm is present in a family or in school, children should be examined frequently for signs so that treatment can be started early. Domestic animals, both large and small affected with the fungus, should be isolated and not handled until a cure has been effected.
Regulations	*Case:* None if case is under treatment and wears protective cap. *Contacts:* None.

SCABIES

In scabies, the skin is infested by a tiny mite.

What to look for	Evidence of scratching. The mite burrows under the skin between the fingers, bend of elbow, or wherever skin touches skin. The small lesions resemble pinholes occurring along a line.
How disease is spread	By direct contact with an infested person—handshaking, contact with clothing or articles used by such a person.
How to prevent	Cases must be treated. All infested members of the family of a case should be treated at the same time.
Regulations	*Case:* Exclude from school until symptoms are gone. *Contacts:* None.

STREPTOCOCCAL INFECTIONS (INCLUDING SCARLET FEVER)

The streptococci are bacteria. Slight attacks of strep throat are just as contagious as severe ones. Scarlet fever and strep throat are the same disease except for the rash. Children should not be in school with a sore throat and should be treated.

What to look for	Strep infections begin suddenly. Headache, fever, sore throat are common. The glands of the neck are swollen. Scarlet fever rash appears within 24 hours—fine, granular to the touch. Symptoms develop 2-5 days after exposure.
How disease is spread	By contact with case or carrier. Discharges from the nose and throat are infectious. Strep infections often spread through the mild, unrecognized case.
How to prevent	Children should not be in school with a sore throat. A physician should be consulted concerning evaluation and treatment of a child with sore throat and to consider treatment of other family members in order to limit spread.
Regulations	*Case:* Exclude from school 48 hours or until symptoms are gone if under treatment. If not under treatment exclude until symptoms are gone—not less than 7 days. *Contacts:* None.

TUBERCULOSIS

Tuberculosis is usually a long-term disease and usually is a disease of the lungs. It is due to a bacterium. It may involve bones or other organs. Primary tuberculosis, which is the kind most often found in children, usually shows no symptoms and is not infectious. When a child is found to have tuberculosis it is rare that he has it in a stage where he could expose other children in school or his playmates.

What to look for	There is no way to observe children for tuberculosis. Once in a while a child will show a low fever and be tired and listless because of tuberculosis, but these symptoms may be due to many things. Such a child should be examined by his physician for his own good, not because he may be a threat to others.
How disease is spread	For all practical purposes, tuberculosis is an air-borne disease spread by inhalation of droplets resulting from coughing, sneezing or talking by persons with active tuberculosis. Children become infected by exposure to an active case most often a parent, grandparent or teacher.
How to prevent	There is no practical immunization. The best prevention is through locating infectious cases, usually adults, and keeping these away from others until treatment with specific antibodies makes them noninfectious. Persons with positive skin test, especially a child, may be advised by his physician to take antituberculous medication. Of special value in preventing TB are skin testing programs. A child with a positive skin test has TB germs in his body and may point the way to an active case and should be seen by a physician for evaluation as to whether specific antituberculous medication is indicated. General good health habits, adequate rest, good nutrition and medical care for illness are important.
Regulations	*Case:* Doctor determines whether child may attend school. When a child is kept out of school because of tuberculosis, it is usually for the good of his own health and not because of danger to others. *Contacts:* None. May attend school. NOTE: A positive tuberculosis skin test alone does not indicate that a child is infectious. It does indicate that the child has been infected, at some time in his life, with tubercle bacilli and should be examined at regular one- to two-year intervals for evidence of active tuberculosis. If he is a young child, his family should be checked to see if there is an active case.

VENEREAL DISEASE

The two most common venereal diseases are syphilis, caused by a spirochete, and gonorrhea, caused by a bacterium. Both are spread by sexual contact.

Syphilis (clinical stages)	1. Primary is manifested by a sore of varying size occurring on skin or mucous membranes approximately three weeks after exposure. Persons are capable of spreading the disease at this stage. Occasionally, persons have syphilis without being aware of the sore.
	2. The secondary stage is manifested by generalized rash within a month or two after primary syphilis if it has not been adequately treated or has gone unnoticed. Persons are infective at this time.
	3. The late stages, noninfectious, result in severe damage to heart, blood vessels, brain and spinal cord.
	Treatment: A person with any possibility of having syphilis or having been exposed should consult a physician.
Gonorrhea	1. In males, it is manifest by a purulent urethral discharge often manifest by burning urination.
	2. In females, it causes a discharge from urethra or vagina or may cause infection in the fallopian tubes or ovaries producing fever and abdominal pain.
	Treatment: A physician should be consulted if any of these symptoms occur or exposure to possible infected person is known.

WHOOPING COUGH (PERTUSSIS)

Whooping cough is most dangerous in infancy. It is especially infectious during the first or second week, before the whoop occurs. Complications can be severe. It is caused by bacteria.

What to look for	Usually not possible to recognize until characteristic whoop appears. Cough is only constant symptom and may be due to many diseases other than whooping cough. Symptoms appear 5-21 days following exposure.
How disease is spread	By contact with a case. Discharges of the nose and throat probably most infectious before whoop appears.
How to prevent	By immunization with whooping cough vaccine. Since these shots are not recommended after five years of age, all children should be immunized in first year of life.
Regulations	*Case:* Exclude from school 21 days after appearance of whoop. *Contacts:* None.

B Immunization requirements for school enrollment 1975-1976

Immunizations required for specific diseases*

	Smallpox	Tetanus	Diphtheria	Whooping cough	Polio	Measles	German measles	Mumps	Tuberculin test	Other
Alabama	†	X	X	X	X	X	X		X	
Alaska		X	X	X	X	X	X		X	
Arizona		†	†	†	†	†	†		†	
Arkansas		X	X	X	X	X	X			
California		X	X	X	X	X	X	X		
Colorado		X	X	X	X	X	X			
Connecticut	‡	X	X	X	§	§	X			
Delaware				X	X	X	X			
Florida		X	X		X	X	X			
Georgia		X	X	X	X	X	X			
Hawaii			X		X	X	X		X	
Idaho										
Illinois			X	X	X	X	X	X		
Indiana‖										
Iowa										
Kansas		X	X	X	X	X	X		X	
Kentucky		X	X	X	X	X			X	
Louisiana			X	X	X	X	X			
Maine										
Maryland		X	X	X	X	X	X			
Massachusetts		X	X	X	X	X				
Michigan		X	X	X	X	X			X	
Minnesota						X	X			
Mississippi	†	†	†	†	†	†	†	†	†	
Missouri			X		X	X	X			

*Adapted from Garcia, E. M.: Immunization requirements for school enrollment by states, 1975-1976, unpublished report, Las Cruces, N.M., 1976, New Mexico State University.
†Optional.
‡Varies within the system and/or states.
§May require.
‖Not required for admission, but upon original entry.

Immunizations required for specific diseases—cont'd

	Smallpox	Tetanus	Diphtheria	Whooping cough	Polio	Measles	German measles	Mumps	Tuberculin test	Other
Montana*		X	X	X	X	X	X			
Nebraska										
Nevada			X	X	X	X	X			†
New Hampshire		X	X	X	X	X	X	‡	X	
New Jersey	X		X		X	X			X	
New Mexico										
New York			X		X	X	X			
North Carolina	X	X	X	X	X	X				
North Dakota		X	X	X	X	X	X	X		
Ohio	X	X	X	X	X	X	X			
Oklahoma		X	X	X	X	X	X		X	
Oregon				X	X	X				
Pennsylvania		X	X		X	X	X		§	
Rhode Island		X	X		X	X	X			
South Carolina		X	X	X	X		X			
South Dakota		X	X	X	X	X	X		X	
Tennessee		X	X	X	X	X	X		X	
Texas		X	X		X	X	X			
Utah		X		X	X	X	X			
Vermont										
Virginia		X	X	X	X	X	X			
Washington		X	X		X	X	X			
West Virginia		X	X	X	X	X	X		X	
Wisconsin		X	X	X	X	X	X			
Wyoming		‖								

*May require.
†D.T. boosters.
‡Optional.
§Not required for admission, but upon original entry.
‖Varies within the system and/or states.

C Criteria for evaluating the elementary school health program

CALIFORNIA STATE DEPARTMENT OF EDUCATION*

Criteria for Evaluating the Elementary School Health Program provides school personnel with a tool to use in making an evaluation of the school health program. The results of such an evaluation reveal the strengths and weaknesses of the program. Where weaknesses are revealed, the school health committee may act to bring all the available forces into action for the express purpose of securing strength in the program where weaknesses exist and for planning ways all other phases of the program may be kept strong.

The criteria are organized into four divisions: I—Administration, II—Health instruction, III—Health services, and IV—Healthful school environment. The criteria are expressed in terms of desirable practices presented in the left column. The evaluation should be made by a representative group of the faculty, including administrators, teachers, and health service personnel. The results should express judgments approved by the evaluation committee as a whole.

Provision is made for the quality of each *provision* or *practice* stated in the criteria to be judged on a four-point scale: *excellent, good, fair,* or *poor*. If the provision is not made, the practice is not followed; or if the quality is fair or poor, there is space for listing changes needed. At the top of each section, space is provided for recording recommended steps to be taken in relation to

the changes needed. Care should be taken to make recommendations that will not have an adverse effect on provisions or practices already judged excellent or good.

SUGGESTED PROCEDURE FOR USING THE CRITERIA FOR EVALUATING THE ELEMENTARY SCHOOL HEALTH PROGRAM

1. Determine the membership of study group to evaluate the program.
2. Determine the need for consultant help.
3. Study thoroughly the criteria and the provisions for making the desired evaluations.
4. Determine whether the program meets each criterion.
5. If the criterion is met, determine the quality of the provision or practice according to the following scale: *excellent* —near perfection; *good*—satisfactory; *fair*—slightly less than satisfactory; *poor* —unsatisfactory.
6. If the criterion is not met—that is, the provision not made or the practice not followed—indicate by a check in the appropriate column.
7. Compile a list of the changes needed and determine how the changes can be secured to best advantage.
8. Set up a priority for accomplishing the changes.
9. Develop recommendations for making the needed changes and record in appropriate space at the top of each section.
10. Submit the recommendations to the administration for action.

---

*Adapted from Criteria for evaluating the elementary school health program, Sacramento, 1962, California State Department of Education.

Criteria for evaluating the elementary school health program

Criteria	Quality of provision or practice					Changes needed
	Excellent (near perfection)	Good (satisfactory)	Fair (slightly less than satisfactory)	Poor (unsatisfactory)	Provision not made or practice not followed	
I. Administration						
A. The policies of the district's governing board provide for a school health program designed to help all pupils achieve the degree of health their potentialities permit through health instruction, health services, a healthful school environment—essentials of the program.	RECOMMENDED STEPS TO BE TAKEN:					
B. A written statement of the school district's point of view regarding the kind and quality of the school health program is available.	RECOMMENDED STEPS TO BE TAKEN:					
C. Responsibility for planning, developing, and administering the district's school health program is delegated by the governing board of the district to the district superintendent of schools. 1. A health committee with a membership that includes school personnel, representatives of community health services, and representatives of the other important segments of the community is assigned advisory responsibilities for the district's school health program.	RECOMMENDED STEPS TO BE TAKEN:					
D. The principal of the school has outlined the practices that are employed in operating the school health program. 1. A health council or committee with a membership that includes an administrator, teachers, health personnel, and, when possible, counselors, custodians, and school lunch personnel is assigned advisory responsibilities for the school health program.	RECOMMENDED STEPS TO BE TAKEN:					
E. Clerical help, equipment, and supplies, in keeping with the pupil population, are provided for the health services program.	RECOMMENDED STEPS TO BE TAKEN:					

Continued.

Criteria for evaluating the elementary school health program—cont'd

Criteria	Quality of provision or practice					Changes needed
	Excellent (near perfection)	Good (satisfactory)	Fair (slightly less than satisfactory)	Poor (unsatisfactory)	Provision not made or practice not followed	
F. Health personnel are adequate in number and specialization to provide needed services.	RECOMMENDED STEPS TO BE TAKEN:					
1. School nurses are available in a ratio of one nurse for each 1,000 to 1,400 pupils. (Distances traveled to visit homes and types of terrain should be considered in determining the desired ratio.)						
2. Physicians are available for consultation and advice.						
3. Dentists are available for consultation and advice.						
G. The professional library and the school library are well supplied with health materials.	RECOMMENDED STEPS TO BE TAKEN:					
H. Each classroom is supplied with the materials needed for use in health instruction.	RECOMMENDED STEPS TO BE TAKEN:					
1. The classrooms for each grade are supplied with the basic textbooks in health.						
2. Each classroom is supplied with health materials, in addition to adopted textbooks, that cover each phase of health.						
3. The scope of the materials in each classroom is sufficient to provide for all the pupils, from the slowest to the fastest learner.						
I. The in-service education program for school personnel provides for health instruction to have the same emphasis as other areas of instruction.	RECOMMENDED STEPS TO BE TAKEN:					
J. The in-service education program for school personnel provides for study of the school health services.	RECOMMENDED STEPS TO BE TAKEN:					

RECOMMENDED STEPS TO BE TAKEN:

A. A course of study for health, a course of study and a teachers guide, or a combination of study and teachers guide is provided by the school district or the office of the county superintendent of schools for use in the school.

B. The course of study contains statements of the purposes of health instruction and the objectives to be sought; an outline of the contents that shows both scope and sequence; units of instruction, lists of materials and sources of materials, and recommended means and procedures for evaluating pupils' progress.

1. The scope of the content for the total program includes the following areas:
   a. Consumer health
   b. Mental-emotional health
   c. Drug use and misuse
   d. Family health (including human sexuality, masculine and feminine qualities, marriage, and family planning)
   e. Oral health, vision, and hearing
   f. Nutrition
   g. Exercise, rest, and posture
   h. Diseases and disorders
   i. Environmental health hazards (including pollution, radiation hazards, accidents, and first aid)
   j. Community health resources

2. The basic program of health instruction is developed through the use of units devoted primarily to health.

3. Health instruction is enriched by making it a correlated phase of units in other subjects, such as science, social studies, and homemaking.

4. Pupils' interests and needs are utilized as motivation for learning.

5. Health instruction is adapted to the pupils' abilities by employing a variety of methods.

6. Instruction is enriched through the use of the up-to-date information that is made available by official and voluntary health agencies and professional associations.

7. Instruction is enriched by the use of up-to-date audiovisual materials, such as films and film strips, charts and pictures, and radio and television programs.

Continued.

Criteria for evaluating the elementary school health program—cont'd

Criteria	Quality of provision or practice					Changes needed
	Excellent (near perfection)	Good (satisfactory)	Fair (slightly less than satisfactory)	Poor (unsatisfactory)	Provision not made or practice not followed	

III. Health services

A. A health services guide is provided by the school district or by the office of the county superintendent of schools.

RECOMMENDED STEPS TO BE TAKEN:

B. A health services committee, preferably a subcommittee of the health council or committee, has advisory responsibility for health services.

RECOMMENDED STEPS TO BE TAKEN:

C. Health services are provided in accordance with the provisions of the guide, provided, however, that the advice of the health services committee is an important consideration in decisions regarding adaptations required to meet special needs of individuals and of the total school population.

RECOMMENDED STEPS TO BE TAKEN:

D. The school health services are of sufficient scope to provide school personnel the information and assistance needed to determine status of, protect, and promote the health of pupils.
1. Guidance and assistance are provided in securing an appraisal of each pupil's health status.
2. School personnel, pupils, and parents are counseled regarding the results of health appraisals and ways to protect and promote one's health.
3. Procedures designed to help prevent and control disease are established.
4. First aid for the injured and emergency care for cases of sudden illness are provided.
5. School health services are coordinated with those provided by professional health agencies in the community.

RECOMMENDED STEPS TO BE TAKEN:

E. School health personnel encourage and guide teacher observation of pupils' health characteristics and accept referrals of pupils whose characteristics are unlike those of the well child.

RECOMMENDED STEPS TO BE TAKEN:

	RECOMMENDED STEPS TO BE TAKEN:
F. School personnel inform and advise parents regarding medical examinations their children should have and assist in making provision for the medical examinations as necessary.	
1. Parents are advised to have medical examinations for their children prior to school entrance.	
2. Provision is made for pupils to have medical examinations as required by existing conditions. (Preferably this provision is made in cooperation with the local medical society.)	
3. Procedures are established for the cumulative health record to follow the pupil from grade to grade and school to school.	
G. School personnel inform parents of the importance of eye examinations for children prior to school entrance, maintain a vision screening program, and inform and advise parents regarding eye conditions of their children that require the attention of a specialist.	RECOMMENDED STEPS TO BE TAKEN:
H. School health personnel provide for all pupils to have group hearing tests at regular intervals, individual tests for pupils discovered with hearing difficulties; inform and advise parents regarding their children's need for examinations by ear specialists; and recommend classroom adjustments for children with hearing difficulties.	RECOMMENDED STEPS TO BE TAKEN:
I. Health services provide for parents to be informed regarding their children's need for regular dental examinations beginning prior to the children's entrance to school, and for parents of children who have defective dental conditions to be informed regarding the undesirable effects of the conditions and advised regarding essential treatment.	RECOMMENDED STEPS TO BE TAKEN:
J. Pupils' growth characteristics are observed to determine deviations in growth patterns that merit special attention.	RECOMMENDED STEPS TO BE TAKEN:
K. Follow-up procedures are taken as necessary—begin when pupils with health difficulties are identified and conclude when the health difficulties have been corrected or their effects minimized.	RECOMMENDED STEPS TO BE TAKEN:
L. Health counseling and guidance is provided.	RECOMMENDED STEPS TO BE TAKEN:

Continued.

Criteria for evaluating the elementary school health program—cont'd

Criteria	Quality of provision or practice					Changes needed
	Excellent (near perfection)	Good (satisfactory)	Fair (slightly less than satisfactory)	Poor (unsatisfactory)	Provision not made or practice not followed	
III. Health services—cont'd						
M. Provisions are made for supplying teachers with health information concerning handicapped pupils and for recommending cases for whom home teaching may be necessary.						
RECOMMENDED STEPS TO BE TAKEN:						
N. The health service program includes provisions for the prevention and control of communicable diseases.						
1. Parents of preschool children are advised by the school to protect their children as early as possible against communicable diseases for which immunization is available.						
2. School personnel cooperate with representatives of the local health department in planning community immunization programs available to pupils.						
3. The school cooperates with local health agencies in conducting a tuberculosis case-finding program for pupils and school personnel.						
RECOMMENDED STEPS TO BE TAKEN:						
O. The health service program provides emergency service for injury and sudden illness and for disasters.						
1. Updated written policies and procedures for first aid and emergency care are provided to all school personnel.						
2. The policies and procedures pertaining to first aid and emergency care are approved by the local medical society or the health department.						
3. Phone numbers of parents and of physicians to call in emergencies are on file for each pupil.						
4. Parents are notified immediately in instances of serious injury or illness.						
5. Teachers are prepared to render first aid.						
6. First-aid kits are available in each classroom and in the principal's office.						
RECOMMENDED STEPS TO BE TAKEN:						

IV. Healthful school environment

A. The school environment is protected by employing personnel whose health is good, requiring all personnel to have regular health examinations, and providing measures that encourage good health practices.

	RECOMMENDED STEPS TO BE TAKEN:		

B. A wholesome emotional climate prevails and essential provisions are made for its maintenance.

1. The morale of teachers is at a high level.

2. The following provisions are made for the maintenance of staff morale at a high level:
   a. Leaves of absence without pay are granted for specified purposes.
   b. Sabbatical leaves for study or travel are granted certificated personnel in accordance with written policies of the district.
   c. Communication is maintained between the administration and teaching personnel.
   d. A teamwork approach is utilized in the prevention and solving of staff problems.

3. The following provisions are employed to create classroom environments that are conducive to learning:
   a. The teachers adapt learning experiences to each child's developmental pattern of growth and needs.
   b. The daily program provides for a balance of quiet and active experiences.
   c. Opportunities are provided for each child to release tension by participating in various types of aesthetic and physical activities.
   d. Teachers discuss required behavior standards with pupils.
   e. Pupils share responsibility for securing desired classroom behavior.
   f. Discipline and grading procedures are fair and consistent.
   g. The teacher-pupil ratio permits the individualization of instruction to the extent required for maximum learning.

4. Pupils are given the following types of opportunities to develop as self-directing individuals:
   a. To share responsibility for solving social problems in the school.
   b. To assume leadership responsibility through participation in classroom and student government activities.
   c. To plan and organize school activities under teacher supervision.

Continued.

Criteria for evaluating the elementary school health program—cont'd

Criteria	Excellent (near perfection)	Good (satisfactory)	Fair (slightly less than satisfactory)	Poor (unsatisfactory)	Provision not made or practice not followed	Changes needed
		Quality of provision or practice				

IV. Healthful school environment—cont'd

5. Teachers are helped by the principal and special school personnel—the school psychologist, counselors, curriculum consultants, and others to solve problems that arise in their classes.

6. School personnel and parents are encouraged in the following ways to work cooperatively in solving the problems that are causing pupils to make less than maximum use of their abilities.

C. The school food services are conducted so that each pupil has opportunity to have a wholesome and nutritionally adequate lunch in an environment that is pleasant and sanitary; and pupils are helped to learn the importance of good eating habits, eating well-balanced meals, using good table manners.

RECOMMENDED STEPS TO BE TAKEN:

1. A Type A lunch, a lunch that meets the nutritional standards of the Type A lunch, or both are served daily.

2. Lunchroom and kitchen facilities are periodically inspected by sanitarians from the local health department.

D. The health service unit provides the required space for each type of activity conducted in the unit and is properly equipped with built-in facilities.

RECOMMENDED STEPS TO BE TAKEN:

E. The school site meets the standards established for schools as set forth in the California Administrative Code, Title 5.

RECOMMENDED STEPS TO BE TAKEN:

1. The size of the elementary school site meets the recommendations set forth in Title 5 of the California Administrative Code. (Five net usable acres plus one additional acre for each 100 pupils of predicted ultimate enrollment, plus one additional acre for each 100 or major fraction of the number of seventh- and eighth-grade pupils for the predicted ultimate maximum enrollment.)

2. The school is centrally located in the geographic area served.

3. The area in which the school is located is relatively free of disturbing noises, noxious odors, and other distractions.

4. Water drains rapidly from outdoor areas.

F. A planned procedure is followed to detect and correct possible unsafe conditions of buildings, grounds, and equipment.

RECOMMENDED STEPS TO BE TAKEN:

G. The buildings and play areas are designed to provide for the successful operation of the school program and kept in good condition.

RECOMMENDED STEPS TO BE TAKEN:

1. All doors providing exit from buildings are equipped with panic bars.

2. Ceilings and walls of classrooms and inside corridors are constructed with sound-absorbing materials.

3. Areas or rooms in which noise-producing activities, such as band practice and playing games, take place are located at points where noises are likely to be least disturbing to classes held in other areas.

4. The enrollments in classes assigned to rooms are not in excess of the number of pupils for which the rooms were originally planned.

H. Essential provisions have been made to secure in each classroom the conditions needed for eye comfort.

RECOMMENDED STEPS TO BE TAKEN:

1. The lighting in classrooms is soft, even, properly distributed, and sufficiently bright for eye comfort.

2. The colors of the walls, ceilings, and chalkboards are conducive to eye comfort.

I. The classrooms and the library are heated or cooled and ventilated as required to provide good working conditions for teachers and pupils.

RECOMMENDED STEPS TO BE TAKEN:

J. Drinking fountains in the building and on the school grounds are sufficient in number, of desirable design, of proper height, conveniently located, and cleaned daily.

RECOMMENDED STEPS TO BE TAKEN:

1. An adequate number of drinking fountains are available (one for each 75 pupils and at least one on each floor of a multi-storied building).

2. The water supply is regularly inspected by health department personnel.

Continued.

Criteria for evaluating the elementary school health program—cont'd

Criteria	Quality of provision or practice					Changes needed
	Excellent (near perfection)	Good (satisfactory)	Fair (slightly less than satisfactory)	Poor (unsatisfactory)	Provision not made or practice not followed	
IV. Healthful school environment—cont'd	RECOMMENDED STEPS TO BE TAKEN:					
K. The handwashing and toilet facilities are sufficient in number and kept clean.						
1. The toilet rooms are readily accessible from classrooms and play areas.						
2. Each toilet room contains at least one wash basin equipped with hot and cold running water for every 50 pupils using the room.						
3. An adequate number of toilets for girls are available (one for each 30 girls).						
4. An adequate number of toilets and urinals are available for boys (one toilet for each 60 boys, one urinal for each 30 boys).						
5. A supply of liquid or powdered soap is available near each wash basin.						
6. The supply of toilet paper and hand towels is replenished each day at specified intervals.						
L. Fire prevention equipment is conveniently located and inspected at regular intervals.	RECOMMENDED STEPS TO BE TAKEN:					
1. All school personnel know the location of fire signal switches in the school and of fire alarm boxes near the school.						
2. Fire extinguishers are of a type approved by the local fire department and are inspected at regular intervals by fire officials.						
M. The procedures to be followed in the case of various types of disasters are known by all school personnel and pupils.	RECOMMENDED STEPS TO BE TAKEN:					
1. Written procedures to be followed in times of disaster are displayed in prominent places throughout the school.						
2. School personnel and pupils have practices and know the procedure to be followed in case of a fire, an earthquake, or other disaster.						
3. Fire drills are held monthly.						
4. Drills for disasters other than might be caused by fire are held at specified intervals throughout the school year.						

D Education for health in the school community setting

A POSITION PAPER*

The school is a community in which most individuals spend at least 12 years of their lives, and more if they have the advantages of early childhood programs, college education, and continuing education for adults. The health of our school-age youth will determine to a great extent the quality of life each will have during the growing and developing years and on throughout the life cycle. Their capacity to function as health educated adults will in turn help each to realize the fullest potential for self, family, and the various communities of which each individual will be a part.

The American Public Health Association believes that health education should be a continuing process, from conception to death, and that such education must be comprehensive, coordinated, and integrated in all community planning for health.

The school, as a social structure, provides an educational setting in which the total health of the child during the impressionable years is of priority concern. No other community setting even approximates the magnitude of the grades K to 12 school educational enterprise, with an enrollment in 1973-1974 of 45.5 million in nearly 17,000 school districts comprising more than 115,000 schools with some 2.1 million teachers. This is to say nothing of the administrative, su-

pervisory, and service manpower required to maintain these institutions. In addition, more than 40% of children aged 3 to 5 are enrolled in early childhood education programs. Thus it seems that the school should be regarded as a social unit providing a focal point to which health planning for all other community settings should relate.

Schools provide an environment conducive to developing skills and competencies that will help the individual confront and examine a complexity of social and cultural forces, persuasive influences, and ever-expanding options as these affect health behavior. Today's health problems do not lend themselves to yesterday's solutions. Specificity of cause is multiple rather than singular. The individual must assume increasing responsibility for solutions to major public health problems and consequently must be educated to do so.

Education for and about health is not synonymous with information. Education is concerned with behavior—a composite of what an individual knows, senses, and values, and of what one does and practices. Factual data are but temporary assumptions to be used and cast aside as new information emerges. Health facts unrenewed can become a liability rather than an asset. The health educated citizen is one who possesses resources and abilities that will last throughout a lifetime, such as critical thinking, problem-solving, valuing, self-discipline, and self-direction, and that lead to a sense of responsibility for community and world concerns.

The school curriculum offers an opportunity to view health issues in an integrated

---

*Adapted from Governing Council of the American Public Health Association: Education for health in the school community setting; a position paper, New Orleans, Oct. 23, 1974, The Council. A "position paper" is defined as a major exposition of the Association's viewpoint on broad issues affecting the public's health.

context. It is designed to help the learner gain insights about the personal, social, environmental, political, and cultural implications of each issue. Planning for health care delivery, for example, is not simply a matter of providing for manpower, services, and facilities. These things must be considered in concert with housing, employment, transportation, cultural beliefs and values, and the rights and dignity of the persons involved. Nor will nutritional practices be improved substantially by programs based on groupings, labeling, or issuing stamps, because food practices and eating patterns are equally influenced by how, when, where, why, and with whom one eats.

APHA is concerned about the traditional crisis approach to health care. The expense involved in treatment, rehabilitation, recuperation, and restoration to health has sent medical costs soaring. More facilities, more services, and more manpower to staff the facilities and to provide the services appear to be the nation's leading health priorities. The alternative is a redirection of the nation's health goals towards a primary preventive—and constructive—approach to health, through education for every individual.

Because of vested interests, political pressures, mass media sensationalism, and health agency structures with categorical interests, health education programs in schools are compelled to deal with a multitude of separate health issues, with only a few of these given priority at any given time. Too frequently, programs developed to deal with crucial issues are eliminated although the problems remain, because another crisis emerges calling for more new crash programs. A revolving critical issue syndrome has been the result, with the same problems considered crucial a decade or more ago emerging once again. Focusing on selected categorical issues has potential value if time, energy, personnel, and money are available to sustain the emphasis and expand such efforts into an integrated and viable health education framework. A broad concept of healthful living that has consideration for psychosocial dimensions should be the basis for health education.

APHA is encouraged by recent developments in an increasing number of states that attest to recognition of the significance of a comprehensive health education program in grades K to 12. Also encouraging are the exemplary programs being established in many school districts and the expressed intention of the federal government to implement an action plan for "better health through education."

Therefore, the American Public Health Association supports the concept of a national commitment to a comprehensive, sequential program of health education for all students in the nation's schools, kindergarten through the twelfth grade. The Association will exert leadership through its sections and affiliates to assure the following for health education:

1. Time in the curriculum commensurate with other subject areas.
2. Professionally qualified teachers and supervisors of health education.
3. Innovative instructional materials and appropriate teaching facilities.
4. Increased financial support at the local, state, and national levels to upgrade the quantity and quality of health education.
5. A teaching/learning environment in which opportunities for safe and optimal living exist, and one in which a well-organized and complete health service is functioning.

E State sources of information on school lunch programs

Alabama: State Department of Education, 410 State Office Building, Montgomery 36104.

Alaska: Alaska Office Building, Juneau 99801.

Arizona: Food and Nutrition Division, Department of Education, 1535 West Jefferson, Phoenix 85007.

Arkansas: School Food Services, State Education Building, Little Rock 72201.

California: Bureau of Food Services, State Department of Education, 721 Capitol Mall, Sacramento 95814.

Colorado: School Food Services, State Department of Education, 210 State Office Building, Denver 80202.

Connecticut: Child Nutrition Programs, Connecticut State Department of Education, P.O. Box 2219, Hartford 06115.

Delaware: School Food Services, Department of Public Instruction, Dover 19901.

District of Columbia: Department of Food Services, Presidential Building, 415 12th St., N.W., Washington 20004.

Florida: Food and Nutrition Services, Florida Department of Education, Tallahassee 32304.

Georgia: School Food Services, State Department of Education, 156 Trinity Ave., Room 211, Atlanta 30303.

Hawaii: Department of Education, Box 2360, Honolulu 96804.

Idaho: Food Service Branch, State Department of Education, State Office Building, Boise 83707.

Illinois: School Lunch Department, Office of Superintendent of Public Instruction, 316 Second St., Springfield 62706.

Indiana: Division of School Lunch, State Office Building, Indianapolis 46204.

Iowa: School Food Service Section, Department of Public Instruction, Grimes State Office Building, Des Moines 50319.

Kansas: School Food Services, State Department of Education, 120 E. 10th St., Topeka 66612.

Kentucky: Division of School Lunch, State Department of Education, Frankfort 40601.

Louisiana: School Food Service, State Department of Education, P.O. Box 44064, Baton Rouge 70804.

Maine: School Nutrition Program, State Education Building, Augusta 04330.

Maryland: Food Service Program, Maryland State Department of Education, P.O. Box 8717, Friendship International Airport, Baltimore 21440.

Massachusetts: Bureau of Nutrition, Education and School Food Services, State Department of Education, 182 Tremont St., Boston 02111.

Michigan: School Food Service Section, Michigan Department of Education, Box 420, Lansing 48902.

Minnesota: School Lunch Section, State Department of Education, Capitol Square Building, St. Paul 55101.

Mississippi: School Food Services, State Department of Education, P.O. Box 771, Jackson 39205.

Missouri: School Lunch Section, State Department of Education, Box 480, Jefferson City 65101.

Montana: School Food Services, Office of State Superintendent, Department of Public Instruction, The Capitol Building, Helena 59601.

Nebraska: School Food Service, State Department of Education, 233 S. 10th St., Lincoln 68509.

Nevada: School Lunch Supervisor, State Department of Education, Carson City 87901.

New Hampshire: Director of Child Feeding Services. State Department of Education, Statehouse Annex, Concord 03301.

New Jersey: Food Program Administration, 225 W. State St., Trenton 08625.

New Mexico: School Food Services Division, State Department of Education, Santa Fe 87501.

New York: Bureau of School Food Management, New York State Education Department, 99 Washington Ave., Albany 12210.

North Carolina: School Food Services, P.O. Box 12197, Raleigh 27605.

North Dakota: School Food Services, Department of Public Instruction, State Capitol, Bismarck 58501.

Ohio: School Food Service Program, Ohio Department of Education, 751 Northwest Blvd., Columbus 43212.

Oklahoma: School Lunch Division, 4545 Lincoln Blvd., N. Terrace, Oklahoma City 73105.

Oregon: School Food and Nutrition Services, Oregon Board of Education, 942 Lancaster Dr., N.E., Salem 97310.

Pennsylvania: Division of Foods and Nutrition Services, Pennsylvania Department of Education, Box 911, Harrisburg 17126.

Rhode Island: School Lunch Service, State Department of Education, Roger Williams Building, Providence 02903.

South Carolina: Director, Office of School Food Services, State Department of Education, Rutledge Building, Columbia 29201.

South Dakota: School Food Services, Division of Elementary and Secondary Education, State Capitol Building, Pierre 57501.

Tennessee: School Food Services, State Department of Education, 111 Cordell Hull Building, Nashville 37219.

Texas: School Lunch Program, Texas Education Agency, 201 E. 11th St., Austin 78701.

Utah: Division of School Food Service, Utah State Board of Education, 136 E. South Temple, Salt Lake City 84111.

Vermont: Education Field Services, Department of Education, Montpelier 05602.

Virginia: School Lunch Program, State Department of Education, Richmond 23216.

Washington: Food Services, Department of Public Instruction, P.O. Box 527, Olympia 98504.

West Virginia: School Food Services, Department of Education, 1900 Washington St., East Building 6, Charleston 25305.

Wisconsin: School Food Service Program, Department of Public Instruction, 126 Langdon St., Madison 53703.

Wyoming: School Lunch Program, State Capitol Building, Cheyenne 82001.

Index*

A

Abrams, R. S., 127
Abrasion, first aid for, 41
Acceptance as individual, 123
Accident(s), 92
  bathroom, 97
  bicycle, 95-96
  boating and water, 98
  classes of, deaths and disabling injuries by, 94t
  classification of, 93-98
    National Safety Council, 94
  comments of pupils about, 159
  home, 96-98
  and mental illness, 125
  motor vehicle, 94-95
  pedestrian, 94
  problem, 92-93
  public, 98
  report form, 103
  school
    changing situation regarding, 100
    liability and responsibility for, 99-101
      understanding of teachers regarding, 100
  of school-age children, 8-10, 92, 98
    home, 9
    motor vehicle, 9
    public nonmotor vehicle, 9
    rate for, 8, 92
    school, 9
    school bus, 9
    in "unorganized activities," 9-10
    work, 9
  statistics, 92-93, 94, 141, 160-161
    source of free or low cost materials on, 367
Accident Facts, 8, 94
Accountability, 378
  carried to extremes, 378
  of parents, 378
  with regard to schools, 378
Achievement, 123
  standards, 237
Action domain, 232
Administrators, role of, in school health, 31
  at superintendency level, 31
Adolescence, 238
Advertising and values, 17
Affective domain, 232-233
Airway, opening, 109, 110
Alcohol
  books for students on, 357t
  education
    games for, 373
    source of free materials on, 368

Alcohol—cont'd
  and health, source of free materials on, 366
  and mental illness, 125, 142
  question of pupils about, 159
  sources of free materials on, 362, 366, 367
  teaching about
    self-test for, 259-260
    techniques for, 258-260
Alcoholism, 13, 125, 142
  and family, source of free materials on, 362
  source of free materials on, 366
Allergy
  signs and symptoms of, 54t
  source of free materials on, 367
Amblyopia, 59
American Journal of Public Health, 26
Amphetamines, use of, in management of hyperkinetic child, 57
Anatomy game, 372
Anatomy/physiology, books for students on, 357t
Anderson, C. L., 391
Anemia, 13
  and mental illness, 126
  sickle cell, 13, 55, 68
    test for, 68
"Angel dust," 11, 142
Anxieties and tensions, handling of, by teacher, 133
Appraisals, 4
  definition of, 47
  frequency of, 48, 49
  medical, 48
  nursing, 48
  psychologic, 74
  reasons for, 49
  role of teacher in, 77-78
  screening, 59-69
Arthritis
  and quackery, source of free materials on, 363
  sources of free materials on, 367
Artificial respiration, 108-109
  administering, 108, 109-111
  most efficient method of, 108
  mouth-to-mouth, 108
  mouth-to-nose, 108
  obstruction to breathing during, 108
  rate of breathing for, 108
  for small child, 108
Asthma, 10
Astigmatism, 59
Athletes, immunizations for, 41
Athletic programs, provisions in, for injuries, 41
Atmosphere, social, 16
Atomic energy, source of free materials on, 369
Attitudes, 151, 233
  importance of, in student health behaviors, 233
  student fire safety, 386

*Numbers followed by t indicate tables; those followed by n indicate footnotes.

Health—cont'd
 education—cont'd
  goal(s) for—cont'd
   modification of, to fit individual differences, 232
  grade placement of, 145-146
  grading in, 380
  health department personnel role in, 360
  implications of growth and development characteristics, 50t-52t
  increasing public acceptance of, in controversial
   areas, 25
  and individual differences, 27
  influence of, 39
  informal, 82; *see also* Counseling, health; Health,
   guidance in
   for parents, 149
  in-service preparation of school personnel in,
   148
  interests and needs as determinants of, 158-162
  materials
   current, advantage of using, 360
   governmental organizations providing, 360
   printed, 355
   provided by professional organizations, 360-361
   provided by publishers, 356
   resource center for, 352
  and maturation of pupil, 238
  methods and materials in, 227-234
  motivation in, 24
  need for, 140
  objectives and evaluation of, 389
  organizing subject matter in, 145-146
  outcomes of, importance of data on, 390
  parent, 148-149
  patterns of instruction in, 147
  periodicals, 370
  problem solving and, 241-242
  program(s) in
   community resource people in, 252
   content of, meaningful, 241
   creative activities in, 247
   discussions in, 247-249
   for early adolescent period, 254
   effect of cultural and social factors on, 236
   evaluation of, 237-238
   excursions and field trips in, 251
   experiments in, 251
   formal phase of, 81
   in intermediate grades, 253-254
   at kindergarten–primary grades, 253
   methods of teaching used in, 245-246
   motivating events usable in, sources of, 254
   motivational role of teachers in, 235
   needs of, 18
   relating knowledge to behavior in, 233-234
   responsibility for, 147-148
   role of teachers in, 147-148, 239
   selecting procedures for, 253
   source of free materials on, 364
   special voluntary, 82
   teaching aids in, 236
   using incident in, 255
  pupil-centered methods in, 245
  purposes of, 257
  resource materials for, 152
  school
   administrative problems in, 144-149

Health—cont'd
 education—cont'd
  school—cont'd
   American Public Health Association's viewpoint
    on, 139
   curriculum needed in, type of, 143
   definition of, 14
   importance of, 139
   position paper on, 415-416
   providing for individual differences in, 26-27
   reasons for, 143
   status of, 18
   teacher's role in, 20-32
   value of, 415
  seasonal events offering opportunities for, 256
  for solving public health problems, 415
  source materials, types of, 354
  for special children, 164t, 165
  spectrum of, 377
  states mandating time for, at junior and senior high
   school levels, 18
  supervisor of, 29-30
  teacher guides to, 241
  teaching methods and materials to use in, 147
  techniques, 245
  time allotment in, 146
  today, 139-150
  unique aspects of, 24
  venereal disease in, 24
  workshops, source of free or low cost materials on,
   367
 emotional, teacher influence on, 74
 endowment fund for, 17
 and environment, 17
 environmental, questions and statement of pupils
  about, 160
 examinations; *see* Examinations, medical
 experiences in upper grades, 254
 eye, source of free materials on, 363
 fair, 257n
 family
  books for students on, 358t
  questions and comments of pupils about, 158, 159
  source of free materials on, 363
  teaching about, techniques for, 292-294
  unit on, 191-197
 fear approach in, 237
 films on, 370-372
 good
  characteristics of, 16-17, 50t
  for pupils, 15-18
  purpose of, 232
 guidance in, 81-91
  coordination in, 84
  definition of, 81-83
  follow-up, 4, 81
  objective(s) of, 81, 82-83
  operation of, principles for, 83-84
  personnel
   assisting in, 90
   responsibility of, 86-87
  problems requiring, 83, 84-85
  procedures used in formal program of, 81
  program(s) in
   contributions of school nurse to, 85-86
   evaluation of, 84
   policy formulation in, 83